Pulmonary Arterial Hypertension

Pulmonary Arterial Hypertension

Diagnosis and Evidence-Based Treatment

Edited by Robyn J. Barst, MD

Professor of Pediatrics (in Medicine),
Columbia University College of Physicians & Surgeons
and Cornell University, New York, NY, USA
Director, New York Presbyterian Pulmonary Hypertension Center,
New York, NY, USA

Provided as a service to medical education
by Gilead Sciences, Inc., committed to
treatment and discovery in pulmonary
arterial hypertension

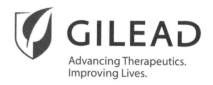

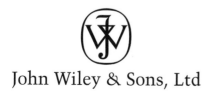

John Wiley & Sons, Ltd

Copyright © 2008   John Wiley & Sons Ltd, The Atrium, Southern Gate, Chichester,
West Sussex PO19 8SQ, England
Telephone   (+44) 1243 779777

Email (for orders and customer service enquiries): cs-books@wiley.co.uk
Visit our Home Page on www.wileyeurope.com or www.wiley.com

Other Wiley Editorial Offices

John Wiley & Sons Inc., 111 River Street, Hoboken, NJ 07030, USA

Jossey-Bass, 989 Market Street, San Francisco, CA 94103-1741, USA

Wiley-VCH Verlag GmbH, Boschstr. 12, D-69469 Weinheim, Germany

John Wiley & Sons Australia Ltd, 42 McDougall Street, Milton, Queensland 4064, Australia

John Wiley & Sons (Asia) Pte Ltd, 2 Clementi Loop #02-01, Jin Xing Distripark, Singapore 129809

John Wiley & Sons Canada Ltd, 6045 Freemont Blvd, Mississauga, Ontario, L5R 4J3

Wiley also publishes its books in a variety of electronic formats. Some content that appears in print may not
be available in electronic books.

Library of Congress Cataloging-in-Publication Data

Pulmonary arterial hypertension : diagnosis and evidence-based treatment /
edited by Robyn J. Barst.
     p. ; cm.
  Includes bibliographical references and index.
  ISBN 978-0-470-72148-3 (alk. paper)
1. Pulmonary hypertension. 2. Evidence-based medicine. I. Barst, Robyn.
  [DNLM: 1. Hypertension, Pulmonary--diagnosis. 2. Hypertension,
Pulmonary--therapy. 3. Evidence-Based Medicine--methods. 4. Pulmonary
Artery--pathology. WG 340 P9813 2008]
  RC776.P87.P838 2008
  616.2'4--dc22
                             2007051228

British Library Cataloguing in Publication Data

A catalogue record for this book is available from the British Library

ISBN: 9780470721483 (H/B)

Typeset in 10.5/12.5 pt Times by Thomson Digital, India
Printed and bound in Great Britain by CPI Antony Rowe, Chippenham, Wiltshire.

Contents

Preface

The consequences of pulmonary arterial hypertension (PAH), i.e. pulmonary vascular disease, although variable with respect to time course and disease progression, are progressive right heart failure and death, if untreated. However, in the past 2 decades, significant advances made in our understanding of its pathobiology have led to exciting developments in therapeutic strategies. And although pulmonary vascular disease is associated with various etiologies, based on similarities in clinical presentation, pathology and mechanistic abnormalities in the pulmonary circulation, similar therapies for the PAH appear to be safe and efficacious in many PAH patients, regardless of the underlying associated condition. With these therapeutic developments, despite an inability to "cure" the pulmonary vascular disease, currently available treatment options have significantly improved the overall quality of life and long-term outcome for many PAH patients. The objectives of this book are: 1) review the current approach to subjects suspected of having pulmonary hypertension, and 2) how best to treat individual patients with PAH based on overall risk-benefit considerations. The book encompasses evaluation, diagnosis and assessment of disease severity, and provides an up-to-date reference source for the current approach to the treatment of pulmonary hypertension. Drug strategies have evolved that include targeting pathways considered instrumental in the development of pulmonary arterial hypertension, e.g. the prostacyclin pathway, the endothelin pathway, and the nitric oxide pathway, which as discussed in the specific chapters on these therapeutic agents, have a significant impact in this challenging disease. We believe this book presents in an authoritative manner the necessary background and clinical review of a rapidly changing field. The book has been written with the busy clinician in mind, particularly those in pulmonary medicine, cardiology, intensive care, and pediatrics.

The book is a combined effort of a distinguished group of investigators heavily invested in the study of pulmonary hypertension from the United States, many parts of Europe, Mexico, and Australia. These authors collectively have contributed to a better understanding of the pathobiology of pulmonary hypertension and to the development of new drug treatments. We structured the book in an attempt to allow each chapter to stand alone, although the order of the chapters is based on the following: suspect pulmonary hypertension, which is first and foremost most important, with subsequent evaluation, diagnosis and assessment of pulmonary hypertension and its associated conditions, and all chapters to follow focusing on clinical management derived from evidence-based data whenever possible, with a closing chapter on a "look to the future."

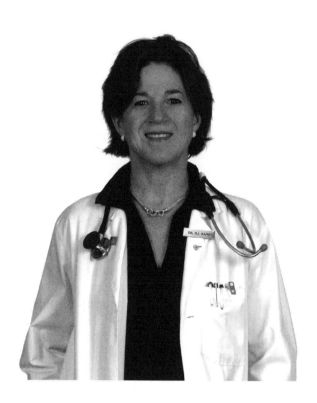

Contributors

David B. Badesch, MD
Professor of Medicine
Divisions of Pulmonary Sciences &
  Critical Case Medicine, and
  Cardiology
Clinical Director, Pulmonary
  Hypertension Center
University of Colorado Health Sciences
  Center
Aurora, CO 80045
USA

Robyn J. Barst, MD
Professor of Pediatrics (in Medicine),
  Columbia University College of
  Physicians & Surgeons and
Cornell University.
Director, New York Presbyterian
  Pulmonary Hypertension Center
New York, NY
USA

Richard N. Channick, MD
University of California
San Diego Medical Center
La Jolla, CA
USA

Ramona Doyle MD
Stanford University Medical Center
300 Pasteur Drive
Stanford, CA 94305
USA

Nazzareno Galiè MD
Institute of Cardiology
University of Bologna
Bologna
Italy

Hossein A. Ghofrani
Medical Clinic II/IV/V
University Hospital Giessen and
  Marburg GmbH
Giessen
Germany

Mardi Gomberg-Maitland MD, MSc
University of Chicago Medical Center
Department of Medicine
S Maryland Ave
Chicago, IL
USA

Friedrich Grimminger
Medical Clinic II/IV/V
University Hospital Giessen
   and Marburg GmbH
Giessen
Germany

Naushad Hirani MD
Division of Respiratory Medicine
University of Calgary
Calgary, Alberta
Canada

Marius Hoeper, MD
Department of Respiratory
   Medicine and Critical Care Medicine
Hannover Medical School
Hannover
Germany

Marc Humbert, MD
Centre des Maladies Vasculaires
   Pulmonaires
Hôpital Antoine-Béclère
Université Paris-Sud
92141 Clamart
France

Anne Keogh, MD
St Vincent's Hospital Darlinghurst
University of New South Wales
Randwick
Sydney
Australia

Alessandra Manes MD PhD
Institute of Cardiology
University of Bologna
Bologna
Italy

Michael D. McGoon, MD
Department of Cardiovascular
   Diseases
Mayo Clinic College of Medicine
Rochester, MN 55905
USA

Robert Naeije MD
Department of Cardiology
Erasme University Hospital
Brussels
Belgium

Ronald J. Oudiz, MD
Mayo Clinic College of Medicine
Rochester, MN 55905
USA

Andrew J. Peacock
Scottish Pulmonary Vascular Unit
Western Infirmary
Glasgow
UK

Stuart Rich MD
University of Chicago
Department of Medicine
S Maryland Ave
Chicago, IL
USA

Lewis J. Rubin MD
University of California
San Diego School of Medicine
La Jolla, CA
USA

Julio Sandoval MD
300 Pasteur Drive
Stanford University
Medical Center
Stanford, CA 94305
USA

Werner Seeger
Medical Clinic II/IV/V
University Hospital Giessen and
    Marburg GmbH
Giessen
Germany

Gérald Simonneau, MD, Phd
Centre National de Référence pour
    l'Hypertension Artérielle Pulmonaire
Hôpital Antoine-Béclère
Université Paris-Sud
92141 Clamart
France

Olivier Sitbon, MD, PhD
Centre National de Référence pour
    l'Hypertension Artérielle Pulmonaire
Hôpital Antoine-Béclère
Université Paris-Sud
92141 Clamart
France

Adam Torbicki, MD
Mayo Clinic College of Medicine
Rochester, MN 55905
USA

1 Introduction

Robyn J. Barst

Professor of Pediatrics (in Medicine),
Columbia University College of Physicians & Surgeons
and Cornell University, New York, NY, USA
Director, New York Presbyterian Pulmonary Hypertension Center,
New York, NY, USA

Pulmonary arterial hypertension (PAH) is a progressive disease characterized by an elevation of pulmonary artery pressure and pulmonary vascular resistance, leading to right ventricular failure and death. Idiopathic PAH (IPAH; formerly termed primary pulmonary hypertension) occurs in the absence of known causes. Estimates of the incidence of IPAH and familial PAH (FPAH) range from 1 to 2 cases per million people in the general population, with at least 6% of these patients having FPAH. Although the incidence of PAH in patients with other illnesses is not known with certainty, from various reports it appears that 2–4% of patients with portal hypertension and 0.1–0.6% of HIV patients have PAH. The incidence of PAH that occurs in patients with connective tissue disease is extremely variable; prevalence ranges from 2 to 35% in patients with the scleroderma spectrum of disease, and may reach as high as 50% of patients with limited scleroderma. PAH has also been reported to occur in 10–45% of patients with mixed connective tissue disease and in 1–14% of cases with systemic lupus erythematosus. The incidence of PAH associated with anorexigens is cyclical in nature and varies depending on the availability of specific appetite suppressants. The link was first identified in the 1960s, when an epidemic of PAH occurred in Switzerland, Austria and Germany that was linked to the anorexigen aminorex fumarate. Use of the anorexigens fenfluramine and dexfenfluramine has also been linked with an increased risk for PAH.

Prior to the development of disease-specific targeted PAH therapies, the median survival for subjects diagnosed with IPAH was reported to be approximately

Pulmonary Arterial Hypertension, Edited by Robyn J. Barst
© 2008 John Wiley & Sons, Ltd

2.8 years. However, 2.8 years likely underestimates current survival, as the course of the disease has been favorably altered by therapeutic advances since that report from the 1980s. Prognosis is also dependent on the underlying etiology of the disease. The prognosis for patients with PAH associated with connective tissue disease appears to be worse than for those with IPAH. Estimates for two-year survival with scleroderma patients with associated PAH are 40% compared with 48% for three-year survival in patients with IPAH. Survival in patients with HIV-associated PAH is similar to that in patients with IPAH. With current HIV therapies, most of the deaths in patients with HIV and associated PAH are now attributed to PAH.

Although Ernst von Romberg, a German physician, described an autopsy in 1891 as 'pulmonary vascular sclerosis,' it is only since 1995 with the introduction of intravenous epoprostenol that disease-specific targeted medical therapies for PAH have become available. In addition, significant advances in the treatment of PAH have occurred during the past decade with six medical therapies now having received regulatory approval worldwide targeting the prostacyclin pathway, the nitric oxide pathway and the endothelin pathway (Plate 1). Furthermore, ongoing clinical trials are evaluating novel therapeutic approaches based on scientific insights gleaned over the past decade in the pathobiology of PAH (Plate 2).

From a therapeutic standpoint, why had it taken from 1891 until 1995 to develop a safe and efficacious therapeutic modality for the treatment of PAH (Figure 1.1)?

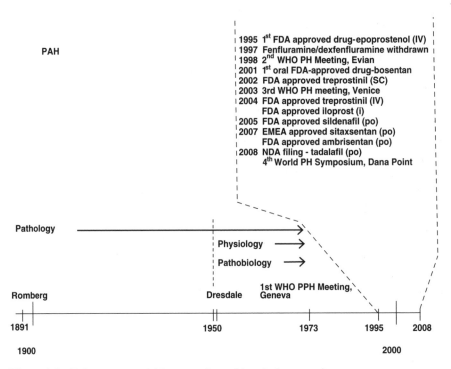

Figure 1.1 Pulmonary arterial hypertension: a historical perspective.

Although several reports of young women dying of right heart failure without a diagnosis were published in 1940, it was not until pulmonary artery pressures could be recorded directly with the introduction of right heart catheterization that the physiology of the pulmonary circulation could be studied. In 1951, Dresdale tested the acute effects of tolzoline in a young woman with IPAH; the tolzoline caused a sudden decrease in pulmonary arterial pressure (PAP) and pulmonary vascular resistance (PVR) without significant systemic effects. Unfortunately, no drugs were available at that time for chronic treatment. However, despite this, there remained little interest in PAH until the epidemic of the aminorex-induced PAH became apparent in the late 1960s. Prompted by the aminorex-induced PAH epidemic in 1973, the World Health Organization (WHO) held its first meeting in Geneva to assess what was known about IPAH and what remained unknown. In 1981, the National Heart, Lung and Blood Institute of the National Institutes of Health in the United States supported a national registry of patients with IPAH which resulted in several reports over the next decade describing clinical features of IPAH and its natural history. Interestingly, despite the fact that IPAH was an orphan disease, significant interest from the scientific community rapidly ensued. Advances in the understanding of the mechanisms involved in the pathobiology of IPAH and PAH associated with other conditions have focused on molecular biology, developmental biology and genetics. Together with epidemiological and natural history studies, collaborative efforts between the scientific community and industry have led to a surge in clinical trials since the mid-1990s: following the approval of intravenous epoprostenol for the treatment of IPAH in 1995, the prostacyclin analogue treprostinil was approved for continuous subcutaneous infusion in 2002, and for continuous intravenous infusion in 2004. In addition, use of the prostacyclin analogue iloprost via inhalation was approved in 2004. In 2001, bosentan, an endothelin ET_A/ET_B receptor antagonist (ERA), was the first oral therapy approved for the treatment of PAH and sildenafil citrate, an oral phosphodiesterase type 5 inhibitor, was approved in 2005. In 2007, the oral ET_A selective ERA ambrisentan was approved in the US, and the oral ET_A selective ERA sitaxsentan was approved in the EU.

Prompted by scientific insights from the 1990s, in 1998 the second WHO meeting was held on the 25th anniversary of the original meeting and, with the dramatic advances over the following five years, the 3rd WHO Symposium on PAH was held in 2003 and the 4th World Symposium on PH will be held in 2008.

Based on the clinical trials to date, current consensus evidence-based guidelines for the treatment of PAH are shown in Figure 1.2. What have we been able to achieve? The disease-specific PAH therapies currently available in conjunction with anticoagulant, diuretic, digitalis and oxygen therapy, have improved exercise capacity, functional capacity, time to clinical worsening, hemodynamic parameters, overall quality of life and survival. However, PAH remains a devastating, life-threatening disorder. In more than 50% of patients, exercise capacity remains significantly limited, approximately 50% of patients remain WHO functional class III or IV, PAH patients continue to have frequent hospitalizations for PAH, right heart function

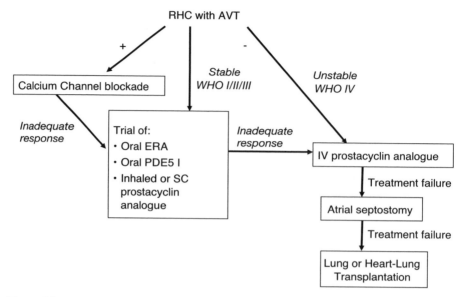

Figure 1.2   Current consensus evidence-based guidelines for the treatment of pulmonary arterial hypertension.

remains significantly impaired in most patients, quality of life is suboptimal, and despite an increase in survival for functional class III and IV patients with IPAH from a predicted survival of 33% (based on the NIH Registry) to 63% with our current therapeutic modalities, the outlook is far from ideal; we need to continue to aggressively pursue furthering our understanding of PAH if we ever hope to give these patients a near-normal life.

The objectives of this book are based on what we currently know about diagnosing and assessing PAH, and what we have learned from the basic science and clinical research that has resulted in the currently approved disease-specific PAH treatments. However, clinical trials in PAH are often difficult to carry out owing to the orphan nature of the disease and the difficulties in determining appropriate assessments that will translate into an improvement in quality of life, symptoms and survival. Despite the achievements to date, patients remain significantly limited. Thus, we must pursue appropriately designed clinical trials in the hope that we will ultimately be able to increase exercise capacity in PAH patients to within 10% of normal, improve functional capacity to class I, increase time to clinical worsening indefinitely, improve hemodynamic parameters and restore right ventricular function and strive to achieve a normal quality of life and normal survival. These hurdles are addressed in this book, which also includes a 'look to the future'. In addition to medical therapeutic interventions for the treatment of PAH, because the outcome for many patients remains suboptimal, palliative interventional procedures have developed, e.g. atrial septostomy (often as a 'bride' to transplantation) and lung transplantation for patients in whom outcome data favors a better outcome with this procedure than with continued medical therapy.

We believe that future developments in vascular biology will improve our understanding of the pathobiology of PAH, and provide rationale and 'proof of concept' for more disease-specific targeted therapies. With the advent of genomic technologies and methods, the necessary tools are now becoming available to begin pinpointing the genes that contribute to disease susceptibility and progression. Candidate gene discovery, involving gene analysis using microarrays, can identify genes that may provide valuable insight into disease biology and may represent an initial step towards the identification of genetic polymorphisms that may help predict efficacy, or lack thereof, with various disease-specific targeted PAH therapeutic modalities. By identifying the genes and gene variants that determine individual disease susceptibility, we might one day be able to identify patients in pre-clinical stages of disease as well as allow for individualized therapies that are most efficacious and least likely to cause side effects. Furthermore, although right ventricular function appears to be the most significant prognostic parameter in PAH, comparatively little attention has been devoted to how right ventricular function and dysfunction can be detected and measured, what specific molecular and cellular mechanisms contribute to the maintenance or failure of right ventricular function, how right ventricular dysfunction evolves structurally and functionally or what interventions might best preserve right ventricular function. In addition, right ventricular–left ventricular interaction, and right ventricular–pulmonary arterial coupling have largely been overlooked as potential targets for investigation and therapy.

Whether cell-based or gene therapy in addition to new drugs, or new combinations of existing drugs, targeting right heart failure in conjunction with PAH specific vasodilator and antiproliferative drugs will improve outcomes in PAH will require further study. Ultimately, as these novel therapeutic options are developed, individualized treatment regimens will evolve. However, many questions remain regarding the treatment of patients with PAH, e.g. identification of patient populations who will most benefit from a specific therapy, determining when treatment should be initiated, and establishing optimal drug sequencing and combinations. We hope that by further increasing our understanding of the pathobiology of PAH, we will one day be able to prevent and cure this disease.

However, in the interim, it is imperative that we base our treatment regimens on evidence-based studies. As stated by Hippocrates in *Precepts* (~440 BCE), 'In Medicine one must pay attention not to plausible theorizing but to experience and reason together . . . I agree that theorizing is to be approved, provided that it is based on facts, and systematically makes its deductions from what is observed . . . But conclusions drawn from unaided reason can hardly be serviceable; only those drawn from observed fact.'

2 Diagnosis and assessment of pulmonary arterial hypertension

Michael D. McGoon, Adam Torbicki and Ronald J. Oudiz

Mayo Clinic College of Medicine, Rochester, MN, USA

The term pulmonary hypertension (PH) refers to elevated blood pressure that is measured within the pulmonary artery. PH is merely an observation, and does not in itself constitute a specific diagnosis, and therefore does not suggest a specific approach to therapy. Rather, the suspicion or detection of PH requires that a comprehensive diagnostic strategy be performed in order to elucidate the clinical context in which it occurs. The diagnosis encompasses two broad objectives: determination of the hemodynamic profile and characterization of the clinical context in which it occurs.

2.1 Hemodynamics of pulmonary hypertension

By consensus, PH refers to the presence of a mean pressure within the pulmonary artery which exceeds 25 mm Hg. PH may be due to abnormalities confined

Pulmonary Arterial Hypertension, Edited by Robyn J. Barst
© 2008 John Wiley & Sons, Ltd

predominantly to the pulmonary arterial blood vessels (pre-capillary PH), to elevation of pulmonary venous pressure (post-capillary PH), to elevated cardiac output or to any combination of these factors. The distinction between these types is a key step in identifying the clinical subtype of PH, and is essential in providing rational and effective treatment as well as avoiding inappropriate treatment.

Pre-capillary pulmonary hypertension is also referred to as pulmonary 'arterial' hypertension (PAH), a term which is also used to describe one of the major clinical subtypes of PH (see below). The hemodynamic hallmarks of PAH include a normal pulmonary venous pressure, which is most commonly assessed by measuring the pulmonary capillary wedge pressure (PCWP), at a value of 15 mm Hg or less. The presence of a high mean pulmonary arterial pressure (mPAP) and a normal PCWP implies that the transpulmonary gradient (mPAP – PCWP) is elevated. Consequently, in the setting of a normal or low cardiac output (CO), the pulmonary vascular (or more accurately, arterial) resistance (PVR) is also elevated. In actuality, it is the presence of a high PVR or low pulmonary arterial capacitance, that produces PAH, though in practice it is the pressure which is measured and the PVR is derived (calculated) from the measurements by the relationship PVR (Wood units[U]) = (mPAP – PCWP)/CO. A PVR > 3 U is considered to be elevated, signifying the presence of PAH. These criteria were used to identify patients for enrollment into the NIH registry of primary pulmonary hypertension (now idiopathic PAH (IPAH)) in the 1980s, though the actual hemodynamic demographics of the registry included a mPAP of 60 ± 18 mm Hg, cardiac index of 2.3 ± 0.9 l/min/m^2 and PCWP of 8 ± 4 mm Hg (Rich et al., 1987).

When PH is associated with an elevated PCWP, the transpulmonary gradient may be normal, a defining characteristic of post-capillary PH or pulmonary venous hypertension. In this situation, the elevated pulmonary pressure may occur owing to back pressure arising from an increased resistance to blood flow anywhere downstream from the pulmonary capillaries, including the pulmonary veins, left heart or even the systemic vasculature. The PVR may be normal, though the total pulmonary resistance (TPR) is elevated. Regardless of the source of the elevated resistance, the workload of the right ventricle is increased.

High cardiac output may produce relatively high pulmonary pressures in situations such as febrile states, anemia, thyrotoxicosis or arteriovenous shunts. Since the pulmonary vasculature is compliant and recruitable, the presence of marked PH can rarely be attributed to high output alone without a contribution by a superimposed vascular defect.

Determining the hemodynamic profile requires invasive evaluation by right heart catheterization, and is the reason that catheterization is pivotal to the evaluation of PH (see below).

2.2 Venice classification

The diagnostic strategy aims to discover whether the presence of PH accounts for the patient's presentation, and if so, whether the PH is a manifestation of an

underlying disease. The physician therefore must have at the outset an understanding of the contexts in which PH occurs. The clinical substrates of PH have
been catalogued based on their pathological characteristics, clinical presentations,
hemodynamic profiles and therapeutic outcomes. The current nosology of PH
has been provided by the consensus of a worldwide symposium of PH specialists
held in Venice in 2003, and is shown in Table 2.1 (Simonneau *et al.*, 2004). The
term PH refers to the presence of abnormally high pulmonary vascular pressure.

Table 2.1　The Venice classification of pulmonary hypertension

1. Pulmonary arterial hypertension (PAH)
　1.1. Idiopathic (IPAH)
　1.2. Familial (FPAH)
　1.3. Associated with (APAH):
　　　1.3.1. Collagen vascular disease
　　　1.3.2. Congenital systemic-to-pulmonary shunts
　　　1.3.3. Portal hypertension
　　　1.3.4. HIV infection
　　　1.3.5. Drugs and toxins
　　　1.3.6. Other (thyroid disorders, glycogen storage disease, Gaucher's disease, hereditary
　　　　　　hemorrhagic telangiectasia, hemoglobinopathies, chronic myeloproliferative dis-
　　　　　　orders, splenectomy)
　1.4. Associated with significant venous or capillary involvement
　　　1.4.1. Pulmonary veno-occlusive disease (PVOD)
　　　1.4.2. Pulmonary capillary hemangiomatosis (PCH)
　1.5. Persistent pulmonary hypertension of the newborn

2. Pulmonary hypertension with left heart disease
　2.1. Left-sided atrial or ventricular heart disease
　2.2. Left-sided valvular heart disease

3. Pulmonary hypertension associated with lung diseases and/or hypoxemia
　3.1. Chronic obstructive pulmonary disease
　3.2. Interstitial lung disease
　3.3. Sleep-disordered breathing
　3.4. Alveolar hypoventilation disorders
　3.5. Chronic exposure to high altitude
　3.6. Developmental abnormalities

4. Pulmonary hypertension due to chronic thrombotic and/or embolic disease (CTEPH)
　4.1. Thromboembolic obstruction of proximal pulmonary arteries
　4.2. Thromboembolic obstruction of distal pulmonary arteries
　4.3. Non-thrombotic pulmonary embolism (tumor, parasites, foreign material)

5. Miscellaneous
　Sarcoidosis, Histiocytosis X, Lymphangiomatosis, compression of pulmonary vessels
　(adenopathy, tumor, fibrosing mediastinitis)

Reproduced from *J Am Coll Cardiol*, **43**, Supplement 1(12), Simonneau *et al.*, S5–S12, Copyright (2004)
with permission from the American College of Cardiology.

PAH is a category of PH (Venice Group 1; Table 2.1); the two terms are not synonymous.

2.3 Overview of the diagnostic process (algorithm)

The management of patients with PH involves (1) detecting the presence of PH, (2) confirming its presence and (3) establishing the specific clinical scenario of the abnormal hemodynamic state, including its severity, the associated or causal conditions, the functional status of the patient and the prognosis (McGoon *et al.*, 2204; McLaughlin and McGoon, 2006). This information is necessary to provide optimal therapy. The algorithm depicted in Figure 2.1 is intended to assure that each component of this process is included in order to screen for PH in symptomatic or high-risk patients, to systematically examine potential underlying conditions with appropriate tests, to delineate predictive factors, to evaluate functional status and to confirm the hemodynamic profile by invasive testing.

Symptoms which require consideration of PH are shown in Table 2.2.

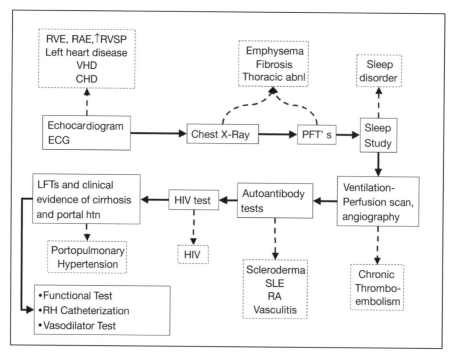

Figure 2.1 The basic diagnostic strategy consists of utilizing appropriate procedures to diagnose or exclude associated underlying diseases. (Reproduced with permission from McLaughlin and McGoon, *Circulation* 2006;**114**(13):1417–31.

Table 2.2 Symptoms requiring consideration of PH in the differential diagnosis

Symptom	Cause

Dyspnea	• Decreased oxygen transport
	   ◦ Hypoxemia
	   ◦ Low cardiac output
	• Low DLCO
	• Low mixed venous oxygen saturation
	• Increased work of breathing

Angina	• Increased myocardial oxygen demand
	   ◦ Elevated right ventricular wall stress (volume, pressure)
	• Inadequate oxygen delivery
	   ◦ Reduced aorta-to-right ventricular systolic gradient
	   ◦ Left main coronary artery compression

Syncope	• Hemodynamic
	   ◦ Systemic vasodilation (exertion, orthostatic, vasodepressor) and low
	      fixed cardiac output due to high pulmonary resistance
	• Arrhythmic
	   ◦ 'Benign' arrhythmias (atrial fibrillation) result in loss of atrial
	      contribution to cardiac output
	   ◦ Malignant arrhythmias provoked by wall stretch, ischemia

Edema	• Right ventricular failure • Tricuspid regurgitation • Sedentary lifestyle • Chronic deep venous insufficiency

Reproduced with permission from McLaughlin and McGoon, *Circulation* 2006;**114**(13):1417–31.

2.4 Screening (identifying a pre-existing risk)

Patients with a sufficiently high risk of developing PH or of having pre-existing but asymptomatic PH should undergo periodic screening. High-risk patients are those who are known to have a condition which predisposes them to PH. Not all patients at increased risk, however, have a high enough risk to warrant screening. High-risk conditions and the likelihood of having PH are shown in Table 2.3. The ACCP Consensus statement (McGoon *et al.*, 2004) recommended Doppler-echocardiographic screening in the first five categories of Table 2.3 because of relatively high detection rates and the disease severity when it develops. Among patients with portopulmonary hypertension being evaluated for orthotopic liver transplantation, screening is necessary in order to identify patients with PAH who are likely to have a poor outcome with surgery (Castro *et al.*, 1996; Tan *et al.*, 2001; Hoeper, Krowka and Strassburg, 2004; Krowka *et al.*, 2004; Krowka, 2005; Krowka, 2004). Screening for PAH associated with drugs or toxins, or PAH associated with HIV infection, has not been recommended because of the low likelihood of discovering PAH; the cost of population-wide screening in these groups is prohibitive. There is

Table 2.3 Patients at risk of developing PH

Patient characteristics	Risk profile
Patients with known genetic mutations predisposing to PH	20% chance of developing PAH
First degree relatives in a FPAH family	10% chance of developing PAH
Scleroderma spectrum of disease	27% prevalence of PAH (RVSP > 40 mm Hg)[a]
Portal hypertension in patients considered for liver transplantation	5% prevalence of PAH (mPAP > 25 mm Hg and PVR > 3.0 U)
Congenital heart disease with systemic to pulmonary shunts	Likely approximately 100% in high flow, nonrestrictive L-R shunts
Used fenfluramine appetite suppressants > 3 months	Prevalence of 136/million users based on odds ratio of 23 times background prevalence of 5.9 IPAH/million[b]
HIV infection	Prevalence 0.5/100
Sickle cell disease	Prevalence 9.0/100 (TRV > 3.0)[c]
Interstitial lung disease	Prevalence 32/100 (mPAP > 35 mm Hg) undergoing RHC)[d]

[a]Wigley et al., 2005; [b]Humbert et al., 2006; [c]Gladwin et al., 2004; [d]Leuchte et al., 2006

no consensus opinion regarding screening in sickle cell disease; although the prevalence is high, most patients have only mild elevation of pulmonary pressure. Nevertheless, even mild PAH in this group appears to have prognostic implications so that early treatment may be warranted (Gladwin *et al.*, 2004). Although PH is relatively common in parenchymal lung disease, the degree is generally not severe in relation to the prognosis and symptomatic consequences of the lung disease alone (Nadrous *et al.*, 2005; Naeije, 2005; Leuchte *et al.*, 2006). Again, however, some progressively symptomatic patients have PH out of proportion to the underlying disease (Nadrous *et al.*, 2005; Naeije, 2005; Leuchte *et al.*, 2006; Thabut, *et al.*, 2005), though the response to vascular targeted therapy has not been defined.

Screening by tests other than direct or noninvasive measurements of pulmonary hemodynamics may be useful in some patients. Those with scleroderma tend to exhibit a progressive trend of worsening diffusing capacity prior to the occurrence of clinically significant PAH (Figure 2.2). The ratio of forced vital capacity (FVC) to the diffusing capacity of the lung for carbon monoxide (DLco) can be measured and a ratio of FVC%/DLco% > 1.8 is predictive of the presence or future development of PAH in scleroderma (Chang *et al.*, 2003).

The question of when to begin screening in patients with the potential for having familial PAH remains open. Patients with more than one family member with PAH related to a BMPR2 mutation might be considered for testing for a BMPR2 mutation, since a negative test would imply that there is no higher than normal risk of developing PAH. However, any testing should be preceded by extensive family and genetic counseling. Since penetrance is low (averaging around 10–20%, but varying

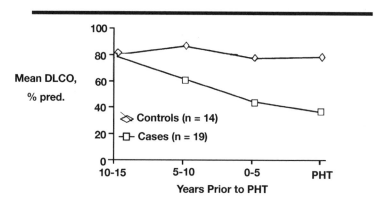

**DLCO (% predicted) in Patients
Who Developed PHT vs Controls**

Figure 2.2 DLCO in patients who developed PHT compared with controls. (Based on Steen & Medsger (2003). Predictors of isolated pulmonary hypertension in patients with systemic sclerosis and limited cutaneous involvement. *Arthritis and Rheumatism*, **48**:516–22. Reproduced courtesy of John Wiley & Sons, Inc.

between families (Loyd, 2002)), the finding of a BMPR2 mutation does not lead to certainty that PAH will develop, though the likelihood that the mutant gene will be transmitted to the next generation is 50%. For patients with a BMPR2 mutation or family members whose genetic status is unknown, the timing for a first echocardiographic screening test is unclear. Because of the phenomenon of genetic anticipation, in which successive generations tend to exhibit the PAH phenotype earlier and more severely (Loyd *et al.*, 1995), screening relatively early in life is probably advisable, though a specific age recommendation has not yet been suggested.

2.5 Detection (discovering pulmonary hypertension)

Screening of high risk asymptomatic patients or evaluation of symptomatic patients requires that there be a clear understanding of what results of testing imply regarding the presence of disease. The use of a specific hemodynamic definition of PH, as outlined above (page 8) does not imply that PH is completely present or completely absent. Like many pathologic processes, PH is a continuum. Moreover, screening tests are subject to errors of specificity and sensitivity. Thus, the presence of 'borderline' or 'mild' PH by echocardiographic examination may not have the same prognostic significance reported for the cohort of symptomatic patients in the NIH registry, who had markedly elevated pulmonary artery pressure and resistance. The presence of mild PH, even if confirmed by right heart catheterization, may not have the same outcome as patients with more significantly abnormal pulmonary hemodynamics. Indeed, suspicious symptoms may not be fully explained by the presence of mild PH. The observation of mild PH may require further evaluation prior to making an unqualified diagnosis of PH. Further examination should include confirmation by right heart catheterization, evaluation of possible end-organ consequences (such as right sided chamber enlargement, right ventricular dysfunction or increased brain natriuretic peptide (BNP) levels, a search for associated diseases and for alternative explanations of symptoms. If resting hemodynamics are inadequate to explain symptoms, an exercise hemodynamic study should be performed (see below). At the very least, the observation of mild PH should prompt careful follow-up to determine whether a trend of worsening hemodynamics develops in the future.

2.6 Definition (diagnosing the clinical context)

The presence of PH requires that a systematic evaluation be undertaken to identify the cause or the presence of associated disease, as represented by the broad differential diagnosis depicted in Table 2.1 utilizing the algorithm shown in Figure 2.1. As opposed to screening for PH in the presence of recognized risk factors, PH may be the first indication of an underlying disease requiring specific treatment. For example, PH may lead to the initial diagnosis of connective tissue disease, severe sleep disorder or previously undetected atrial septal defect. A more detailed description of specific tests used in the evaluation of PH is provided below.

2.7 Prediction (estimating prognosis)

The results of a full evaluation are used to provide a prediction of natural history which in turn determines the type and aggressiveness of therapy. The first predictive index was based on a regression equation derived from hemodynamic measurements obtained in the NIH Registry. The probability of survival $P(t)$ at one, two or three years after baseline can be estimated as $P(t) = H(t)^{A(x,y,z)}$, where $H(t) = 0.88 - 0.14t + 0.01t^2$, $A(x,y,z) = e^{(0.007325x + 0.0526y - 0.3275z)}$, $t =$ years, $\times =$ mean pulmonary arterial pressure (mPAP, mm Hg), $y =$ mean right atrial pressure (mm Hg), and $z =$ cardiac index (l/min/m^2) (D'Alonzo et al., 1991). Other logistic regression equations have been reported to predict survival or death within one year (Okada et al., 1999; Sandoval et al., 1994) The significance of the NIH formula is not that it has been useful in predicting individual survival, but it has provided a quasi-control population for patients on newer therapies. By comparing actual survival of a population on treatment with their expected survival based on baseline hemodynamics, the purported degree of survival benefit of several medications has been publicized (Figure 2.3).

Other factors of survival have been identified which may be useful in assessing the severity and implications of PH in patients (Figures 2.4–2.8). In addition,

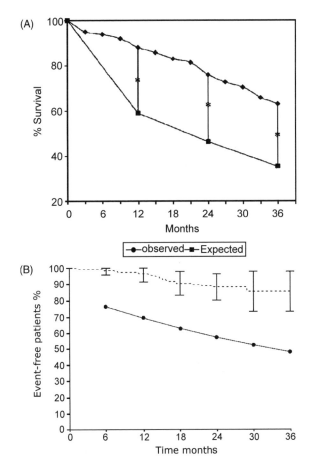

Figure 2.3 Observed survival compared to predicted survival with: (A) Epoprostenol (Reproduced with permission from McLaughlin *et al. Circulation* 2002; **106**:1477–82.) (B) Bosentan. ------: observed survival; ——: predicted survival. (Reproduced with permission from McLaughlin *et al.* (2005) *Eur Respir J.* **25**:244–9. ©European Respiratory Journals Ltd.)

elevated right atrial pressure is consistently identified as having adverse predictive value for survival (D'Alonzo *et al.*, 1991; McLaughlin, Shillington and Rich, 2002; Sitbon *et al.*, 2002). Early response to vascular targeted therapy is also predictive of survival. Patients who achieve an NYHA status of I or II, 6-minute walk distance greater than 380 meters, peak VO2 > 10.4 ml/kg/min, peak SBP > 120 mm Hg, or cardiac index >2.2 l/min/m2 have better survival than those who do not achieve these levels with treatment (D'Alonzo *et al.*, 1991; McLaughlin, Shillington and Rich, 2002; Sitbon *et al.*, 2002; Wensel *et al.*, 2002; Hoeper *et al.*, 2005).

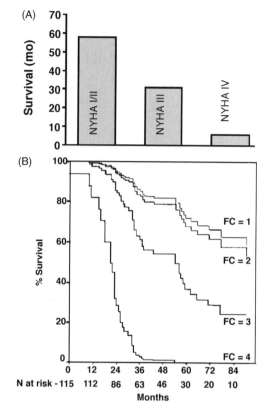

Figure 2.4 Predictors of survival: Functional Status. A. (Reproduced from D'Alonzo *et al.*, *Annals of Internal Medicine* 1991, **115**:343–349, with permission from the American College of Physicians.) B. (Reproduced with permission from McLaughlin *et al. Circulation* 2002; **106**:1477–82.) C. (Reproduced from *J Am Coll Cardiol*, **40**, Sitbon *et al.*, 780–8, Copyright (2002), with permission from the American College of Cardiology.) D. (Reproduced with permission from Miyamoto *et al.* (2000), Clinical correlates and prognostic significance of six-minute walk test in patients with primary pulmonary hypertension. *Am J Resp Crit Care Med*, **161**: 487–92. ©American Thoracic Society.)

2.8 Principles of follow-up (evaluating and responding to outcome)

The importance of treatment response emphasizes the need for continued scrupulous follow-up and reassessment of clinical status in patients with PH who are being managed with any of the currently available medications. The goal of therapy is to achieve a level of symptomatic, functional and hemodynamic improvement in which long-term outlook is predictably optimized. Failure to achieve an adequate degree of benefit warrants continuing efforts to adjust the medical regimen or to consider other interventions, such as lung transplantation. The best means of

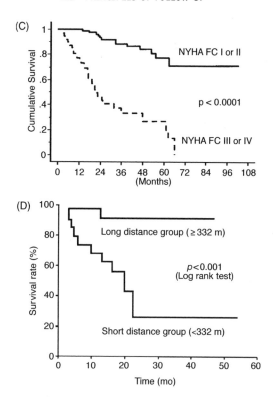

Figure 2.4 *(Continued)*

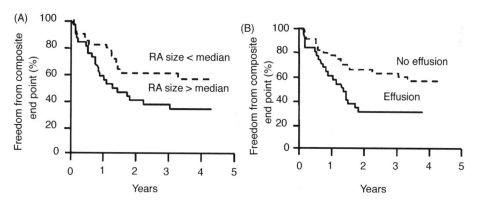

Figure 2.5 Echocardiographic predictors of outcome. Freedom from clinical progression of disease: (A) Right atrial size, (B) Pericardial effusion, (C) Eccentricity index. Survival: (D) Right atrial size, (E) Pericardial effusion, (F) Eccentricity index. (Reproduced from *American Journal of Cardiol*, **39**, Raymond *et al.*, 1214–9, Copyright (2002), with permission from the American College of Cardiology.)

(Continued)

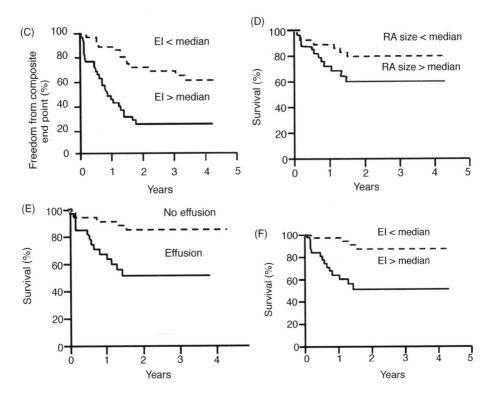

Figure 2.5   *(Continued)*

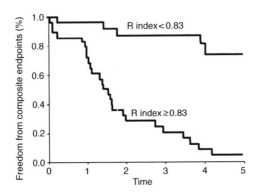

Figure 2.6   Right ventricular index of myocardial performance prediction of outcome. (Reproduced from *American Journal of Cardiology*, **81**, Yeo *et al* 1157–61, Copyright 1998, with permission from Elsevier.)

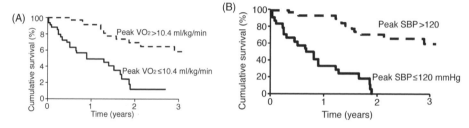

Figure 2.7 Cardiopulmonary exercise predictors of survival. (A) Peak VO$_2$. (B) Peak systemic systolic blood pressure. (Reproduced with permission from Wensel *et al.*, *Circulation* 2002; **106**:319–24.)

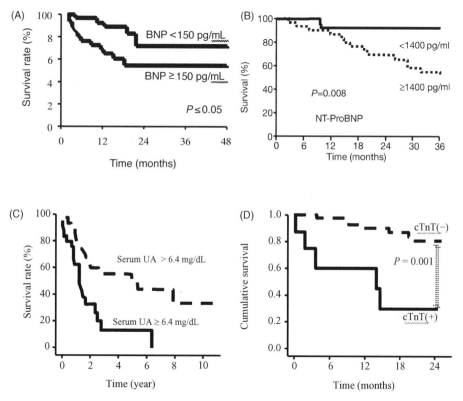

Figure 2.8 Prediction of survival by biomarkers. (A) BNP. (Reproduced with permission from Nagaya *et al.*, *Circulation* 2000; **102**(8):865–70.) (B) N-terminal ProBNP. (Adapted from Fijalkowska *et al.*, *Chest* 2006;**129**(5):1313–21 and reproduced with permission from American College of Chest Physicians.) (C) Uric acid (Reproduced with permission from Nagaya *et al.* (1999), Serum uric acid levels correlate with the severity and mortality of primary pulmonary hypertension. *Am J Resp Crit Care Med*, **160**:487–92. ©American Thoracic Society.) (D) Troponin (Reproduced with permission from Torbicki *et al.*, *Circulation* 2003; **108**(7):844–848.)

reassessment remains under debate, and is necessarily somewhat context driven. Some centers repeat invasive hemodynamic measurements on a regular basis while others rely on echocardiographic parameters. There is general consensus that careful repeated determination of symptomatic functional status and exercise capacity as measured by cardiopulmonary exercise testing or 6-minute walk distance is advisable in patients who are not limited by other factors, such as musculoskeletal problems. BNP appears likely to be a meaningful criterion of progress or progression as well.

The frequency of follow-up depends on the general status of the patient, with higher risk or unstable patients requiring more frequent re-assessment. However, repeat evaluation in less than three months is unlikely to detect meaningful trends in most patients, since intrinsic variability of testing measurements may exceed the ability to detect true changes over short durations.

2.9   Specific tests in the evaluation of pulmonary hypertension

Evaluation and re-assessment of patients mandates proper performance and balanced interpretation of key medical tests. Some tests are required in all patients in order to obtain a meaningful understanding of the state of the disease. Other tests are reserved for those situations in which the clinical situation and early tests warrant additional evaluation.

Required

Physical examination Findings on physical examination which are important for detecting PH and guiding further evaluation are shown in Table 2.4. The importance

Table 2.4   Physical findings pertinent to PH and their significance
Physical signs that indicate pulmonary hypertension

Sign	Implication
Accentuated pulmonary component of S2 (audible at apex in over 90%)	High pulmonary pressure increases force of pulmonary valve closure
Early systolic click	Sudden interruption of opening of pulmonary valve into high-pressure artery
Midsystolic ejection murmur	Turbulent transvalvular pulmonary outflow
Left parasternal lift	High right ventricular pressure and hypertrophy present
Right ventricular S4 (in 38%)	High right ventricular pressure and hypertrophy present
Increased jugular 'a' wave	High right ventricular filling pressure

Table 2.4 *(Continued)*

Physical signs that indicate severity of pulmonary hypertension

Sign	Implication
Moderate to severe pulmonary hypertension	
Holosystolic murmur that increases with inspiration	Tricuspid regurgitation
Increased jugular 'v' waves	Tricuspid regurgitation
Pulsatile liver	Tricuspid regurgitation
Diastolic murmur	Pulmonary regurgitation
Hepatojugular reflux	High central venous pressure
Advanced pulmonary hypertension with right ventricular failure	
Right ventricular S3 (in 23%)	Right ventricular dysfunction
Marked distention of jugular veins	Right ventricular dysfunction or tricuspid regurgitation or both
Hepatomegaly	Right ventricular dysfunction or tricuspid regurgitation or both
Peripheral edema (in 32%)	Right ventricular dysfunction or tricuspid regurgitation or both
Ascites	Right ventricular dysfunction or tricuspid regurgitation or both
Low blood pressure, diminished pulse pressure, cool extremities	Reduced cardiac output, peripheral vasoconstriction

Physical signs that detect possible underlying cause or associations of pulmonary hypertension

Sign	Implication
Central cyanosis	Hypoxemia, right-to-left shunt
Clubbing	Congenital heart disease, pulmonary venopathy
Cardiac auscultatory findings, including systolic murmurs, diastolic murmurs, opening snap and gallop	Congenital or acquired heart or valvular disease
Rales, dullness or decreased breath sounds	Pulmonary congestion or effusion or both
Fine rales, accessory muscle use, wheezing, protracted expiration, productive cough	Pulmonary parenchymal disease
Obesity, kyphoscoliosis, enlarged tonsils	Possible substrate for disordered ventilation
Sclerodactyly, arthritis, rash	Connective tissue disorder
Peripheral venous insufficiency or obstruction	Possible venous thrombosis

of physical signs, coupled with close attention to the medical history and symptoms, cannot be overstated in promoting timely suspicion and pursuit of appropriate evaluation. However, signs of PH may be subtle and potentially overlooked, so that the absence of definite findings does not exclude the possibility of clinically significant PAH. An accentuated pulmonary component of the second heart sound is heard at the apex in over 90% of patients with IPAH (suggesting high pulmonary pressure increasing the force of pulmonary valve closure) and a right ventricular S4 is present in 38% (Rich *et al.*, 1987) Physical signs may also point to the consequences of PAH, such as the diastolic murmur of pulmonary regurgitation, the systolic murmur and jugular vein V waves of tricuspid regurgitation as evidenced by a diastolic murmur, and the S3 gallop, pulsatile hepatomegaly, edema and ascites of right ventricular failure.

Finally, the physical examination also provides clues to causal or associated conditions, including central cyanosis of hypoxemia related to right-to-left shunt, low cardiac output, a markedly depressed diffusing capacity, digital clubbing associated with congenital heart disease or pulmonary veno-occlusive disease (Holcomb *et al.*, 2000), and murmurs of valvular disease. Findings of rales, dullness or decreased breath sounds may suggest pulmonary congestion or effusion or both; and fine rales, accessory muscle use, wheezing or protracted expiration imply pulmonary parenchymal disease. Obesity, kyphoscoliosis and a crowded oropharynx owing to enlarged tonsils are possible substrates for disordered ventilation. Scleroderma skin changes or other rashes, nail fold capillary abnormalities, arthritis and other stigmata are suggestive of an underlying connective tissue disorder. Peripheral venous insufficiency or obstruction can be found in the setting of venous thrombosis and pulmonary thromboembolic disease.

Chest X-ray (CXR) The CXR imparts information relevant to the detection of PH and its causes, but is nonspecific and qualitative (Figure 2.9). Efforts to construct quantitatively predictive indices have been made, but are seldom employed clinically because of more focused noninvasive test availability. For example, an index has been described based on the ratio of the summed horizontal measurements of the pulmonary arteries from midline to their first divisions divided by the transverse chest diameter (Lupi *et al.*, 1975): an index of ≤ 0.38 is associated with a pressure < 30 mm Hg, whereas an index ≥ 0.38 was associated with a higher (10%) probability of a pulmonary arterial systolic pressure > 45 mm Hg. Radiographic signs suggestive of pulmonary hypertension are enlarged main and hilar pulmonary arterial shadows with concomitant attenuation of peripheral pulmonary vascular markings ('pruning') (Rich *et al.*, 1987). Right ventricular enlargement is evidenced by extension of the right ventricular silhouette into the retrosternal clear space on the lateral CXR. Findings of underlying disease may be observed, such as pulmonary venous congestion (pulmonary venous hypertension, pulmonary veno-occlusive disease, pulmonary capillary hemangiomatosis), hyperinflation (chronic obstructive pulmonary disease), or kyphosis (restrictive pulmonary disease). Common findings in chronic thromboembolic pulmonary

hypertension (CTEPH) are generalized cardiomegaly (86%), right ventricular enlargement (68%), mosaic oligemia (68%), right descending pulmonary arterial enlargement (55%), chronic volume loss (27%), atelectasis or effusion (23%), and pleural
thickening (14%) (Woodruff *et al.*, 1985). Other radiographic studies report high
prevalence in patients with confirmed CTEPH of pulmonary trunk and central pulmonary arterial dilation (Schmidt *et al.*, 1996). With the possible exception of clear-
cut oligemia, these findings are not specific to CTEPH and are found in many
patients with PAH of any cause. There is no definite correlation between radiographic abnormalities and severity of pulmonary hypertension.

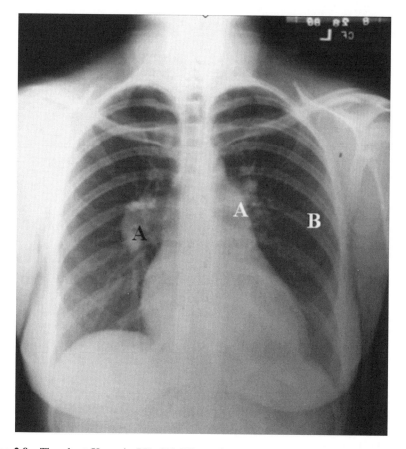

Figure 2.9 The chest X-ray in PH. (A) Hilar pulmonary artery prominence; (B) Peripheral
attenuation of vascular markings; (C) Right Ventricular enlargement; (D) Left heart disease suggested by Kerley B lines, pulmonary venous hypertension, pulmonary congestion and pleural
effusions; (E) Interstitial fibrosis (scleroderma); (F) Hyperinflation of chronic obstructive lung
disease (emphysema).

(Continued)

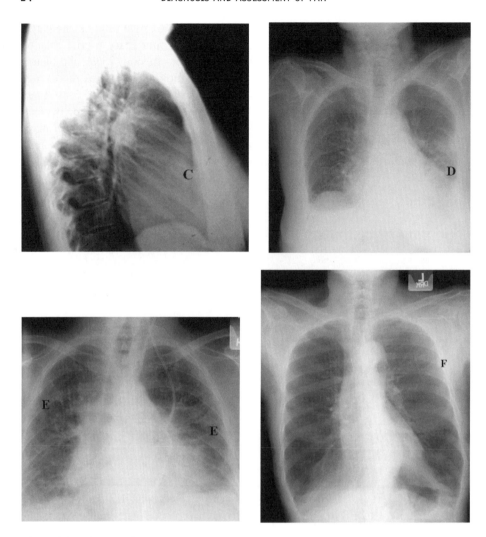

Figure 2.9   *(Continued)*

Electrocardiography Right ventricular hypertrophy and right axis deviation are present in 87% and 79% respectively of patients with IPAH (Rich *et al.*, 1987). Electrocardiogram (ECG) findings considered suggestive of PAH producing right ventricular hypertrophy are right axis deviation, right ventricular strain and right atrial enlargement (Figure 2.10). The ECG has inadequate sensitivity (55–73%) and specificity (70%) to be an effective sole screening tool for the detection of PH (Ahearn *et al.* 2002). Some features of the ECG in patients with IPAH may have prognostic value: a P wave amplitude in lead II of ≥ 0.25 mV predicts a 2.8-times greater risk of death over a six-year follow-up period, and each additional 1 mm of

A. Right axis deviation (>100°)
B. Right ventricular hypertrophy (a tall R
   wave and small S wave with R/S ratio >
   1 in lead V1; qR complex in lead V1)
C. Right ventricular strain (ST-T wave
   depression and inversion are often
   present in the right precordial leads)
D. Right atrial enlargement (P wave ≥ 2.5
   mm in leads II, III, and aVF and frontal P
   axis of ≥ 75°, large terminal negative
   deflection in V1)

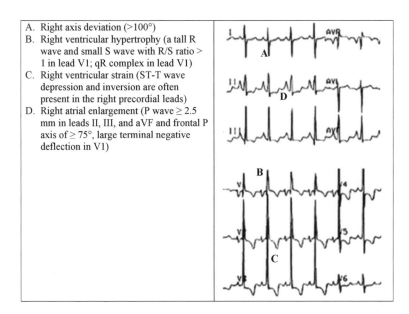

Figure 2.10   The electrocardiogram in PH.

P wave amplitude in lead III corresponds with a 4.5-fold increase in risk of death
(Bossone *et al.*, 2002).

   **Echocardiography with "cavitation" study (also known as "bubble" or
"contrast" study)** Echocardiography is among the most important tests in patients
with suspected or confirmed PH. It permits noninvasive insight into the morphology,
function and hemodynamics of the right heart using multiple, often unrelated and
independent, echocardiographic and Doppler signs.

   Variables useful for assessing pulmonary artery pressure and making the noninvasive diagnosis of PH are different from those which correlate with prognosis in
patients diagnosed to have PH. Increased peak velocity of the tricuspid regurgitant
jet indicating increased systolic pressure gradient between right ventricular and
right atrium (TIPG) is a noninvasive hallmark of PH. Based on data collected in
healthy subjects and reported correlations between right heart catheterization (RHC)
and Doppler measurements, a peak jet velocity between 2.8 and 3.4 m/sec (corresponding to systolic PAP 36–50 mm Hg according to the modified Bernoulli equation) should raise suspicion of mild PH (Mukerjee *et al.*, 2004; McQuillan *et al.*,
2001). Unfortunately, unequivocal noninvasive diagnosis of PH with this method is
not possible. It does not allow calculation of mPAP and requires an assumption of
the right atrial pressure. A trial evaluating the reliability of prospective screening of
patients with scleroderma based on increased tricuspid regurgitant pressure gradient, found that 45% of cases of echocardiographic diagnoses of PH are falsely positive when compared with RHC (Hachulla *et al.*, 2005). Other variables that might
reinforce echocardiographic suspicion of mild PH include increased velocity of

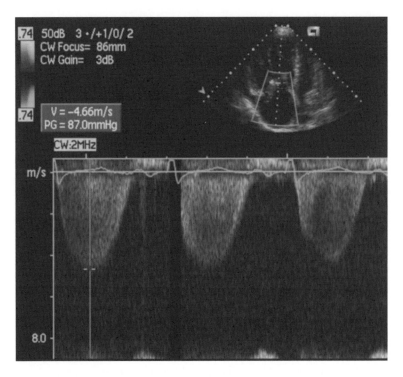

Figure 2.11 Doppler measurement of peak velocity of tricuspid regurgitation used for estimation of pulmonary artery systolic pressure. In this particular case $V_{max} = 4.66$ m/sec predicts a tricuspid insufficiency pressure gradient (TIPG) of 87 mm Hg.

pulmonary valve regurgitation and short acceleration time of RV ejection to pulmonary artery. Doppler-calculated systolic pulmonary arterial pressure (sPAP) > 50 mm Hg can be considered as a reasonably reliable sign of PH (Figure 2.11) (Mukerjee *et al.*, 2004).

Once the diagnosis of PH is made, echocardiography can be helpful in detecting its cause. Congenital shunts can be searched for with the help of two-dimensional Doppler and bubble contrast examinations. Resting and exercise pulse oximetry and its response to supplemental oxygen is helpful when choosing the strategy for contrast examinations. High pulmonary flow in the absence of detectable shunt, or significant dilatation of proximal pulmonary arteries despite only moderate PH, may warrant transesophageal examination or magnetic resonance imaging (MRI) to exclude atypically positioned defects, such as sinus venosus or anomalous pulmonary venous return.

While echocardiography may help in detecting systolic left ventricular (LV) dysfunction as a potential cause of PH it might miss some cases with diastolic LV failure, again underscoring the need for RHC (Galie *et al.*, 2004).

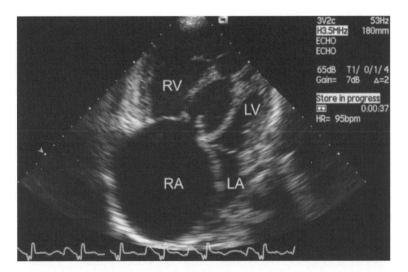

Figure 2.12 Typical echocardiographic appearance of the heart in a patient with severe PAH: marked dilatation of right heart chambers contrasting with under-filled slit-like left heart chambers. RA: right atrium; LA: left atrium; RV: right ventricle; LV: left ventricle.

While useful for noninvasive assessment of sPAP, tricuspid jet velocity may be misleading as a follow-up marker, especially in severe pulmonary hypertension. Tricuspid jet velocity may actually drop, not because of decreased afterload, but because of increasing right atrial pressure and/or further deterioration of RV systolic function. Therefore clinical decision-making based predominantly on Doppler estimates of sPAP should be discouraged

Echocardiographic variables with confirmed adverse prognostic value can be classified into morphological and functional. The former are represented by pericardial effusion, leftward interventricular septum shift and increased right atrial area (Figure 2.12) (Raymond *et al.*, 2002). The latter consist of high 'index of global RV dysfunction' known also as the Tei index, and low tricuspid annulus plane systolic excursion (TAPSE) (Tei *et al.*, 1996; Yeo *et al.*, 1998).

In a retrospective study involving 53 IPAH patients, although the Tei index of myocardial dysfunction, combining information contained in RV systolic and diastolic time intervals, was independent of heart rate, RV pressure, dilation or tricuspid regurgitation, it did correlate with survival (Yeo *et al.*, 1998). TAPSE has also been reported to predict survival rates in consecutive patients with PH who were referred for right heart catheterization (Forfia *et al.*, 2006). Among 47 patients with pulmonary arterial hypertension, survival estimates at two years for those with TAPSE > 1.8 cm were 88% contrasting with 50% in the remaining subjects (Figure 2.13). Those two functional prognostic markers seem more interesting as potential follow-up tools. Unfortunately data on the cost-effectiveness and reliability

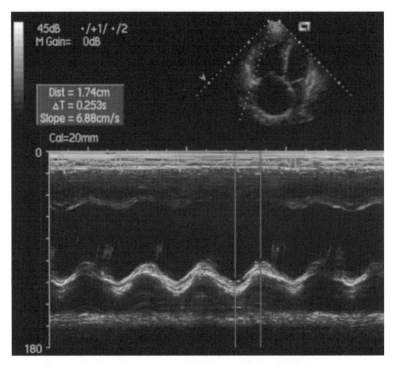

Figure 2.13   Measurement of tricuspid annulus plane systolic excursion: TAPSE = 1.74 cm. TAPSE has been found to be of prognostic significance, with values below 1.8 cm indicating worse long-term outcomes.

of echocardiographic follow-up are limited. In our experience, serial monitoring with echocardiography is possible, but requires assessment of multiple variables, and preferably the same experienced operator using a standardized methodology in order to limit the operator-dependent variability of reported results.

Ventilation–perfusion scintigraphy Because of its high sensitivity, ventilation-perfusion (V/Q) scintigraphy is widely used to screen for CTEPH (Figure 2.14) (Worsley, Palevsky and Alavi, 1994; Fedullo *et al*., 2001). While segmental or larger perfusion defects suggest CTEPH, further imaging including computed tomography and/or pulmonary angiography with RHC is mandatory for final diagnosis, staging and qualification for surgical treatment (Fedullo *et al*., 2001). This is particularly important since a V/Q scan, showing redistribution rather than absolute volume of flow to various regions, can significantly underestimate the hemodynamic significance of post-embolic intravascular structures (Ryan *et al*., 1988); unless the V/Q report is within normal limits, further studies should be done to rule out CTEPH.

The relative character of data acquired with a V/Q scan is best exemplified after successful thromboendarterectomy. Often areas apparently well perfused prior to thromboendarterectomy present as perfusion defects at post-surgical follow-up scans.

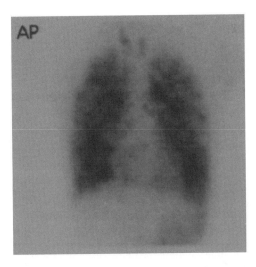

Figure 2.14   Diffuse subsegmental perfusion defects often found at lung scintigraphy in patients with PAH.

This is most likely due to redistribution of flow to surgically re-opened areas of pulmonary vascular bed which were previously protected from high pressure and flow and maintained normal pulmonary vascular resistance (Olman *et al.*, 1990).

Less-frequent causes of significant V/Q mismatch evidenced by lung scan which may be misleading include intravascular tumors, most often sarcomas, Takayasu arteritis, fibrosing mediastinitis, lung and mediastinal tumors and/or adenopathy and other space occupying structures compressing the pulmonary arterial bed and affecting regional lung perfusion. Among patients with PAH, those with pulmonary veno-occlusive disease (PVOD) may present with larger and asymmetric defects mimicking thromboembolic disease (Sola *et al.*, 1993). Many of the remaining PAH patients have multiple small subsegmental perfusion defects uniformly spread within the lungs.

Scintillations recorded over systemic organs suggest right-to-left shunting, either due to congenital heart disease (Johnson and Worsley, 1996) with Eisenmenger syndrome or from intrapulmonary anastomoses such as pulmonary arterial–venous fistulas as seen in the Osler Weber Rendu syndrome, i.e. hereditary hemorrhagic telangiectasia.

Pulmonary function testing Pulmonary function tests (PFTs) are a required component of the PAH workup and can be useful in the workup of unexplained dyspnea. Evidence of significant airway restriction and/or obstruction suggests an alternative diagnosis, which may lead to an entirely different treatment approach. While PFTs are essential for excluding significant hypoxic lung disease as a cause for PH, lung mechanics are commonly abnormal in PAH, albeit usually only mildly so.

The degree of the PFT abnormalities correlates with the severity of the disease in IPAH patients (Sun *et al.*, 2003). In patients with IPAH, there is a reduction in forced vital capacity (FVC), forced expiratory volume in one second (FEV1), maximum voluntary ventilation (MVV), total lung capacity (TLC), and effective alveolar volume (VA´) in proportion to NYHA class or aerobic capacity; however, the magnitude of the reduction in these measures is small, and most IPAH patients' symptoms and hemodynamic findings are out of proportion to the degree of PFT abnormalities.

The diffusing capacity of the lung for carbon monoxide (DLco) is also reduced in proportion to IPAH disease severity, with most patients falling below the lower limits of normal (Figure 2.15) (Sun *et al.*, 2003). The magnitude of this reduction in DLco is often large, in keeping with the significant loss of pulmonary capillary bed found in these patients.

In APAH patients, particularly those with connective tissue diseases such as scleroderma, PFT abnormalities may help differentiate an isolated pulmonary vasculopathy out of proportion to the degree of pulmonary fibrosis from that of pulmonary hypertension resulting from more severe parenchymal lung disease. Chang and coworkers found that patients with a predominant pulmonary vasculopathy had FVC/DLCO ratios of > 1.8, whereas those with pure fibrotic disease and secondary pulmonary hypertension had FVC/DLCO ratios closer to 1.0 (Chang *et al.*, 2003).

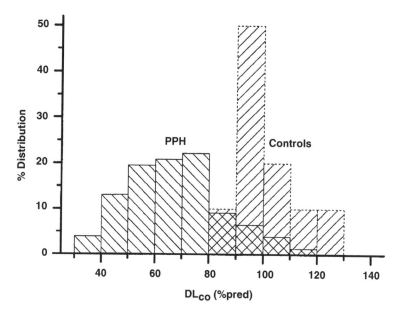

Figure 2.15 Distribution of values for gas transfer index or diffusing capacity for carbon monoxide (DLCO) in 79 IPAH patients (lines from upper left to lower right) and 20 normal controls (lines from lower left to upper right). Values are divided by deciles of percent predicted (%pred). For these measurements, all individuals below 80% of predicted are below the normal 95% confidence limits. Approximately 75% of the PPH patients have a reduced DLCO. (Adapted from *J Am Coll Cardiol*, **41**(6), Sun *et al.*, 1027–35, Copyright (2003) with permission from the American College of Cardiology.)

Overnight oximetry Nocturnal hypoxemia is common in patients with IPAH (Rafanan *et al.*, 2001); however, the oxygen desaturation occurs independently of the presence of apneas or hypopneas. Thus, overnight oximetry may be useful as a screening tool for detection of sleep apnea, which may contribute to or exacerbate pulmonary hypertension, and may also be useful for detecting nocturnal hypoxemia associated with PAH.

Antinuclear antibodies PAH association with connective tissue diseases (CTD) is well documented and recognized. However, severity of PAH often has little correlation with the severity of CTD. Indeed, often serologic abnormalities are the only signs of the disease, and therefore antinuclear antibody (ANA) screening is part of the evaluation of patients with PH. An ANA titer > 1:80 should be followed by a search of disease-specific antinuclear antibodies using a standard diagnostic panel.

HIV PAH may be associated with HIV infection (de Chadarevian *et al.*, 1994; Mani and Smith, 1994; Mesa *et al.*, 1998; Mette *et al.*, 1992; Nunes *et al.*, 2003; Pellicelli *et al.*, 2001; Petitpretz *et al.*, 1994; Petrosillo *et al.*, 2001; Polos *et al.*, 1992; Speich *et al.*, 1991; Zuber *et al.*, 2004). Therefore an HIV serologic screening should be obtained and if positive, confirmed by Western blot analysis.

Liver function tests PAH can be associated with portal hypertension (Castro *et al.* 1996; Krowka *et al.*, 2004; Kawut *et al.*, 2004; Edwards *et al.*, 1987; Robalino and Moodie, 1991; Krowka, 1997; Ramsay *et al.*, 1997; Auletta *et al.*, 2000; Yang *et al.*, 2001; Halank *et al.*, 2006; Michael *et al.*, 2006). Therefore, it is important to search for markers of liver disease, which could lead to a diagnosis of cirrhosis. Assessment of hepatic transaminases, bilirubin, serum proteins and clotting factors are useful in screening for liver disease. Tests for viral hepatitis should be considered in the presence of abnormal liver function markers. However, liver imaging, portal vein ultrasonography or even assessment of transhepatic gradient during right heart catheterization by wedging the catheter in the hepatic vein may be needed to differentiate between secondary liver congestion and portal hypertension.

6-minute walk test The 6-minute walk (6MW) distance is a simple, inexpensive measure of the functional limitation in patients with cardiovascular and/or lung disease. The 6MW test is used as a measure of functional capacity in patients with heart disease (Guyatt *et al.*, 1985). It has prognostic significance in PAH (Sitbon *et al.*, 2002; Miyamato *et al.*, 2000; Paciocco *et al.*, 2001), and has been used in most randomized controlled trials of PAH therapies as the primary endpoint to demonstrate efficacy (Channick *et al.*, 2001; Rubin *et al.*, 2002; Galie *et al.*, 2002; Simonneau *et al.*, 2002; Barst *et al.*, 2003; Olschewski *et al.*, 2002; Langleben *et al.*, 2002).

While useful as a crude measure of aerobic capacity, the 6MW distance does not aid the clinician in confirming the diagnosis of suspected PAH, as it does not differentiate the nature of a patient's exercise limitation. In fact, in most patients, factors such as stride length, body weight and walking skills may be more important determinants of 6MW distance than aerobic capacity (Guyatt *et al.*, 1985). According to guidelines prepared by the American Thoracic Society, the information provided by a

6MW test should be considered complementary to cardiopulmonary exercise testing (see below), not a replacement for it (ATS Statement 2002).

Right heart catheterization The standard for confirming and characterizing PAH is right heart catheterization. By definition, PAH requires demonstration of a mean PAP of $\geq$ 25 mm Hg at rest, or $\geq$ 30 mm Hg with exercise, a normal left ventricular end diastolic pressure (LVEDP) or PCWP and a pulmonary vascular resistance of $>$ 3 Wood units (Rubin and Rich, 1996). This can only be demonstrated via invasive hemodynamic monitoring, using a balloon flotation catheter to document pulmonary hemodynamics. Careful attention must be given to the PCWP tracing, as the pressure waveforms are often misinterpreted if the catheter is not in the proper position.

Hemodynamics are prognostic in PAH (Rich et al., 1987), but, more importantly, serve to confirm the suspicion of PAH and exclude other secondary etiologies of pulmonary hypertension. In particular, the inability of echocardiography to measure PCWP (and thus LVEDP) bears important clinical significance, since it is essential to exclude pulmonary venous hypertension when making the diagnosis of PAH. The consensus among PAH experts is the requirement to obtain at least one diagnostic and confirmatory right heart catheterization in PAH patients.

The prognostic value of pulmonary hemodynamic measurements is illustrated by the finding that patients with IPAH whose mean right atrial pressure is $<$ 10 mm Hg have a median survival of nearly 50 months without pulmonary vasodilator therapy, whereas those with a mean right atrial pressure (RAP) of $\geq$ 20 mm Hg survive less than three months (D'Alonzo et al., 1991). RAP has also been shown to be prognostic in patients with systemic sclerosis (Mukerjee et al., 2003).

Realizing that the symptoms of PAH are mainly exertional, investigators have recently begun to focus upon exercise hemodynamics as a measure of hemodynamic exertional impairment (James et al., 2000; Raeside et al., 1998; Raeside et al., 2000). However, technical limitations to measuring exercise hemodynamics during catheterization include the lack of a standardized exercise protocol, practical mechanical difficulties in exercising subjects with invasive catheters in place, and pressure wave artifacts related to chest wall motion and intrathoracic pressure variations during exercise. Implantable devices designed to continuously measure pulmonary hemodynamics may overcome for some of these potential inaccuracies and are currently under investigation (Karamanoglu et al., 2007).

Context Driven

High resolution computed tomography (HRCT) This technique is particularly useful in patients with pulmonary hypertension and suspected interstitial lung disease suggested by abnormal pulmonary function tests and/or associated connective tissue disease. HRCT also supports a diagnosis of CTEPH when a mosaic pattern can be seen in the presence of pulmonary hypertension, indicating areas of preserved regional perfusion (King et al., 1994). One of the important described patterns relates to pulmonary capillary hemangiomatosis and pulmonary veno-occlusive disease, which until recently was rarely diagnosed pre-mortem without a lung biopsy or autopsy. These rare conditions can be suspected in the presence of local signs of congestion

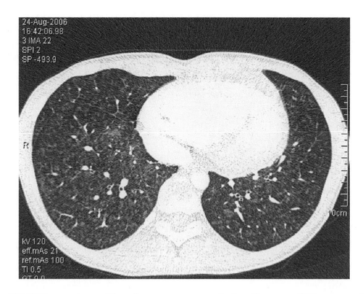

Figure 2.16 HRCT in a patient with pulmonary veno-occlusive disease – diffuse ground glass opacities and thickened septal lines.

presenting as thickening of the septae and centrilobular ground glass attenuations on HRCT (Figure 2.16) (Dufour *et al.*, 1998). HRCT can also detect regional emphysema and/or parenchymal changes more precisely than CXR, explaining some of the perfusion defects seen at lung scintigraphy. Expiratory imaging might also be useful for detection of air-trapping, suggesting the lungs and not the heart as the primary cause of dyspnea and exercise limitation.

Arterial blood gas Arterial blood gas measurements may be useful in the evaluation of PH when hypoxic pulmonary hypertension is suspected, when acid–base disturbances are present or suspected, and/or when precise quantitation of left-to-right shunt is required.

CT angiogram In patients with PH, CT angiography is useful to clarify the cause of abnormal perfusion detected by a lung perfusion scan. The potential presence of intravascular tumors, Takayasu arteritis, fibrosing mediastinitis, lung and mediastinal tumors and/or adenopathy can also be assessed with angio CT. However, its major role is in defining the site and proximal extension of intrapulmonary lesions of CTEPH, while acknowledging that there is a 7% false negative rate for CTEPH using CT angiogram alone without pulmonary angiography (Bergin *et al.*, 1996). Multi-segmental tomographs with modern software permit three-dimensional reconstruction of more distal pulmonary arteries and increasingly precise visualization of intraluminal post-embolic residua (Figure 2.17). Virtual angiography using automatic lumen tracing options became feasible with the new generation of CT machines, but has not been validated for clinical use. There is no consensus on the importance of assessment of bronchial arteries for the diagnosis and surgical qualification of CTEPH.

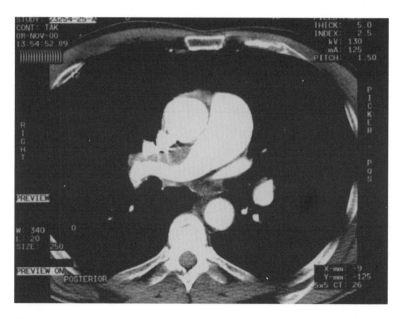

Figure 2.17   Large mural organized thrombus in proximal right pulmonary artery in a patient with chronic thromboembolic PH.

CT angiography can also provide information about the dimensions of central pulmonary arteries. While generally such dimensions correlate with mPAP, an occasional patient with PH may develop a large pulmonary artery aneurysm which might be prone to dissection and/or rupture with fatal consequences (Figure 2.18). Whether rules applying to monitoring of aortic aneurysm dimensions apply also to the pulmonary artery is not clear, but progressive increase in dimensions can suggest impending rupture and consideration of surgical intervention based on an overall risk–benefit assessment (Wekerle *et al.*, 1998).

Pulmonary angiography   While the pulmonary angiogram has been largely replaced by CT angiography in diagnosis of acute pulmonary embolism, it is still recommended as a part of the assessment of patients with CTEPH. It is indicated in all patients with pulmonary hypertension and segmental or larger perfusion defects at lung scintigraphy. Angiography can be performed directly after right heart catheterization. Also, if clear hemodynamic and angiographic indications for thromboendarterectomy are found a caval filter may be introduced during the same session and using the same vascular approach.

Pulmonary angiography is not contra-indicated in severe PH. However, patients with PAH seem to tolerate angiography less well and therefore it should be the last imaging method applied to patients with suggestive signs of CTEPH at lung scan and/or CT. Safety measures should be respected, with special precautions taken in patients with right atrial pressures > 20 mm Hg, indicating right ventricular failure. The flow rate and volume of injected contrast material, preferably nonionic and

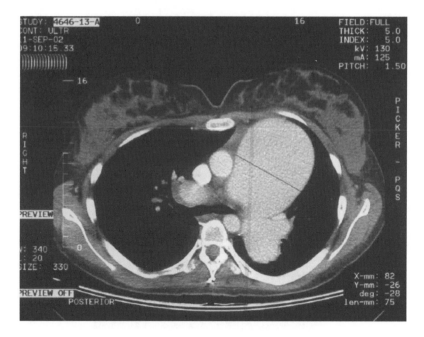

Figure 2.18   Main pulmonary artery aneurysm in a patient with PAH.

low-osmotic should be decreased in patients with significant restriction of pulmonary arterial bed, as judged from lung scintigraphy and angio CT, and with decreased pulmonary flow, as indicated by right heart catheterization (Pitton *et al.*, 2006; Pitton *et al.* 1996).

Angiographic appearance is specific for CTEPH. While sometimes complete vascular occlusions are seen as in acute PE, they are accompanied by irregular outlines of contrast-filled arterial contours, pouches, webs and bands representing partly recanalized thromboembolic material (Figure 2.19) (Auger, Fedullo and Moser, 1992).

In the near future, the new developments in CT and magnetic resonance imaging (MRI) technology may obviate the need for invasive contrast studies in a growing proportion of patients considered for pulmonary thromboendarterectomy.

Coagulation profile Blood testing to screen for evidence of hypercoagulability is commonly performed in patients with suspected or confirmed PH. The presence of a coagulation disorder in these patients may be suggestive of thromboembolism, which could lead to CTEPH. However, in one study of 13 patients undergoing thromboendarterectomy for CTEPH, only 38% had an identifiable coagulation disorder.

Current consensus recommendations for the medical treatment of PAH support the use of anticoagulation, usually with warfarin. Obtaining a baseline coagulation profile in these patients is recommended before initiating the anticoagulation medication.

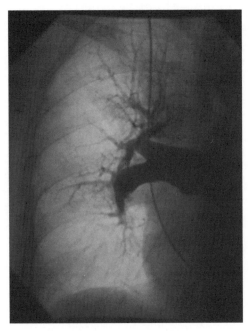

Figure 2.19 Typical angiographic changes in a patient with chronic thromboembolic PH: progressive narrowing of right intermediate artery with almost complete absence of perfusion to lower and medial lobe.

Cardiopulmonary exercise test with gas exchange measurements A noninvasive, comprehensive assessment of cardiopulmonary function can be obtained with the use of formal cardiopulmonary exercise testing (CPET). CPET also has prognostic significance (Guyatt *et al.*, 1985), because it measures both cardiovascular and ventilatory performance during exercise. It has the advantage of aiding the clinician in determining the physiologic nature of a patient's limitation (i.e. determining the cause of unexplained dyspnea) (Wasserman *et al.*, 2004., Oudiz and Sun, 2002; Markowitz and Systrom, 2004). Interestingly, the peak systolic blood pressure (SBP) during cardiopulmonary exercise testing has been shown to be an independent predictor of mortality in untreated patients with IPAH, with a peak SBP of less than 120 mm Hg correlating with a higher mortality than a peak SBP more than 120 mm Hg (Wensel *et al.*, 2002).

In patients with PAH, CPET can quantitate PAH severity by assessing cardiovascular impairment and ventilatory inefficiency (Sun *et al.*, 2001) The reduction in peak oxygen consumption (peak $\dot{V}O_2$) and increased ventilatory inefficiency ($\dot{V}E/\dot{V}O_2$) are proportional to PAH disease severity reflecting the inability of PAH patients to adequately increase pulmonary (and therefore systemic) blood flow during exercise (Sun *et al.*, 2001). Early lactic acidosis in PAH, resulting from impaired blood flow to tissues, causing increased CO_2 output and ventilatory drive, is also best quantitated with CPET, measured as a decrease in the anaerobic threshold or AT.

Additional useful CPET parameters include O_2 pulse ($\dot{V}O_2/HR$) and the ratio of the change in oxygen consumption with change in work rate ($\Delta \dot{V}O_2/\Delta WR$). The O_2 pulse reflects the capacity of the heart to deliver oxygen per beat, and is equal to the product of stroke volume and arterial–mixed venous O_2 difference. A decreasing O_2 pulse as work rate increases signifies a decreasing stroke volume. In normal patients, $\Delta \dot{V}O_2/\Delta WR$ is approximately 10 ml/min/W. In patients who are unable to increase their cardiac output in response to exercise, this ratio decreases proportional to the severity of the impairment in cardiac output with exercise.

Transesophageal echocardiography (TEE) This procedure should be considered in patients in whom clinical and imaging data suggest shunt as the cause of PH, but transthoracic echocardiography fails to document it or is inconclusive. Therefore TEE should be considered when the right heart chambers and proximal pulmonary arteries are dilated out of proportion to the severity of PH, and/or pulmonary artery flow seems increased when assessed with Doppler. Sinus venosus atrial septal defect (ASD) (an atypically situated ASD), abnormal pulmonary venous drainage or patent ductus arteriosus should be specifically searched for during TEE (Figure 2.20) (Pruszczyk *et al.*, 1997).

TEE can be also used for visualization of organized proximal thrombi in main pulmonary arteries, though with modern CT equipment this is rarely necessary. However, even in the presence of angiographic findings that may suggest intravascular tumors, Takayasu arteritis or other non-thrombotic causes of vascular obstruction, TEE may still provide contributing information and may help in decision-making (Pruszczyk *et al.*, 1997).

Exercise hemodynamic echocardiogram Contrast-enhanced exercise Doppler echocardiography was suggested for early detection of patients with normal tricuspid

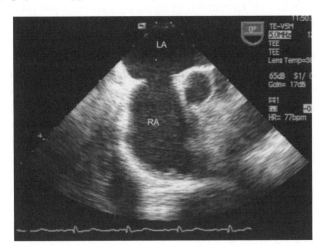

Figure 2.20 Large atrial septal defect in the upper part of the interatrial septum revealed at transesophageal echocardiography (TEE) in a patient with moderate PH. LA – left atrium, RA – right atrium.

jet velocities at rest in the late 1980s (Himelman 1989). This method, however, did not gain popularity, probably because technical difficulties resulted in a significant proportion of inconclusive results. More recently, Doppler echocardiography during supine bicycle exercise was reported useful for identification of persons susceptible to high altitude pulmonary edema. The cut-off used was an sPAP value of 45 mm Hg at work rates less than 150 W (Grunig et al., 2000a, 2000b).

The same group reported an increase in sPAP out of proportion to the amount of work performed in some asymptomatic family members of IPAH patients. The increase was found to be linked to genotype. A normal response to exercise was arbitrarily defined as maximal sPAP < 40 mm Hg (Grunig et al., 2000a). A multi-center trial has been designed to provide external validation of those findings. Standardized protocols and thresholds, which can be useful for interpretation of an exercise echocardiographic test in high-risk asymptomatic subjects or patients with PH, remain to be established.

Vasodilator testing Most PAH experts suggest that acute vasodilator testing be performed at least once when PAH is diagnosed to determine acute pulmonary vasoreactivity. Usually this is done during the confirmatory right heart catheterization (see above). Pulmonary vasoreactivity is defined as a decrease in PAP with a concomitant increase in cardiac output, and a decrease in pulmonary vascular resistance PVR after the administration of a selective pulmonary vasodilator (vasodilator 'challenge'). Until recently, a 'significant' response, i.e. one that would suggest clinical benefit from long-term high-dose calcium channel blockers, was defined as a decrease in mean PAP and/or PVR, by at least 20% (Sandoval et al., 1994; Rich, Kaufmann and Levy, 1992; Weir et al., 1989., Sitbon et al., 1998). However, this practice has recently been challenged in recommendations made by the European Society of Cardiology, suggesting that only patients whose mPAP drops by $\geq$ 10 mm Hg to a target level of $\geq$ 40 mm Hg (with an increased or unchanged cardiac output) after an acute vasodilator challenge may benefit from high-dose calcium channel blockers (Sitbon et al., 2005). The agents of choice with a short half-life for determining acute pulmonary vasoreactivity include intravenous epoprostenol, intravenous adenosine, inhaled nitric oxide and inhaled iloprost. While these agents appear to elicit similar responses when used in an acute challenge, they are not identical (Nootens et al., 1995). However, the clinical implications of this variability in acute pulmonary vasoreactive responses are unclear. The decision to perform subsequent acute vasodilator testing with a calcium channel blocker in patients demonstrated to be acute responders with the short acting agents stated above, before considering long-term calcium channel blocker treatment remains controversial. However, what is not controversial is that calcium channel blocker acute testing and/or chronic treatment is contraindicated in patients with an increased RAPm, i.e. $\leq$ 20 mm Hg.

Genetic testing Bone morphogenetic protein receptor-2 (BMPR2) coding sequence mutations account for approximately 55% of cases of familial PAH (and are present in 11–40% instances of IPAH) (Humbert et al., 2002; Koehler et al., 2004;

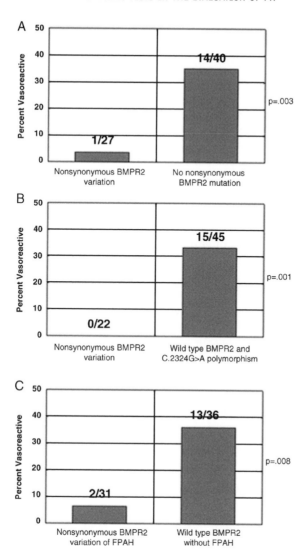

Figure 2.21 (A) BMPR2 nonsynonymous variations are associated with a negative test for vasoreactivity. (B) This remains true when the 5 patients in the study with a BMPR2 variation (c. 2324 G>A) found in unrelated northern Europeans with a genotype frequency of 5 percent, were included with the 40 patients who did not have BMPR2 nonsynonymous variations. (C) The result also was not altered by assuming that deleterious variants were present in all 15 patients with familial pulmonary arterial hypertension (FPAH). Vasoreactivity was defined by ≥ 10 mmHg decrease of mean pulmonary artery pressure to ≤ 40 mmHg. The numbers represent number of vasoreactive patients (numerator) and total number of patients in each category (denominator). The p values represent results of Fisher's exact test. (Reproduced with permission from Elliott *et al.*, *Circulation* 2006; **13**:2509–15.)

Thomson *et al.*, 2000). The presence of a mutation confers a susceptibility to, but not a certainty of, developing PAH (Deng *et al.*, 2000; Lane *et al.*, 2000; Machado *et al.*, 2001; Morse, 2002; Morisaki *et al.*, 2004). Although BMPR2 mutation status does not directly affect the treatment strategy for the patient, it may have importance in terms of family planning and also for the intensity of follow-up assessment of the individual to detect early signs of PAH. The penetrance of BMPR2 mutations averages about 10–20% among affected kindreds, suggesting that other genetic or environmental factors may be needed for phenotypic expression (Newman *et al.*, 2001). There is also an unexplained tendency for IPAH to be more severe and develop at earlier ages in subsequent generations, i.e. genetic anticipation (Loyd *et al.*, 1995).

Some studies have suggested that patients with BMPR2 mutations are unlikely to exhibit pulmonary vasoreactivity with acute vasodilator testing (Figure 2.21) (Rosenzweig *et al.*, 2006; Elliot *et al.*, 2006), and therefore may be less likely to benefit from long-term treatment with calcium channel blockade. However, based on the available data at the time of this writing, the presence of a BMPR2 mutation in a PAH patient should not replace acute vasodilator testing.

The ACCP guidelines previously recommended that genetic counseling and BMPR2 testing be offered only when at least one other family member is affected; however, with the recent increase in identification of BMPR2 mutations in IPAH, these recommendations may need to be reconsidered. The process of testing and counseling individual subjects for genetic mutations should be considered as part of a comprehensive program that includes thorough pre-test and post-test genetic counseling to discuss risks, benefits and the limitations of the test results. For genetic testing and counseling, molecular testing for the mutation should only be performed in a clinically approved and certified molecular genetics laboratory (Clinical Laboratory Improvement Amendments certified).

References

Ahearn GS., Tapson VF., Rebeiz A., Greenfield JC. (2002) Electrocardiography to define clinical status in primary pulmonary hypertension and pulmonary arterial hypertension secondary to collagen vascular disease. *Chest*;**122**:524–7.

ATS Statement. (2002) Guidelines for the six-minute walk test. *Am J Respir Crit Care Med*; **166**:111–117.

Auger WR., Fedullo PF., Moser KM. (1992) Chronic major-vessel thromboembolic pulmonary artery obstruction: appearance at angiography. *Radiology*;**182**:393–8.

Auletta M., Oliviero U., Iasiuolo L. *et al.* (2000) Pulmonary hypertension associated with liver cirrhosis: an echocardiographic study. *Angiology*;**51**:1013–20.

Barst RJ., McGoon MD., McLaughlin VV. *et al.* (2003) Beraprost therapy for pulmonary arterial hypertension. *J Am Coll Cardiol*;**41**(12):2119–25.

Bergin CJ., Rios G., King MA. *et al.* (1996) Accuracy of high-resolution CT in identifying chronic pulmonary thromboembolic disease. *Am J Roentgenol*;**166**(6):1371–7.

Bossone E., Paciocco G., Iarussi D., *et al.* (2002) The prognostic role of the ECG in primary pulmonary hypertension. *Chest*;**121**:513–8.

Castro M., Krowka MJ., Schroeder DR., *et al.* (1996) Frequency and clinical implications of increased pulmonary artery pressures in liver transplant patients. *Mayo Clin Proc*; **71**:543–51.

Chang B., Wigley FM., White B., Wise RA. (2003) Scleroderma patients with combined pulmonary hypertension and interstitial lung disease. *J Rheumatol*;**30**(11):2398–405.

Channick RN., Simonneau G., Sitbon O., *et al.* (2001) Effects of the dual endothelin-receptor antagonist bosentan in patients with pulmonary hypertension: a randomised placebo-controlled study. *Lancet*;**358**:1119–23.

D' Alonzo GE., Barst RJ., Ayres SM., *et al.* (1991) Survival in patients with primary pulmonary hypertension: results from a national prospective registry. *Ann Int Med*;**115**:343–9.

de Chadarevian JP., Lischner HW., Karmazin N. *et al.* (1994) Pulmonary hypertension and HIV infection: new observations and review of the syndrome. *Mod Path*;**7**:685–89.

Deng Z., Morse JH., Slager SL., *et al.* (2000) Familial primary pulmonary hypertension (gene PPH1) is caused by mutations in the bone morphogenetic protein receptor-II gene. *Am J Hum Genet*;**67**:electronically published.

Dufour B., Maitre S., Humbert M. *et al.* (1998) High-resolution CT of the chest in four patients with pulmonary capillary hemangiomatosis or pulmonary venoocclusive disease. *Am J Radiol*;**171**: 1321–4.

Edwards BS., Weir K., Edwards WD. *et al.* (1987) Coexistent pulmonary and portal hypertension: morphologic and clinical features. *J Am Coll Cardiol*;**10**:1233–8.

Elliot CG., Glissmeyer EW., Havlena GT., *et al.* (2006) Relationship of BMPR2 mutations to vasoreactivity in pulmonary arterial hypertension. *Circ*;**113**:2509–15.

Fedullo PF., Auger WR., Kerr KM., Rubin LJ. (2001) Chronic thromboembolic pulmonary hypertension. *N Engl J Med*;**345**:1465–72.

Fijalkowska A., Kurzyna M., Torbicki A., *et al.* (2006) Serum N-Terminal Brain Natriuretic Peptide as a Prognostic Parameter in Patients With Pulmonary Hypertension. *Chest*;**129**(5):1313–21.

Forfia PR., Fisher MR., Mathai SC., *et al.* (2006) Tricuspid Annular Displacement Predicts Survival in Pulmonary Hypertension. *Am J Respir Crit Care Med*:200604–547OC.

Galie N., Humbert M., Vachiery J., *et al.* (2002) Effects of beraprost sodium, an oral prostacyclin analogue, in patients with pulmonary arterial hypertension: a randomized, double-blind, placebo-controlled trial. *J Am Coll Cardiol*;**39**:1496–502.

Galie N., Torbicki A., Barst R., *et al.* (2004) Guidelines on diagnosis and treatment of pulmonary arterial hypertension. The task force on diagnosis and treatment of pulmonary arterial hypertension of the European Society of Cardiology. *Eur Heart J*;**25**:2243–78.

Gladwin M., Sachdev V., Jison M., *et al.* (2004) Pulmonary hypertension as a risk factor for death in patients with sickle cell disease. *N Engl J Med*;**350**(9):886–95.

Grunig E., Janssen B., Mereles D., *et al.* 2000a Abnormal pulmonary artery pressure response in asymptomatic carriers of primary pulmonary hypertenson gene. *Circ*;**102**:1145–50.

Grunig E., Mereles D., Hildebrandt W., *et al.* 2000b Stress Doppler echocardiography for identification of susceptibility to high altitude pulmonary edema. *J Am Coll Cardiol*;**35**(4):980–7.

Guyatt GH., Sullivan MJ., Thompson PJ., Fallen EL., Pugsley SO., Taylor DW., Berman LB. (1985) The 6-minute walk: a new measure of exercise capacity in patients with chronic heart failure. *Can Med Assoc J*;**132**:919–23.

Hachulla E., Gressin V., Guillevin L., *et al.* (2005) Early detection of pulmonary arterial hypertension in systemic sclerosis: a French nationwide prospective multicenter study. *Arthritis Rheumatism*;**52**(12):3792–800.

Halank M., Ewert R., Seyfarth H-J., Hoeffken G. (2006) Portopulmonary hypertension. *J Gastroenterol*;V41(9):837–47.

Himelman RB., Stulbarg M., Kircher B., *et al.* (1989) Non-invasive evaluation of pulmonary artery pressure during exercise by saline-enhanced Doppler echocardiography in chronic pulmonary disease. *Circ*;**79**:863–71.

Hoeper M., Krowka M., Strassburg C. (2004) Portopulmonary hypertension and hepatopulmonary syndrome. *Lancet*;**363**:1461–8.

Hoeper MM., Markevych I., Spiekerkoetter E. *et al.* (2005) Goal-oriented treatment and combination therapy for pulmonary arterial hypertension. *Eur Respir J*;**26**(5):858–63.

Holcomb BW., Jr., Loyd JE., Ely W. *et al.* (2000) Pulmonary veno-occlusive disease: a case series and new observations. *Chest*;**118**:1671–79.

Humbert M., Deng Z., Simonneau G., *et al.* (2002) BMPR2 germline mutations in pulmonary hypertension associated with fenfluramine derivatives. *Eur Respir J*;**20**(3):518–23.

Humbert M., Sitbon O., Chaouat A., *et al.* (2006) Pulmonary arterial hypertension in France: results from a national registry. *Am J Respir Crit Care Med*;**173**:1023–30.

James KB., Maurer J., Wolski K., *et al.* (2000) Exercise hemodynamic findings in patients with exertional dyspnea. *Tex Heart Inst J*;**27**:100–5.

Johnson RD., Worsley DF. (1996) Patent ductus arteriosus causing infradiaphragmatic activity on perfusion lung scintigraphy. *Clin Nucl Med*;**21**(10):812–4.

Karamanoglu M., McGoon M., Frantz RP., Benza RL., Bourge RC., Barst RJ., Kjellstrom B., Bennett TD. (2007) Right ventricular pressure waveform and wave reflection analysis in patients with pulmonary arterial hypertension. *Chest*; **132**:37–43.

Kawut SM., Taichman DB., Ahya VN., *et al.* (2005) Hemodynamics and survival of patients with portopulmonary hypertension. *Liver Transpl*;**11**(9):1107–11.

King MA., Bergin CJ., Yeung DW., *et al.* (1994) Chronic pulmonary thromboembolism: detection of regional hypoperfusion with CT. *Radiology*;**191**(2):359–63.

Koehler R., Grunig E., Pauciulo MW., *et al.* (2004) Low frequency of BMPR2 mutations in a German cohort of patients with sporadic idiopathic pulmonary arterial hypertension. *J Med Genet*;**41**(12):e127.

Krowka M. (1997) Hepatopulmonary syndrome and portopulmonary hypertension: distinctions and dilemmas. *Hepatology*;**25**:1282–4.

Krowka M. (2004) Portopulmonary hypertension: understanding pulmonary hypertension in the setting of liver disease. *Adv Pulm Hypertension*;**3**(2):4

Krowka M. (2005) Portopulmonary hypertension and the issue of survival (editorial). *Liver Transpl*;**11**:1026–7.

Krowka MJ., Frantz RP., McGoon MD., Wiesner RH.,(2006) Portopulmonary hypertension: Results from a 10-year screening algorithm. *Hepatology*;**44**(6):1502–10.

Krowka M., Mandell M., Ramsay M., *et al.* (2004) Hepatopulmonary syndrome and portopulmonary hypertension: A report of the multicenter liver transplant database. *Liver Transpl*;**10**(2): 174–82.

Lane KB., Machado RD., Pauciulo MW., *et al.* (2000) Heterozygous germline mutations in BMPR2, encoding a TGF-beta receptor, cause familial primary pulmonary hypertension. The International PPH Consortium. *Nature Genetics*;**26**(1):81–4.

Langleben D., Christman B., Barst RJ., *et al.* (2002) Effects of the thromboxane synthetase inhibitor and receptor antagonist terbogrel in patients with primary pulmonary hypertension. *Am Heart J*;**143**(5)(May 2002):E4.

Leuchte HH., Baumgartner RA., Nounou ME., *et al.* (2006) Brain Natriuretic Peptide Is a Prognostic Parameter in Chronic Lung Disease. *Am J Respir Crit Care Med*;**173**(7):744–50.

Loyd JE. (2002) Genetics and gene expression in pulmonary hypertension. *Chest*;**121**:46S–50S.

Loyd JE., Butler MG., Foroud TM. *et al.* (1995) Genetic anticipation and abnormal gender ratio at birth in familial primary pulmonary hypertension. *Am J Respir Crit Care Med*;**152**:93–7.

Lupi E., Dumont C., Tejada V. *et al*. (1975) A radiologic index of pulmonary arterial hypertension. *Chest*;**68**:28–31.

Machado R., Pauciulo MW., Thomson J., *et al*. (2001) BMPR2 haploinsufficiency as the inherited molecular mechanism for primary pulmonary hypertension. *Am J Hum Genet*;**68**:92–102.

Mani S., Smith GW. (1994) HIV and pulmonary hypertension: a review. *Southern Med J*;**87**:357–62.

Markowitz DH., Systrom DM. (2004) Diagnosis of pulmonary vascular limit to exercise by cardiopulmonary exercise testing. *J Heart Lung Transpl*;**23**:88–95.

McGoon MD., Fuster V., Freeman WK. *et al.*. (1996) The heart and the lungs: pulmonary hypertension, in *Mayo Clinic Practice of Cardiology*, 3rd edn (eds ER. Guiliani, BJ. Gersh, MD. McGoon, DL. Hayes, HV. Schaff), Mosby Yearbook 1996:1815–36.

McGoon MD., Gutterman D., Steen V., *et al*. (2004) Screening, early detection, and diagnosis of pulmonary arterial hypertension: ACCP evidence-based clinical practice guidelines. *Chest*;**126**(Supplement 1):14S-34S.

McLaughlin V., Sitbon O., Badesch DB., *et al*. (2005) Survival with first-line bosentan in patients with primary pulmonary hypertension. *Eur Respir J*;**25**:244–9.

McLaughlin VV., McGoon MD. (2006) Pulmonary Arterial Hypertension. *Circ*;**114**(13):1417–31.

McLaughlin VV., Shillington A., Rich S. (2002) Survival in primary pulmonary hypertension: the impact of epoprostenol therapy. *Circ*;**106**:1477–82.

McQuillan BM., Picard MH., Leavitt M., Weymann AE. (2001) Clinical correlates and reference intervals for pulmonary artery systolic pressure among echocardiographically normal subjects. *Circ*;**104**:2797–802.

Mesa R., Edell E., Dunn WF., Edwards WD. (1998) Human immunodeficiency virus infection and pulmonary hypertension: two new cases and a review of 86 reported cases. *Mayo Clin Proc*; **73**:37–45.

Mette SA., Palevsky HI., Pietra GG., *et al*. (1992) Primary pulmonary hypertension in association with human immunodeficiency virus infection: a possible viral etiology for some forms of hypertensive pulmonary arteriopathy. *Rev Resp Dis*;**145**:1196–200.

Miyamoto S., Nagaya N., Satoh T., *et al*. (2000) Clinical correlates and prognostic significance of six-minute walk test in patients with primary pulmonary hypertension: comparison with cardiopulmonary exercise testing. *Am J Respir Crit Care Med*;**161**:487–92.

Morisaki H., Nakanishi N., Kyotani S., *et al*. (2004) BMPR2 mutations found in Japanese patients with familial and sporadic primary pulmonary hypertension. [erratum appears in Hum Mutat. (2004) Sep;**24**(3):275]. *Human Mutation*;**23**(6):632.

Morse JH. (2002) Bone morphogenetic protein receptor 2 mutations in pulmonary hypertension. *Chest*;**121**:50S-3S.

Mukerjee D., St. George D., Coleiro B., *et al*. (2003) Prevalence and outcome in systemic sclerosis associated pulmonary arterial hypertension: application of a registry approach. *Ann Rheumatol Dis*;**62**:1088–93.

Mukerjee D., St. George D., Knight C., *et al*. (2004) Echocardiography and pulmonary function as screening tests for pulmonary arterial hypertension in systemic sclerosis. *Rheumatology (Oxford)*;**43**(4):461–6.

Nadrous H., Pellikka PA., Krowka M., *et al*. (2005) The impact of pulmonary hypertension on survival in patients with idiopathic pulmonary fibrosis. *Chest*;**128**:616–7.

Naeije R. (2005) Pulmonary hypertension and right heart failure in chronic obstructive pulmonary disease. *Proc Am Thoracic Soc*;**2**:20–2.

Nagaya N., Nishikimi T., Uematsu M., *et al*. (2000) Plasma brain natriuretic peptide as a prognostic indicator in patients with primary pulmonary hypertension. *Circ*;**102**(8):865–70.

Nagaya N., Uematsu M., Satoh T., *et al*. (1999) Serum uric acid levels correlate with the severity and mortality of primary pulmonary hypertension. *Am J Respir Crit Care Med*;**160**: 487–92.

Newman JH., Wheeler L., Lane K., *et al.* (2001) Mutation in the gene for bone morphogenetic protein receptor II as a cause of primary pulmonary hypertension in a large kindred. *N Engl J Med*;**345**(5):319–24.

Nootens M., Schrader BJ., Kaufmann E. *et al.* (1995) Comparative acute effects of adenosine and prostacyclin in primary pulmonary hypertension. *Chest*;**107**:54–7.

Nunes H., Humbert M., Sitbon O., *et al.* (2003) Prognostic factors for survival in human immunodeficiency virus-associated pulmonary arterial hypertension. *Am J Respir Crit Care Med*;**167**(10): 1433–9.

Okada O., Tanabe N., Yasuda Y. *et al.* (1999) Prediction of life expectancy in patients with primary pulmonary hypertension. A retrospective nationwide survey from 1980–1990. *Int Med*;**38**:12–6.

Olman MA., Auger WR., Fedullo PF., *et al.* (1990) Pulmonary vascular steal in chronic thromboembolic pulmonary hypertension. *Chest*;**98**(6):1430–4.

Olschewski H., Simonneau G., Galie N., *et al.* (2002) Inhaled iloprost for severe pulmonary hypertension. *N Engl J Med*;**347**:322–9.

Oudiz R., Sun XG. (2002) Abnormalities in exercise gas exchange in primary pulmonary hypertension, in *Cardiopulmonary Exercise Testing and Cardiovascular Health*, (ed. K. Wasserman) Futura;179–90.

Paciocco G., Martinez F., Bossone E. *et al.* (2001) Oxygen desaturation on the six-minute walk test and mortality in untreated primary pulmonary hypertension. *Eur Respir J*;**17**:647–52.

Pellicelli AM., Palmieri F., Cicalini S., Petrosillo N. (2001) Pathogenesis of HIV-related pulmonary hypertension. *Ann N Y Acad Sci*;**946**:82–94.

Petitpretz P., Brenot F., Azarian R., *et al.* (1994) Pulmonary hypertension in patients with human immunodeficiency virus infection: comparison with primary pulmonary hypertension. *Circ*;**89**:2722–27.

Petrosillo N., Pellicelli AM., Boumis E., Ippolito G. (2001) Clinical manifestation of HIV-related pulmonary hypertension. *Ann N Y Acad Sci*;**946**:223–35.

Pitton MB., Duber C., Mayer E., *et al.* (1996) Hemodynamic effects of nonionic contrast bolus injection and oxygen inhalation during pulmonary angiography in patients with chronic major-vessel thromboembolic pulmonary hypertension. *Circ*;**94**(10):2485–90.

Pitton MB., Kemmerich G., Herber S., *et al.* (2006) Hemodynamic effects of monomeric nonionic contrast media in pulmonary angiography in chronic thromboembolic pulmonary hypertension. *Am J Roentgenol*;**187**(1):128–34.

Polos PG., Wolfe D., Harley RA. *et al.* (1992) Pulmonary hypertension and human inmunodeficiency virus infection: two reports and a review of the literature. *Chest*;**101**:474–78.

Pruszczyk P., Torbicki A., Pacho R., *et al.* (1997) Noninvasive diagnosis of suspected severe pulmonary embolism: transesophageal echocardiography vs spiral CT. *Chest*;**112**(3):722–8.

Raeside DA., Chalmers G., Clelland J. *et al.* (1998) Pulmonary artery pressure variation in patients with connective tisuue disease: 24 hour ambulatory pulmonary artery pressure monitoring. *Thorax*;**53**:857–62.

Raeside DA., Smith AL., Brown A., *et al.* (2000) Pulmonary artery pressure measurement during exercise testing in patients with suspect pulmonary hypertension. *Eur Respir J*;**16**:282–7.

Rafanan AL., Golish JA., Dinner DS. *et al.* (2001) Nocturnal hypoxemia is common in primary pulmonary hypertension. *Chest*;**120**:894–9.

Ramsay M., Simpson B., Nguyen A. *et al.* (1997) Severe pulmonary hypertension in liver transplant candidates. *Liver Transplant Surg*;**3**(5):494–500.

Raymond RJ., Hinderliter AL., Willis PW., *et al.* (2002) Echocardiographic predictors of adverse outcomes in primary pulmonary hypertension. *J Am Coll Cardiol*;**39**:1214–9.

Rich S., Dantzker DR., Ayres SM., *et al.* (1987) Primary pulmonary hypertension: a national prospective study. *Ann Int Med*;**107**:216–23.

Rich S., Kaufmann E., Levy PS. (1992) The effect of high doses of calcium-channel blockers on survival in primary pulmonary hypertension. *N Engl J Med*;**327**:76–81.

Robalino BD., Moodie DS. (1991) Association between primary pulmonary hypertension and portal hypertension: analysis of its pathophysiology and clinical, laboratory and hemodynamic manifestatons. *J Am Coll Cardiol*;**17**:492–8.

Rosenzweig EB., Morse JH., Knowles JA., *et al.* (2006) Acute Pulmonary Vasoreactivity and BMPR2 Mutations in IPAH/FPAH Children and Adults. European Society of Cardiology.

Rubin L., Rich S., (eds) (1996) *Primary Pulmonary Hypertension*, M. Dekker.

Rubin LJ., Badesch DB., Barst RJ., *et al.* (2002) Bosentan therapy for pulmonary arterial hypertension. *N Engl J Med*;**346**:896–903.

Ryan KL., Fedullo PF., Davis GB. *et al.* (1988) Perfusion scan findings understate the severity of angiographic and hemodynamic compromise in chronic thromboembolic pulmonary hypertension. *Chest*;**93**:1180–5.

Sandoval J., Baurle O., Palomar A. *et al.* (1994) Survival in primary pulmonary hypertension: validation of a prognostic equation. *Circ*;**89**:1733–44.

Schmidt H., Kauczor H., Schild H., *et al.* (1996) Pulmonary hypertension in patients with chronic pulmonary thromboembolism: chest radiograph and CT evaluation before and after surgery. *Eur Radiol*;**6**:817–26.

Simonneau G., Barst RJ., Galie N., *et al.* (2002) Continuous subcutaneous infusion of treprostinil, a prostacyclin analogue, in patients with pulmonary arterial hypertension. *Am J Respir Crit Care Med*;**165**:800–4.

Simonneau G., Galiè N., Rubin L., *et al.* (2004) Clinical classification of pulmonary hypertension. *J Am Coll Cardiol*;**43**, Supplement 1(12):S5-S12.

Sitbon O., Humbert M., Jagot JL., *et al.* (1998) Inhaled nitric oxide as a screening agent for sagely identifying responders to oral calcium-channel blockers in primary pulmonary hypertension. *Eur Respir J*;**12**:265–70.

Sitbon O., Humbert M., Jais X., *et al.* (2005) Long-term response to calcium channel blockers in idiopathic pulmonary arterial hypertension. *Circ*;**111**:3105–11.

Sitbon O., Humbert M., Nunes H., *et al.* (2002) Long-term intravenous epoprostenol infusion in primary pulmonary hypertension: prognostic factors and survival. *J Am Coll Cardiol*;**40**: 780–8.

Sola M., Garcia A., Picado C., *et al.* (1993) Segmental contour pattern in a case of pulmonary venoocclusive disease. *Clin Nucl Med*;**18**(8):679–81.

Speich R., Jenni R., Opravil M. *et al.* (1991) Primary pulmonary hypertension in HIV infection. *Chest*;**100**:1268–71.

Steen V., Medsger T. (2003) Predictors of isolated pulmonary hypertension in patients with systemic sclerosis and limited cutaneous involvement. *Arthritis Rheumatism*;**48**(2):516–22.

Sun XG., Hansen JE., Oudiz R., Wasserman K. (2003) Pulmonary function in primary pulmonary hypertension. *J Am Coll Cardiol*;**41**(6):1027–35.

Sun XG., Hansen JE., Oudiz RJ., Wasserman K. (2001) Exercise pathophysiology in patients with primary pulmonary hypertension. *Circ*;**104**:429–35.

Tan H., Markowitz J., Montgomery R., *et al.* (2001) Liver transplantation in patients with severe portopulmonary hypertension treated with preoperative chronic intravenous epoprostenol. *Liver Transpl*;**7**:745–9.

Tei C., Dujardin KS., Hodge DO., *et al.* (1996) Doppler echocardiographic index for assessment of global right ventricular function. *J Am Soc Echo*;**9**:838–47.

Thabut G., Dauriat G., Stern JB., *et al.* (2005) Pulmonary hemodynamics in advanced COPD candidates for lung volume reduction surgery or lung transplantation. *Chest*;**127**: 1531–6.

Thomson JR., Machado RD., Pauciulo MW., *et al.* (2000) Sporadic primary pulmonary hypertension is associated with germline mutations of the gene encoding BMPR-II., a recepor member of the TGF-ß family. *J Med Genet*;**37**:741–5.

Torbicki A., Kurzyna M., Kuca P., *et al.* (2003) Detectable Serum Cardiac Troponin T as a Marker of Poor Prognosis Among Patients With Chronic Precapillary Pulmonary Hypertension *Circ*;**108**(7):844–8.

Wasserman K., Hansen JE., Sue DY. *et al.* (eds) (2004) *Principles of Exercise Testing and Interpretation*, Lippincott Williams and Wilkins.

Weir EK., Rubin LJ., Ayres SM., *et al.* (1989) The acute administration of vasodilators in primary pulmonary hypertension: experience from the National Institutes of Health Registry on Primary Pulmonary Hypertension. *Am Rev Respir Dis*;**140**:1623–30.

Wekerle T., Klepetko W., Taghavi S., Birsan T. (1998) Lung transplantation for primary pulmonary hypertension and giant pulmonary artery aneurysm. *Ann Thorac Surg*; **65**(3):825–7.

Wensel R., Opitz CF., Anker SD., *et al.*2002 Assessment of survival in patients with primary pulmonary hypertension: importance of cardiopulmonary exercise testing. *Circ*;**106**:319–24.

Wigley FM., Lima JA., Mayes M. *et al.* (2005) The prevalence of undiagnosed pulmonary arterial hypertension in subjects with connective tissue disease at the secondary health care level of community-based rheumatologists (the UNCOVER study). *Arthritis Rheumatism*;**52**(7):2125–32.

Woodruff W., Hoeck B., Chitwood W., Lyerly H., Sabiston DC., Chen JTT. (1985) Radiographic findings in pulmonary hypertension from unresolved embolism. *Am J Radiol*;**4**:681–6.

Worsley DF., Palevsky HI., Alavi A. (1994) Ventilation-Perfusion lung scanning in the evaluation of pulmonary hypertension. *J Nuc Med*;**35**:793–96.

Yang YY., Lin HC., Lee WC., *et al.* (2001) Portopulmonary hypertension: distinctive hemodynamic and clinical manifestations. *J Gastroenterol*;**36**:181–6.

Yeo TC., Dujardin KS., Tei C. *et al.* (1998) Value of a Doppler-derived index combining systolic and diastolic time intervals in predicting outcome in primary pulmonary hypertension. *Am J Cardiol*;**81**:1157–61.

Zuber JP., Calmy A., Evison JM., *et al.* (2004) Pulmonary arterial hypertension related to HIV infection: improved hemodynamics and survival associated with antiretroviral therapy. *Clin Infect Dis*;**38**:1178–85.

3 Conventional therapy in pulmonary arterial hypertension

Richard N. Channick

San Diego Medical Center, University of California, La Jolla, USA

Defining 'conventional therapy' for pulmonary arterial hypertension (PAH) is challenging, because by the time this chapter is published, what is 'conventional' is likely to have changed. In addition, what is 'conventional' to one clinician might not be 'conventional' to another. Historically, supportive treatments and calcium channel blockers were considered 'conventional' therapy. Thus, the first clinical trial in PAH, i.e. the pivotal randomized controlled intravenous epoprostenol trial, compared 'conventional therapy alone' with 'intravenous epoprostenol plus conventional therapy.' The rationale for treatment with conventional therapies is based on uncontrolled observational studies rather than randomized controlled trials. However, with the availability now of at least six approved PAH therapies, what one should consider 'conventional' may change with time.

Nevertheless, for the sake of this chapter, we will still define 'conventional' therapy as that which has been used for patients with PAH in the years prior to the clinical development of disease-specific 'targeted' PAH treatments with randomized controlled clinical trials, i.e. prostanoids, PDE-5 inhibitors and endothelin receptor antagonists, all of which are covered in subsequent chapters. Thus, the 'conventional' therapies we will discuss in this chapter include calcium channel blockers (CCBs), warfarin, diuretics,

Pulmonary Arterial Hypertension, Edited by Robyn J. Barst
© 2008 John Wiley & Sons, Ltd

supplemental oxygen and inotropes. In addition to discussing such therapies, the chapter will outline general measures in the management of PAH patients.

Once the diagnostic process in a patient with PH is complete, and the patient is characterized as having PAH (WHO Group 1), therapy should be initiated. But how does one decide which medication(s) to begin? Does the subtype of PAH affect this decision? With new studies and agents rapidly emerging, these are not easy questions to answer. Personal preference no doubt plays a role. However, it is preferable to follow the adage: know the data. Are there prospective, controlled studies, or only retrospective data that are potentially biased? In what patient populations have the therapies been studied? What are the short- and long-term efficacy data? What safety concerns are present with the therapies? Are there published guidelines in which experts have evaluated the quality of evidence and issued a 'grade' for the therapy? We will discuss 'conventional' therapies with these perspectives in mind.

3.1 Calcium channel antagonists

In 1958, Paul Wood first defined the clinical entity of PH with reference to the 'vasoconstrictive factor' (Wood, 1958). It is not surprising, then, that a search for pulmonary vasodilators as effective therapies ensued. Agents including phentolamine (Froom and Ortiz, 1979), tolazine (Weir *et al.*, 1989), captopril (Leier *et al.*, 1983), and hydralazine (Rubin and Peter, 1980) were evaluated in uncontrolled reports. Results, although variable, were not overwhelmingly favorable. No systematic studies of these medications were carried out.

Out of the myriad of oral antihypertensive agents emerged CCBs. Ostensibly, this class of agents 'made sense' for treating pulmonary hypertension. CCBs have acceptable side effect profiles and are potent pulmonary vasodilator agents as well as systemic vasodilator agents. The role of intracellular cytosolic calcium in the vasoconstriction of pulmonary artery smooth cells was well established. Thus, blocking influx of calcium into the cells seemed desirable. And early reports suggested benefits with CCBs, e.g. diltiazem and nifedipine, in some patients with pulmonary hypertension (Rich and Brundage, 1987).

Then, in a highly quoted paper, Rich and colleagues described favorable survival in a subgroup of idiopathic PAH (IPAH) patients treated with either diltiazem or nifedipine (Rich, Kaufmann and Levy, 1992). In that study, patients manifesting acute pulmonary vasoreactivity with CCBs, defined as an acute decrease in mean pulmonary arterial pressure and pulmonary vascular resistance of at least 20%, had a five year survival of 94% (Figure 3.1); in contrast, patients who did not have an acute response had only a 55% five year survival. In addition, predicted survival for the 'acute responders', using an equation based on hemodynamics at time of diagnosis, was significantly worse than the observed survival. Although not a placebo-controlled study, these data suggested a benefit with CCBs in some IPAH patients.

The Rich study, although seminal, likely led to overuse of CCBs, not only for IPAH but for other forms of PAH as well. However, CCBs are not selective pulmonary vasodilators. In addition, CCBs have potential negative inotropic effects

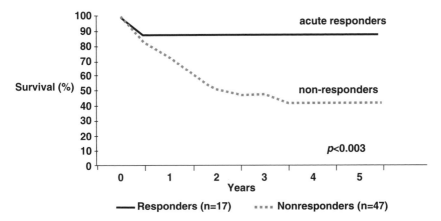

Figure 3.1 Kaplan–Meier curves for survival in adult patients with IPAH, acute responders
— (*n* = 17) vs non-responders •••• (*n* = 47) treated with long-term CCB. Survival rates were 94%
at five years in the acute responders vs 55% in the non-responders (*p* < 0.003). (Reproduced
from Rich *et al.*, *N Engl J Med* 1992;**327**:76–81. Copyright ©[2004] Massachusetts Medical
Society. All rights reserved.)

(Packer, Medina and Yushak, 1984). Thus, in patients with minimal or no acute
pulmonary vasoreactivity, the negative effects of CCBs can become predominant,
with potential for catastrophic consequences.

A recent, large retrospective study by Sitbon and coworkers has further narrowed
the role of CCBs in IPAH patients (Sitbon *et al.*, 2005). In that study, 557 IPAH
patients were tested for acute pulmonary vasoreactivity using either intravenous
prostacyclin, e.g. epoprostenol, or inhaled nitric oxide. Seventy patients (~13%) had
an acute response (at least 20% fall in mean pulmonary artery pressure and pulmonary vascular resistance), and were treated with CCBs. However, only half of
those 'acute responders' (~7% of the total) did 'well' long term on CCBs, defined as
being alive and in functional class I or II at five years follow-up (Figure 3.2). The
long-term survivors had less severe disease as assessed by hemodynamics at baseline and had reached a lower mean pulmonary artery pressure with acute vasodilator challenge than the long-term CCB failures (33 mm Hg vs 46 mm Hg). In other
words, rather than the percentage drop in mean pulmonary artery pressure during an
acute test, the absolute mean pulmonary artery pressure reached appeared to be better in defining the patients that would benefit long term with CCBs. These data have
been codified into evidence-based guidelines (Badesch *et al.*, 2007; Galie *et al.*,
2004), which define potential CCB candidates as IPAH patients in whom, during an
acute pulmonary vasoreactivity test, the mean pulmonary artery pressure decreases
by at least 10 mm Hg to a level below 40 mm Hg, with no decrease in cardiac output.

The method for performing acute pulmonary vasoreactivity testing varies
among PH centers. Most frequently, one of three short-acting pulmonary
vasodilators is used in the cardiac catheterization laboratory, i.e. inhaled nitric
oxide, intravenous adenosine or intravenous epoprostenol. Using a short-acting

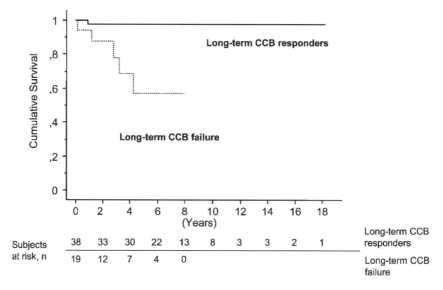

Figure 3.2 Kaplan–Meier estimates in the 57 of 70 adult acute responder patients with IPAH who survived after one year onward on CCB. The number of patients included in the long-term CCB failure subgroup was only 19 of 32, with the 13 remaining patients being dead ($n = 6$), transplanted ($n = 4$), or lost to follow-up ($n = 3$, considered 'dead' in the analysis) within the first year. The difference between the group of long-term CCB responders (solid line) and that of patients who failed on CCB (dashed line) was highly significant ($p = 0.0007$ by Cox–Mantel log-rank test) (Reproduced with permission from Sitbon *et al.*, *Circulation* 2005;**111**:3105–11).

agent prevents refractory systemic hypotension, which could result when a PAH patient with minimal pulmonary vasoreactivity is given a systemic vasodilator. A distinct advantage of inhaled nitric oxide is the absence of systemic hemodynamic effects, the very rapid 'on/off' properties of the drug, i.e. half-life 20 s, and the absence of side effects. With inhaled nitric oxide, an acute pulmonary vasoreactivity test with repeat hemodynamic measurements can be accomplished in less than 20 min.

It should be noted that, as limited as the data are regarding the use of CCBs in IPAH, there is even less guidance in other forms of PAH. It is generally acknowledged that in PAH associated with connective tissue diseases and congenital systemic-to-pulmonary shunts, clinically significant acute pulmonary vasoreacitivity, and thus CCB candidacy, is rare. For that reason, performing acute testing in these subgroups may not be mandatory.

However, one subgroup of IPAH patients that seems to have a higher rate of acute pulmonary vasoreactivity is children. In a study by Barst and others, children ≤ 8 years of age had a 40–70% rate of acute pulmonary vasoreactivity, defined as a decrease in mean pulmonary artery pressure of at least 20%, no decrease in cardiac output and a decrease in the ratio of pulmonary vascular resistance to systemic

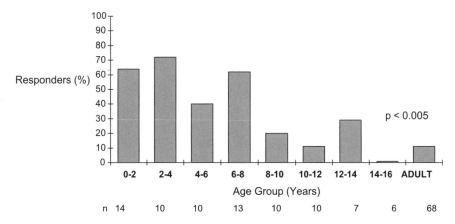

Figure 3.3 Response to short-term acute vasodilator testing by age. The younger the child at the time of testing, the greater the likelihood of eliciting acute pulmonary vasodilation ($p < 0.005$). (Reproduced with permission from Barst *et al.*, *Circulation* 1999;**99**:1197–208).

vascular resistance (Barst, Maislin and Fishman, 1999) (Figure 3.3). However, with longer follow-up, loss of acute pulmonary vasoreactivity appeared to predict treatment failure with CCBs (at least in pediatric IPAH patients) (Yung *et al.*, 2004) (Figure 3.4).

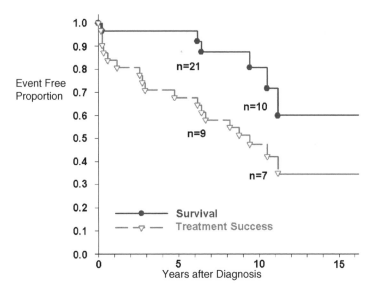

Figure 3.4 Kaplan–Meier curves for survival and treatment success in acute responders on CCB ($n = 31$). Survival rates at 1, 5, and 10 years were 97%, 97% and 81%, respectively; treatment success rates at 1, 3, 5, and 10 years were 84%, 71%, 68% and 47%, respectively (Reproduced with permission from Yung *et al.*, *Circulation* 2004;**110**(6):660–5).

Thus, although CCBs were the first agents systematically evaluated in PAH, they continue to be frequently used inappropriately, often causing more harm than benefit. Only a very small subset of IPAH patients benefit from these agents. In addition, empirically using CCBs to treat PAH, without first performing acute vasoreactivity testing in the cardiac catheterization laboratory, is extremely risky and should not be done.

3.2   Diuretics

Diuretics have long been a mainstay of therapy for heart failure, including right ventricular failure. Both total body and intravascular volume overload are common in PAH patients. In pivotal trials of PAH drugs, the majority of patients entered the studies on chronic diuretic therapy (Barst et al., 1996; Rubin et al., 2002; Galie et al., 2005).

In addition to causing symptomatic peripheral edema, volume overload of the right ventricle can cause compression of the left ventricle, and contribute to decreased cardiac output and prerenal azotemia. Thus, it is a common observation that, in decompensated PAH patients, aggressive diuresis leads to clinical and physiologic improvements. Despite the benefits of diuretics in PAH patients, there are no controlled studies to guide the clinician in using these agents.

A loop diuretic is frequently employed first. Although furosemide is often the loop diuretic of choice, there is some evidence that torsemide might be more efficacious without increased side effects (Murray et al., 2001). In addition, in patients with marked extravascular fluid accumulation and poor intestinal absorption, intravenous diuretic therapy is frequently needed. Anti-aldosterone drugs (e.g. spironalactone) are commonly combined with loop diuretics in PAH patients. Whether data suggesting a morbidity and mortality benefit of spironolactone in left side heart failure (Pitt et al., 1999) can be extrapolated to right side heart failure is not known.

In some cases, addition of a thiazide diuretic to the regimen is appropriate. The combination of metolazone and furosemide has been found by the author to be effective in effecting a brisk diuresis. However, marked hypokalemia can occur with this regimen.

Although it is possible that, in some PAH patients, the right ventricle is preload dependent and therefore overdiuresis can be detrimental, this has not been the author's experience. More often, aggressive diuresis (1–3 l negative fluid balance per day) leads to improvement in renal function and blood pressure, consistent with improved cardiac output.

3.3   Warfarin

There is strong rationale for the use of anticoagulants in PAH. Many of the endothelial cell abnormalities that predispose patients to pulmonary arteriopathy also increase thrombosis (Eisenberg *et al.*, 1990; Christman *et al.*, 1992). The presence of heart failure and/or an indwelling central venous catheter are independent risk factors for thromboembolic events, which are poorly tolerated by patients with an already marginal pulmonary vascular reserve. In addition, microscopic thrombotic lesions in the pulmonary vasculature are well appreciated in PAH patients (Moser *et al.*, 1995; Wagenvoort and Mulder, 1993; Palevsky *et al.*, 1989).

Warfarin is the anticoagulant most frequently used in patients with PAH. In clinical trials with PAH drugs, between ~50% and ~85% of patients are on anticoagulants at study entry. However, anticoagulation has risks, i.e. bleeding, as well as the need for frequent monitoring. What is the data to justify the use of warfarin in PAH?

Three studies have examined the effects of warfarin in IPAH or anorexigen-induced PAH (Rich, Kaufmann and Levy, 1992; Fuster *et al.*, 1984; Frank *et al.*, 1997). All three were retrospective analyses with some patients on warfarin. All three demonstrated better survival in patients on warfarin than those not anticoagulated. In an early study by Fuster and coworkers, 120 patients with a clinical diagnosis of IPAH were studied (Fuster *et al.*, 1984); anticoagulation improved survival at three years (49% vs 21%). However, of note, the overall five year survival for the entire cohort was only 21%. In addition, 57% of the patients in whom autopsy was performed had predominantly thrombotic lesions noted, raising the question of whether some of these 'IPAH' patients may have been misdiagnosed and actually had chronic thromboembolic pulmonary hypertension (Figure 3.5). In the study by Rich and coworkers (Rich, Kaufmann and Levy, 1992), which primarily looked at the long-term benefit of CCBs in IPAH, a survival benefit with warfarin was noted predominantly in patients who were 'non-responders' to CCBs (Figure 3.5). The third retrospective study, by Frank and coworkers, compared survival in aminorex-induced PAH and IPAH with and without anticoagulation (Frank *et al.*, 1997). In both groups, the use of oral anticoagulant therapy was associated with better survival, with the longest mean survival observed in anticoagulated aminorex-PAH patients (8.3 years vs 6.1 years for non-anticoagulated aminorex-PAH patients).

Although these three retrospective studies all suggest a survival benefit with warfarin in PAH, it is important to note that none of the studies was conducted during the 'modern' era of effective, targeted PAH therapies, which are already associated with better survival than that seen in these 'historical' studies (McLaughlin *et al.*, 2005; McLaughlin, Shillington and Rich, 2002; Sitbon *et al.*, 2002; Barst *et al.*, 2006). Whether warfarin further improves outcome in patients on these therapies, e.g. ERAs, PDE-5 inhibitors, prostanoids, remains unclear.

Despite the serious limitations in the existing data, published guidelines recommend, with a 'B' grade, that patients with IPAH be treated with warfarin (Badesch *et al.*, 2004). There is less guidance regarding the use of anticoagulation in other forms of PAH, such as that associated with congenital systemic-to-pulmonary shunts or with connective tissue diseases. There may be specific cases where warfarin would be indicated, such as in patients with advanced heart failure, indwelling central venous catheters or erythrocytosis. On the other hand, if there are patients at increased

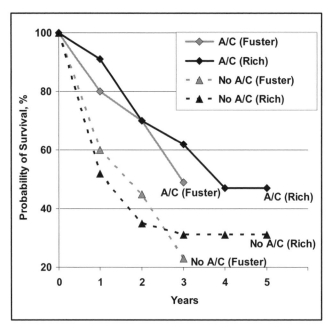

Figure 3.5 Observed survival with and without anticoagulant treatment in patients with idiopathic PAH. In both the study by Fuster and coworkers and the study by Rich and coworkers, survival rates were better among the patients who received oral anticoagulants (solid lines) than among those who did not (dashed lines) (Fuster: $p = 0.02$; Rich: $p = 0.025$). Only non-responders to acute vasodilator testing are included in the Rich *et al.* data in this figure. (Data sourced from Rich, Kaufmann and Levy, 1992 and Fuster *et al.*, 1984).

risk for bleeding (thrombocytopenia, history of hemoptysis or gastrointestinal bleeding) withholding anticoagulation, given the limited data, may be prudent.

The target level of anticoagulation in PAH patients is not known. In general, maintaining an international normalized ratio (INR) of 2–3 seems reasonable, although some experts target a lower INR (1.5–2).

Furthermore, the use of other anticoagulant drugs such as heparin or antiplatelet agents has not been studied. These agents have biological effects that could be beneficial (i.e. anti-proliferative effects). Further studies are warranted.

3.4 Supplemental oxygen

The benefits of supplemental oxygen in PAH patients, unlike patients with PH associated with lung diseases such as COPD (Medical Research Council, 1981; Nocturnal Oxygen Therapy Trial Group, 1980), are not clear. In fact, most PAH patients are not hypoxemic, at least at rest. Mild hypoxemia, when present, is likely on the basis of reduced mixed venous oxygen saturation caused by low cardiac output with mild ventilation/perfusion inequality. The presence of more profound hypoxemia in a PAH patient should raise suspicion for underlying parenchymal lung disease, systemic-to-pulmonary shunting, pulmonary veno-occlusive disease (PVOD), pulmonary capillary hemangiomatosis (PCH), or pulmonary arterial–venous malformations as seen in patients with Osler Weber Rendu associated PAH.

Although oxygen is a pulmonary vasodilator (Roberts *et al.*, 2001), there are no long-term studies supporting its efficacy. However, the consensus is that if systemic arterial oxygen pressure is less than 60 mm Hg or systemic arterial O_2 saturation is less than 90% at rest, supplemental oxygen is indicated. One exception to this approach is in patients with Eisenmenger syndrome, with hypoxemia due to right-to-left shunting. In this group, the use of supplemental oxygen remains controversial (Sandoval, Aguirre and Pulido, 2001; Bush *et al.*, 1986). There is no general agreement about whether exercise-only systemic arterial O_2 desaturation warrants oxygen supplementation. In addition, the 'stigma' of nasal cannulae for a PAH patient often limits compliance outside the home.

3.5 Inotropic therapy

The survival and clinical course of PAH patients is primarily dependent on right ventricular function (D'Alonzo *et al.*, 1991). Although right ventricular failure is initially due to increased right ventricular afterload, decreased right ventricular contractility and perfusion due to increased right ventricular end diastolic pressure decreasing right coronary artery perfusion pressure result in right ventricular ischemia and worsening function. From a cellular point of view, there is data to suggest that the right and left ventricular myocardial cells respond similarly to adrenergic stimulation (Schmidt, Hoppe and Hedenreich, 1979). Thus, agents that enhance contractility and increase systemic blood pressure may be efficacious in PAH patients with severe RV failure.

While copious data exist regarding inotropic therapy in left ventricular dysfunction, little data exist with right heart failure. In practice, inotropic agents, especially adrenergic agents such as dobutamine and dopamine, are used in PAH patients with significant right heart failure.

Dobutamine, primarily a β1 agonist with inotropic and systemic vasodilatory effects, is one option for acute decompensated right ventricular failure. In the setting of acute decompensated right ventricular failure, dobutamine has been shown to improve right ventricle–pulmonary artery coupling and increase cardiac output (Kerbaul *et al.*, 2004). One limitation of dobutamine is systemic hypotension. In addition, decompensated patients are also often receiving intravenous epoprostenol, which also has systemic effects. Thus, maintaining adequate systemic blood pressure is important. Nevertheless, in individual cases, clinicians have found dobutamine to be useful.

Dopamine, an α, β and dopaminergic receptor agonist, may be a better choice in decompensated PAH. The α agonist effects can maintain blood pressure, the β receptor activation improves cardiac output and the dopaminergic stimulation can moderate increased renal blood flow. At UCSD Medical Center, we use dopamine at 'low doses' (1–3 μg/kg/min) as chronic adjunctive therapy in patients on epoprostenol infusion (Batolome *et al.*, 2006). And in patients already on epoprostenol, with intravascular volume overload, maximized on diuretics (pre-renal azotemia), dopamine infusion at low dose appears to increase urine output in response to diuretics, improving renal function and functional status. In this group, chronic dopamine may be considered as a bridge to lung transplantation.

Milrinone, a phosphodiesterase-3 inhibitor, when given either via inhalation or intravenously, has been reported to improve right ventricular function in patients following cardiac surgery (Lamarche *et al.*, 2007; Oztekin *et al.*, 2007). However, no data exist regarding milrinone use in PAH patients.

Nesiritide (brain natriuretic peptide) has also been used in patients with acute decompensated right heart failure. However, unlike the data with left ventricular failure, very limited published data exists with right ventricular failure. One study showed a modest benefit with nesiritide and concomitant sildenafil (Klinger *et al.*, 2006).

The role of digoxin in the treatment of right ventricular dysfunction also remains unclear. The only study that looked at this reported modest acute effects on right ventricular function in PAH patients (Rich *et al.*, 1998).

3.6 General measures

Exercise and physical activity

There is no evidence-based guidance regarding physical activity or exercise in PAH. Patients should avoid activities which lead to undue symptoms such as severe dyspnea, chest pain, lightheadedness or syncope. However, low to moderate levels of exercise to prevent deconditioning and improve mental outlook are appropriate.

One study demonstrated that exercise and respiratory training are safe and result in measurable improvements in subjective and objective parameters (Mereles, Ehlken and Kreuscher, 2006); Mereles and coworkers randomized 30 patients (23 PAH, 7 CTEPH) to exercise training vs no change in treatment. In addition to being safe, patients in the exercise training group had improved quality of life scores, functional class, maximal oxygen consumption and increased exercise capacity assessed by 6-minute walk test, i.e. a 111 meter treatment effect (Mereles, Ehlken and Kreuscher, 2006).

Altitude

Hypobaric hypoxia causes pulmonary vasoconstriction and, thus, can worsen the PH in PAH patients. Patients with PAH not infrequently report symptomatic worsening when traveling to elevations above 3000 feet. It is therefore generally recommended that patients flying on commercial airliners (pressurized to ~5000–7500 feet) or traveling to elevations above 5000 feet, use supplemental oxygen. Not surprisingly, patients with severe PAH residing at high elevations often improve if they move to sea level.

Pregnancy

Pregnancy, and especially delivery, are extremely risky in patients with PAH (Nelson *et al.*, 1983). Although there are rare case reports of patients managed with epoprostenol and undergoing successful pregnancies and deliveries (Nootens and Rich, 1993; Bendayan *et al.*, 2005), it is strongly recommended that women of childbearing potential use appropriate methods of birth control to avoid pregnancy. In terms of which birth control method is preferable, no consensus exists. Some experts recommend avoiding estrogen-containing hormonal contraceptives. Depoprovera is an effective, convenient agent commonly used in PAH patients. It should be noted that in patients on endothelin-receptor antagonists, such as bosentan or ambrisentan, an additional barrier method of birth control should be used.

Anemia

Because PAH patients appear to be more sensitive to the adverse effects of even mild anemia, most experts advocate a lower hematocrit threshold for transfusion (30%), especially for patients in right heart failure. Iron deficiency should also be avoided.

Endocrinopathies

Patients with PAH often develop endocrine disorders, especially hypo- (Badesch *et al.*, 1993) and hyper- (Arroglia, Dweik and Rafanan, 2000) thyroidism. Intercurrent hyperthyroidism can lead to severe decompensation and right ventricular failure. Thus, in any PAH patient, especially if doing poorly, serial thyroid function testing is advisable. In fact, some patients with 'presumed' PAH have complete resolution of the 'PAH' by treating the hyperthyroidism; thus rather than using PAH therapy, thyroid suppression should be undertaken.

3.7 Conclusions

The management of PAH patients has evolved over the past several decades. However, with 'conventional therapy alone,' mean survival for PAH patients remains unacceptable, i.e. less than three years. But there are now effective targeted therapies available which have improved the outcome and clinical course of PAH. Thus, the 'conventional,' adjunctive therapies outlined in this chapter may be most useful by enhancing the effects of the disease-specific PAH targeted treatments. Unfortunately, there are no prospective data to guide the clinician in the use of these conventional therapies. Until such data are available, experience, logic and judgment must be used.

References

Arroglia AC., Dweik RA., Rafanan AL. (2000) Primary pulmonary hypertension and thyroid disease. *Chest*, **118**:1224–5.

Badesch DB., Abman SH., Ahearn GS. *et al.* (2004) Medical therapy for pulmonary arterial hypertension: ACCP evidence-based guidelines. *Chest*, **126**:35S-62S.

Badesch DB., Abman SH., Simonneau G. *et al.* (2007) Medical therapy for pulmonary arterial hypertension: updated ACCO evidence-based clinical practice guidelines. *Chest*, **131**:1917–28.

Badesch DB., Wynne KM., Bonvallet S. *et al.* (1993) Hypothyroidism and primary pulmonary hypertension: an autoimmune pathogenetic link? *Ann Intern Med*, **119**:44–6.

Barst RJ., Maislin G., Fishman AP. (1999) Vasodilator therapy for primary pulmonary hypertension in children. *Circulation*, **99**:1197–208.

Barst RJ., Rubin LJ., Long WA. *et al.* (1996) A comparison of continuous intravenous epoprostenol (prostacyclin) with conventional therapy for primary pulmonary hypertension. The Primary Pulmonary Hypertension Study Group. *N Engl J Med*, **334**:296–302.

Barst RJ., Galie N., Naeije R. *et al.* (2006) Long-term outcome in pulmonary arterial hypertension patients treated with subcutaneous treprostinil. *Eur Respir J*, **28**:1195–203.

Bartolome SD., Channick RN., Williamson TL. *et al.* (2006) Low dose dopamine infusion as outpatient therapy in pulmonary arterial hypertension patients failing intravenous epoprostenol. *Am J Respir Crit Care Med*, Abstract.

Bendayan D., Hod M., Oron G. *et al.* (2005) Pregnancy outcome in patients with pulmonary arterial hypertension receiving prostacyclin therapy. *Obstet Gynecol*, **106**:1206–10.

Bush A., Busst C., Booth K. *et al.* (1986) Does prostacyclin enhance the selective pulmonary vasodilator effect of oxygen in children with congenital heart disease? *Circulation*, **74**(1):135–44.

Christman BW., McPherson CD., Newman JH. *et al.* (1992) An imbalance between excretion of thromboxane and prostacyclin metabolites in pulmonary hypertension. *N Engl J Med*, **327**:70–5.

D'Alonzo GE., Barst RJ., Ayres SM. *et al.* (1991) Survival in patients with prinary pulmonary hypertension. Results from a national prospective registry. *Ann Intern Med*, **115**:343–9.

Eisenberg PR., Lucore C., Kaufman L. *et al.* (1990) Fibrinopeptide A levels indicative of pulmonary vascular thrombosis in patients with primary pulmonary hypertension. *Circulation*, **82**:841–7.

Frank H., Miczoch J., Huber K. *et al.* (1997) The effect of anticoagulant therapy in primary and anorectic drug-induced pulmonary hypertension. *Chest*, **1132**:714–21.

Froom P., Ortiz C. (1979) Primary pulmonary hypertension and oral phentolamine. *Ann Intern Med*, **91**:495–6.

Fuster V., Steele PM., Edwards WD. *et al.* (1984) Primary pulmonary hypertension: natural history and the importance of thrombosis. *Circulation*, **70**:580–7.

Galie N., Seeger W., Naeije R. *et al.* (2004) Comparative analysis of clinical trials and evidence-based treatment algorithm in pulmonary arterial hypertension. *J Am Coll Cardiol*, **43**:81S-88S.

Galie N., Ghofrani HA., Torbicki A. *et al.* (2005) Sildenafil citrate therapy for pulmonary arterial hypertension. *N Engl J Med*, **353**:2148–57.

Kerbaul F., Rondelet B., Motte S. *et al.* (2004) Effects of norepinephrine and dobutamine on pressure load-induced right ventricular failure. *Crit Care Med*, **32**:1035–40.

Klinger JR., Thaker S., Houtchens J. *et al.* (2006) Pulmonary hemodynamic responses to brain natriuretic peptide and sildenafil in patients with pulmonary arterial hypertension. *Chest*, **129**:417–25.

Lamarche Y., Perrault LP., Maltais S. *et al.* (2007) Preliminary experience with inhaled milrinone in cardiac surgery. *Eur J Cardiothoracic Surg*, **31**:1081–7.

Leier CV., Bambach D., Nelson S. *et al.* (1983) Captopril in primary pulmonary hypertension. *Circulation*, **67**:155–61.

McLaughlin VV., Shillington A., Rich S. (2002) Survival in primary pulmonary hypertension: the impact of epoprostenol therapy. *Circulation*, **106**:1477–82.

McLaughlin VV., Sitbon O., Badesch DB. *et al.* (2005) Survival with first-line bosentan in patients with primary pulmonary hypertension. *Eur Respir J*, **25**:244–9.

Medical Research Council (1981) Long term domiciliary oxygen therapy in chronic hypoxic cor pulmonale complicating chronic bronchitis and emphysema. Report of the Medical Research Council Working Party. *Lancet*, i:681–6.

Mereles D., Ehlken N., Kreuscher S. (2006) Exercise and respiratory training improve exercise capacity and quality of life in patients with severe chronic pulmonary hypertension. *Circulation*, **114**:1448–9.

Moser KM., Fedullo PF., Finkbeiner WE. *et al.* (1995) Do patients with primary pulmonary hypertension develop extensive central thrombi? *Circulation*, **91**:741–5.

Murray MD., Deer MM., Ferguson JA. *et al.* (2001) Open-label randomized trial of torseide compared with furosemide therapy for patients with heart failure. *Am J Med*, **111**:513–20.

Nelson DM., Main E., Crafford W. *et al.* (1983) Peripartum heart failure due to primary pulmonary hypertension. *Obstet Gynecol*, **62**:58s-63s.

Nocturnal Oxygen Therapy Trial Group (1980) Continuous or nocturnal oxygen therapy in hypoxemic chronic obstructive lung disease: a clinical trial. *Ann Intern Med*, **93**:391–8.

Nootens M., Rich S. (1993) Successful management of labor and delivery in primary pulmonary hypertension. *Am J Cardiol*, **71**:1124–5

Oztekin L., Yazici S., Oztekin DS. *et al.* (2007) Effects of low-dose milrinone on weaning from cardiopulmonary bypass and after in patients with mitral stenosis and pulmonary hypertension. *Yakuzaku Zasshi*, **127**:375–83.

Packer M., Medina N., Yushak M. (1984) Adverse hemodynamic and clinical effects of calcium channel blockade in pulmonary hypertension secondary to obliterative pulmonary vascular disease. *J Am Coll Cardiol*, **4**:890–901.

Palevsky HI., Schloo BL., Pietra GG. *et al.* (1989) Primary pulmonary hypertension. Vascular structure, morphometry, and responsiveness to vasodilator agents. *Circulation*, **80**:1207–21.

Pitt B., Zannad F., Remme WJ. *et al.* (1999) The effect of spironolactone on morbidity and mortality in patients with severe heart failure. Randomized Aldactone Evaluation Study Investigators. *N Engl J Med*, **341**:709–17.

Rich S., Brundage BH. (1987) High-dose calcium channel-blocking therapy for primary pulmonary hypertension: evidence for long-term reduction in pulmonary arterial pressure and regression of right ventricular hypertrophy. *Circulation*, **76**:135–41.

Rich S., Kaufmann E., Levy PS. (1992) The effect of high doses of calcium-channel blockers on survival in primary pulmonary hypertension. *N Engl J Med*, **327**:76–81.

Rich S., Seidlitz M., Dodin E. *et al.* (1998) The short-term effects of digoxin in patients with right ventricular dysfunction from pulmonary hypertension. *Chest*, **114**:787–92.

Roberts DH., Lepore JJ., Maroo A. *et al.* (2001) Oxygen therapy improves cardiac index and pulmonary vascular resistance in patients with pulmonary hypertension. *Chest*, **120**:1547–55.

Rubin LJ., Peter RH. (1980) Oral hydralazine therapy for primary pulmonary hypertension. *N Engl J Med*, **302**:69–73.

Rubin LJ., Badesch DB., Barst RJ. *et al.* (2002) Bosentan therapy for pulmonary arterial hypertension. *N Engl J Med*, **346**:896–903.

Sandoval J., Aguirre JS., Pulido T. (2001) Nocturnal oxygen therapy in patients with the Eisenmenger syndrome. *Am J Respir Crit Care Med*, **164**:1682–7.

Schmidt HD., Hoppe H., Hedenreich L. (1979) Direct effects of dopamine, orciprenaline, and norepinephrine on the right and left ventricle of isolated canine hearts. *Cardiology*, **64**:133–48.

Sitbon O., Humbert M., Nunes H. *et al.* (2002) Long-term intravenous epoprostenol infusion in primary pulmonary hypertension : prognostic factors and survival. *J Am Coll Cardiol*, **40**:780–8.

Sitbon O., Humbert M., Jais X. *et al.* (2005) Long-term response to calcium channel blockers in idiopathic pulmonary arterial hypertension. *Circulation*, **111**:3105–11.

Wagenvoort CA., Mulder PG. (1993) Thrombotic lesions in primary plexogenic arteriopathy. Similar pathogenesis or complication? *Chest*, **103**:844–9.

Weir EK., Rubin LJ., Ayres SM. *et al.* (1989) The acute administration of vasodilators in primary pulmonary hypertension. Experience from the National Institutes of Health Registry on Primary Pulmonary Hypertension. *Am Rev Respir Dis*, **140**:1623–30.

Wood P. (1958) Pulmonary hypertension with special reference to the vasoconstrictive factor. *Br Heart J*, **20**:557–70.

Yung D., Widlitz AC., Rosenzweig EB. *et al.*, (2004) Outcomes in Children with Idiopathic Pulmonary Arterial Hypertension. *Circulation*, **110**(6):660–5.

4 Prostanoid treatment for pulmonary arterial hypertension

Olivier Sitbon and Gérald Simonneau

Centre National de Référence pour l'Hypertension Artérielle Pulmonaire, Université Paris-Sud, Clamart, France

Prostaglandins are a family of lipid compounds derived from arachidonic acid. Initially described in 1976 by Moncada and Vane, Prostaglandin I_2 or prostacyclin (PGI_2) is the major metabolite of arachidonic acid in vascular endothelium and is formed via the cyclooxygenase pathway (Moncada *et al.*, 1976). It is released from the phospholipid of endothelial cell membranes of the vascular intima. Prostacyclin has a very short half-life of about 3 min. It is a potent systemic and pulmonary vasodilator and powerful inhibitor of platelet aggregation that is produced by endothelial cells (Moncada and Vane, 1979; Rubin *et al.*, 1982). Prostacyclin causes relaxation of vascular smooth muscle through binding to its membrane-associated, G-protein-coupled receptor, subsequent activation of adenylate cyclase and increased production of intracellular cyclic adenosine monophosphate (cAMP). Prostacyclin is the most potent endogenous inhibitor of platelet aggregation and thrombus formation; it also promotes dispersion of pre-existing platelet aggregates. These effects are also mediated by an increase in intracellular levels of cAMP. Furthermore, PGI_2 has other properties that are not

Pulmonary Arterial Hypertension, Edited by Robyn J. Barst
© 2008 John Wiley & Sons, Ltd

Table 4.1   Main properties of prostacyclin

Systemic and pulmonary vasodilatation (relaxation of vascular smooth muscle cells)
Inhibition of platelet aggregation and dispersion of platelet aggregates
Inhibition of vascular cell migration and proliferation
Prevention from ischemic cell injury ('cytoprotective' effect)
Reduction of margination and adherence of white cells
Weak fibrinolytic activity
Improvement in pulmonary clearance of endothelin-1
Possible inotropic effect
Possible improvement in peripheral oxygen consumption by skeletal muscles

---

yet clearly understood but that may play an important role in its activity (Table 4.1). Thus, there is evidence that PGI_2 has an antiproliferative activity, PGI_2 analogs having demonstrated *in vitro* inhibition of vascular smooth muscle cell growth (Clapp *et al.*, 2002).

Other properties of PGI_2 include prevention from ischemic injury ('cytoprotective' effect), reduction of margination and adherence of white cells and a weak fibrinolytic activity (Jones, 1996). Finally, PGI_2 seems to be a protective factor against excessive vasoconstriction by improving the pulmonary clearance of endothelin-1 (Langleben *et al.*, 1999). In addition, PGI_2 inhibits the production and secretion of endothelin-1 from cultured endothelial cells (Prins *et al.*, 1994). In addition to vasodilatation and antiproliferative activity, PGI_2 might have positive inotropic effects as was shown in a small series of 19 patients with pulmonary hypertension secondary to left heart diseases (Montalescot *et al.*, 1998). However, it was not clear whether this reflected a direct inotropic effect of PGI_2 or was caused by enhanced sympathetic activity linked to the baroreceptor reflex stimulated by the fall in systemic vascular resistance. Finally, the marked improvement in exercise capacity observed in patients with pulmonary arterial hypertension (PAH) treated with long-term PGI_2 cannot be explained by the relatively small hemodynamic effect and might be the result of a better peripheral oxygen consumption by skeletal muscles (Galiè, Manes and Branzi, 2001). The main properties of PGI_2 are summarized in Table 4.1.

Vasoconstriction, cellular proliferation, and *in situ* thrombosis are the main mechanisms involved in the development and progression of PAH. A dysregulation of the PGI_2 metabolic pathway has been demonstrated in patients with PAH. An imbalance in arachidonic acid metabolism with a reduction of PGI_2 urinary metabolites and an increase of thromboxane-A2 urinary metabolites has been demonstrated in patients with idiopathic PAH (IPAH) (Christman *et al.*, 1992). Moreover, PGI_2 synthase expression is reduced in pulmonary arteries of patients with PAH (Tuder *et al.*, 1999). Overexpression of PGI_2 synthase in transgenic mice protects against development of hypoxic pulmonary hypertension (Geraci *et al.*, 1999) and monocrotaline-induced pulmonary hypertension (Tahara *et al.*, 2004).

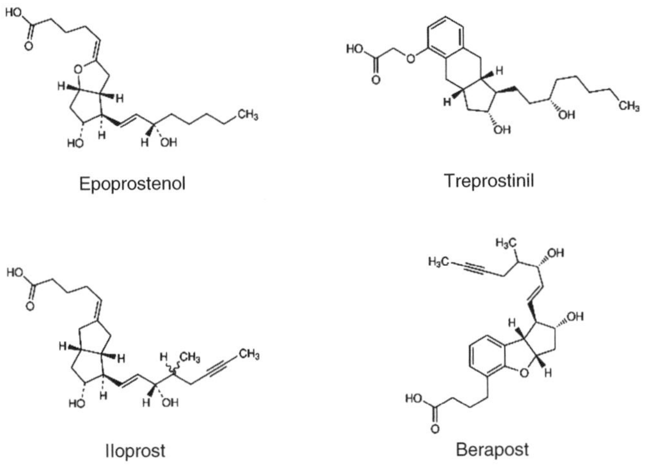

Figure 4.1 Chemical structure of available prostacyclin analogues.

Even if it is not clear whether the dysregulation of the PGI$_2$ metabolic pathway has a causative role or is a consequence of PH, these findings represent a convincing rationale for the therapeutic use of PGI$_2$ in patients with PAH.

The clinical use of PGI$_2$ has been made possible by the development of stable analogues that possess different pharmacokinetic properties but share similar pharmacodynamic effects (Galiè, Manes and Branzi, 2002). These PGI$_2$ analogues can be delivered by intravenous (epoprostenol, treprostinil, iloprost), subcutaneous (treprostinil), inhaled (iloprost, treprostinil) or oral (beraprost, treprostinil) routes. The chemical structures of available prostanoids are shown in Figure 4.1.

4.1 Epoprostenol

Epoprostenol is the synthetic form (sodium salt) of the natural prostaglandin derivative PGI$_2$. The pharmacokinetic properties of epoprostenol are dominated by the lability of the molecule in aqueous biological fluids at physiologic pH values. The stability in solution is dependent on the pH being maintained in the alkaline region (~10 in glycine buffer). The *in vitro* half-life of epoprostenol in human blood at physiologic temperature and pH is ~6 min. There is no chemical assay available to reliably study epoprostenol pharmacokinetics in humans. In blood, epoprostenol undergoes rapid biotransformation through both spontaneous hydrolysis and enzymatic degradation but it does not undergo appreciable metabolism at the pulmonary level. The primary metabolite is 6-keto-PGF$_{1\alpha}$, but a number of other metabolites have been identified. All metabolites are inactive or less active than epoprostenol (Herner and Mauro, 1999). The elimination half-life in humans has been estimated to be 3–5 min, necessitating administration via continuous i.v. infusion.

Clinical use of epoprostenol in idiopathic pulmonary arterial hypertension

Epoprostenol (Flolan®, GSK, UK) was first used to treat IPAH (formerly called primary pulmonary hypertension) in the early eighties (Higenbottam et al., 1984). In this 1984 report, Higgenbottam and coworkers reported for the first time a dramatic and persistent improvement in exercise capacity and hemodynamics in a woman with severe IPAH treated with continuous intravenous epoprostenol infusion. Since then epoprostenol has proved to be life-saving in a large number of patients with PAH of various origins. In 1987, Jones and coworkers described 10 patients with severe IPAH (NYHA class III or IV) and pronounced disability who were unresponsive to oral vasodilators (Jones, Higgenbottam and Wallwork, 1987). They reported subjective and clinical improvement and enhancement of exercise tolerance after 1 to 25 months of treatment. In 1990, Rubin and coworkers reported the results of the first randomized unblinded trial with intravenous epoprostenol in 24 patients with IPAH (Table 4.2) (Rubin et al., 1990). An improvement in hemodynamics was shown after two months in patients treated with intravenous epoprostenol, whereas patients deteriorated on conventional therapy. A sustained improvement in exercise capacity and hemodynamics after 6 and 12 months on epoprostenol was demonstrated in 18 patients enrolled in the open-label uncontrolled trial following that study (Barst et al., 1994). Interestingly, the absence of an acute hemodynamic response to intravenous epoprostenol did not preclude improvement with long-term therapy.

Table 4.2 Summary of randomized controlled, open-label trials with intravenous epoprostenol (compared to conventional therapy)

	Idiopathic PAH[a]	Idiopathic PAH[b]	SSc-PAH[c]
Patients (n)	23	81	111
Duration of trial (months)	2	3	3
NYHA functional class II : III : IV (%)	9 : 65 : 26	0 : 75 : 25	5 : 78 : 17
Conventional therapy subtracted treatment effect:			
6-min walk change	+ 45 m (NS)	+ 47 m ($p < 0.003$)	+ 94 m ($p < 0.001$)
Haemodynamics (PVR)	Improved ($p = 0.087$)	Improved ($p < 0.001$)	Improved (p value: NA)
Clinical events[d]	No change	Reduced (improved survival)	No-change

Adapted from Galiè (2004).
NHYA: New York Heart Association; SSc: systemic sclerosis; PVR: pulmonary vascular resistance; NS: not significant; NA: not available.
[a]Rubin et al., (1990).
[b]Barst et al., (1996).
[c]Badesch et al., (2000).
[d]Clinical events are defined as death or lung transplantation in the study by Barst et al.; only death in the studies by Rubin et al., and Badesch et al.

On the basis of this experience, a second prospective, randomized open trial was conducted in North American pulmonary vascular centers (Table 4.2). In this pivotal study, 81 patients displaying IPAH in NYHA functional class III or IV were randomly assigned to receive either intravenous infusion of epoprostenol or conventional therapy (Barst *et al.*, 1996). After 12 weeks of therapy there was a clinically relevant functional improvement with epoprostenol as demonstrated by the increase in the 6-minute walk distance (an increase by 32 m in the epoprostenol group compared to a decrease by 15 m in the conventional therapy group). During the same period of time, a slight improvement in hemodynamics was shown in the epoprostenol-treated group: mean pulmonary artery pressure (mPAP) was reduced by 5 mm Hg on epoprostenol whereas it increased by 2 mm Hg on conventional therapy, and cardiac index increased by 0.3 l/min/m^2 in the epoprostenol group whereas it decreased by 0.2 l/min/m^2 in the conventional therapy group. A significant improvement in survival with epoprostenol treatment was demonstrated in this 12-week unblinded study: eight patients in the conventional therapy group died during the study whereas no death was reported on epoprostenol (Barst *et al.*, 1996). After this study, intravenous epoprostenol was approved by the United States Food and Drug Administration and the French Authorities of Health for the treatment of patients with IPAH in NYHA functional class III or IV. In an observational study of 27 IPAH patients treated with epoprostenol for an average of 16 months, McLaughlin and coworkers also reported significant improvements in haemodynamics (mainly cardiac output and pulmonary vascular resistance), which in general exceeded those observed with acute adenosine challenge. Thus, this study indicated that long-term infusion of epoprostenol may afford benefits which go beyond immediate vasodilation, possibly by reversing the vascular lesions of PH (McLaughlin *et al.*, 1998).

Shapiro and colleagues described significantly improved survival in a retrospective analysis of 69 patients with IPAH treated with epoprostenol over a five-year period, as compared to a historical group of patients from the US National Institute of Health Registry (Shapiro *et al.*, 1997). In this study, the one-, two- and three-year survival rates were 80%, 76% and 49%, respectively, in patients on long-term epoprostenol, as compared with 10- (88%), 20- (56%) and 30-month (47%) survival rates, respectively, in historical control subjects. Similar results were observed in our epoprostenol-treated IPAH cohort established in 1992 ($n = 178$): the overall survival at one, two, three and five years was 85%, 70%, 63% and 55%, respectively (Sitbon *et al.*, 2002) (Figure 4.2A). In this study, we demonstrated that survival was primarily related to simple baseline clinical parameters such as NYHA functional class and 6-minute walk distance. In addition, both clinical and hemodynamical responses to long-term epoprostenol therapy appeared to be major predictors of survival in this patient population (Table 4.3). Indeed, patients whose symptoms had improved such that they could be reclassified in NYHA functional class I or II after three months on epoprostenol had a markedly improved probability of survival as compared to patients persisting in functional class III or IV. In these patients, the survival rates at one, two and three years were 100%, 93% and 88%, respectively, as compared to 77%, 46% and 33%, respectively, in patients

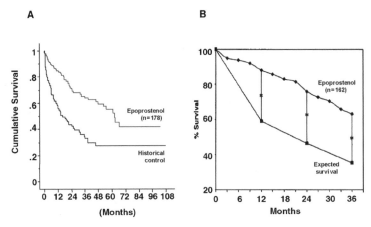

Figure 4.2   Kaplan-Meier survival estimates in two large cohorts of IPAH patients treated with long-term epoprostenol infusion. Three-year survival was identical in the two cohorts (63%). (A) In the French cohort of 178 patients with IPAH, survival was compared to that of a historical group of 135 patients with IPAH matched for NYHA functional class, and who never received epoprostenol therapy. In the population of patients treated with epoprostenol, overall survival rates at one, two, three and five years were 85%, 70%, 63% and 55%, respectively, as compared to 58%, 43%, 33% and 28% in the historical control group. (Reproduced from *J Am Coll Cardiol*, 40, Sitbon *et al.*, 780-8, Copyright (2002), with permission from the American College of Cardiology.) (B) In the cohort from the United States, survival of 162 patients with IPAH was compared to the predicted survival based on the NIH Registry equation (D'Alonzo *et al.*, 1991). Observed survival rates at one, two and three years were 88%, 76% and 63%, respectively, in patients treated with epoprostenol, as compared to the predicted survival rates of 59%, 46% and 35%, respectively, based on the NIH registry equation. (Reproduced from McLaughlin *et al.*, *Circulation* 2006; 106:1477–82.)

persisting in class III or IV (Figure 4.3A). Moreover, significant long-term response to epoprostenol, which can be measured by the fall in pulmonary vascular resistance (PVR) greater than 30% relative to baseline value after a three-month treatment period, appeared to be a major prognostic factor (Sitbon *et al.*, 2002). The combined end-point of a NYHA functional class I or II and a decrease in PVR of more than 30% was associated with a survival of 90% at five years, while survival rate was 40% for the remaining patients.

Another single-center series of 161 consecutive IPAH class III and IV patients treated with epoprostenol also demonstrated the benefits of this therapy on long-term survival (McLaughlin, Shillington and Rich, 2002). Observed survival rates in patients treated with epoprostenol were 88%, 76% and 63% at one, two and three years, respectively (Figure 4.2B). These results were significantly better than the predicted survival rates of 59%, 46% and 35%, at one, two and three years, respectively, based on the NIH registry equation (D'Alonzo *et al.*, 1991; McLaughlin, Shillington and Rich, 2002). In this study, baseline NYHA functional class as well as functional class after 17 months of epoprostenol therapy were strong indicators of patient's outcome (Figure 4.3B).

Table 4.3 Variables associated with a poor survival in patients with severe idiopathic PAH treated with long-term epoprostenol (Multivariate stepwise selection procedure based on the Cox model)

Before starting epoprostenol
History of right heart failure
After 3 months on epoprostenol
NYHA functional class III or IV
Mean pulmonary artery pressure <59 mm Hg
Absence of a 30% fall in pulmonary vascular resistance
vs prior to starting epoprostenol

Reproduced from *J Am Coll Cardiol*, **40**, Sitbon *et al.*, 780–8,Copyright (2002), with permission from the American College of Cardiology.

Initially proposed as a bridge to lung transplantation, intravenous epoprostenol is now considered as a first line therapy and an alternative to lung transplantation in patients with severe PAH. In a survey collected from 19 centers in the US it was shown that more than two-thirds of patients with PAH treated with long-term epoprostenol were sufficiently improved to defer or avoid lung transplantation (Robbins *et al.*, 1998). In another study, 70% of lung transplantation candidates were removed from the active waiting list because of clinical improvement with intravenous

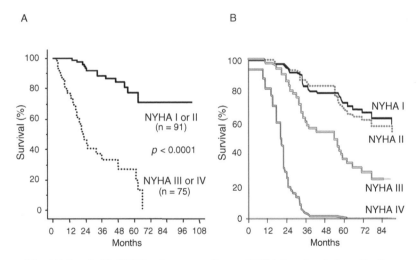

Figure 4.3 (A) Survival in IPAH patients according to NYHA functional class after three months of treatment with intravenous epoprostenol. Survival rates for patients reclassified as NYHA functional class I (solid line) or II (dash-dot-dash-dot) were 100%, 93%, and 88% at one, two and three years, respectively, as compared to 77%, 46% and 33%, respectively, for patients persisting in NYHA class III or IV (dashed line). (Reproduced from *J Am Coll Cardiol*, 40, Sitbon *et al.*, 780–8, Copyright (2002), with permission from the American College of Cardiology.) (B) Subsequent survival in IPAH patients stratified by NYHA functional class (FC) after 17 ± 15 months of treatment with intravenous epoprostenol. $p < 0.001$ for FC IV vs FC III and for FC III vs FC I and FC II. (Reproduced from McLaughlin *et al.*, *Circulation* 2006; 106:1477-82.)

epoprostenol (Conte *et al.*, 1998). However, some patients do not benefit from epoprostenol infusion and in these cases the only therapeutic option remains lung transplantation. There is a need to identify factors that enable early prediction of failure of epoprostenol therapy in order to place these patients on a waiting list for lung transplantation at the earliest possible opportunity. In a recent study, we suggest that such a subset of patients may be identified as those who remain in NYHA functional class III or IV and/or who do not achieved a 30% fall relative to baseline in total pulmonary resistance after three months of epoprostenol therapy (Sitbon *et al.*, 2002).

Dosing of epoprostenol

The optimal dosing of epoprostenol remains undefined, and varies among patients and among PAH centers. In a survey collected in 19 centers in the United States, the doses of epoprostenol were systematically increased at scheduled intervals by two-thirds of the investigators (Robbins, 1998). In all cases, the dose was increased in response to worsening symptoms. In this survey, epoprostenol doses were reported to range from 0.5 to 270 ng/kg/min. MacLaughlin and coworkers reported a mean dose of 40 ± 15 ng/kg/min after a mean of 17 months. The same authors suggested the optimal dose range of epoprostenol to be 22 to 45 ng/kg/min: lower doses appeared to result in diminished effectiveness whereas higher doses resulted in inappropriately high levels of cardiac output leading to clinical deterioration (Rich and McLaughlin, 1999). In those patients with a high cardiac output related to epoprostenol overdose, it was possible to reduce the doses under hemodynamic guidance (Rich and McLaughlin, 1999). In our experience in 340 patients with PAH, mainly IPAH, epoprostenol therapy is initiated during hospital stay at a dose of 1 ng/kg/min, and the dose is increased by 1 ng/kg/min every 12 hours up to 10 ng/kg/min (Sitbon, Humbert and Simonneau, 2002; Humbert, Sitbon and Simonneau, 2004). After this dose is achieved, patients are discharged from the hospital. Dose adjustments are made according to a systematic increase during the first three months of treatment (14 ± 4 ng/kg/min at three months). Thereafter, dose adjustments are based on the following assessment: clinical symptoms consistent with clinical deterioration or the occurrence of adverse events, distance walked during the 6-minute exercise test and hemodynamic measurements. The mean dose of epoprostenol achieved was 21 ± 7 ng/kg/min after one year of treatment, and 32 ± 10 ng/kg/min after 41 ± 17 months (Sitbon, Humbert and Simonneau, 2002).

Practical issues and adverse events

Epoprostenol can only be administered by continuous intravenous infusion since its half-life in circulation is brief and it is inactivated at low pH. A permanent central venous access is required for the infusion of epoprostenol. Venous access is obtained by the insertion of a permanent tunneled central venous catheter, most often via a subclavian or jugular vein. Epoprostenol is infused continuously with the use of a portable infusion pump. Patients are trained in pump programming, drug preparation, sterile technique and catheter care. Frequent side effects attributable to epoprostenol include jaw pain, headache, diarrhea, flushing, leg pain and nausea/vomiting. These side effects are generally mild and dose-related. More serious complications may occur and are generally related to the delivery system (mainly catheter-related infections or thromboembolic events). The incidence of catheter-related bacteremia has been reported to be between 0.1 and 0.4 per patient-year (Barst *et al.*, 1996; McLaughlin *et al.*, 1998). In a recent observational study, the rate of catheter-related infection in patients with PAH receiving epoprostenol was 0.26 per 1000 catheter days (Oudiz *et al.*, 2004). In this study including 192 patients from 1987 to 2000 (335#285 catheter days, mean 1325 ± 74), there were 88 clinical catheter infections with 51 blood culture-positive infections, necessitating catheter removal in 38. *Staphylococcus aureus* was the most frequent pathogen isolated. Surprisingly, *Micrococcus* spp was the second most common etiologic agent, and should not be viewed as a contaminant, but rather as a true pathogen (Oudiz *et al.*, 2004). In our experience with 178 patients with IPAH, 76 episodes of catheter-related bacteremia occurred in 53 patients (0.19 catheter-related infections per patient-year). In four patients, severe catheter-related sepsis was directly responsible for death, including three nosocomial infections which were acquired in the intensive care unit where patients were hospitalized for severe right heart failure. Pump failure or dislocation of the central venous catheter may lead to interruption in drug supply. Because epoprostenol has a very short half-life, the interruption of infusion may be life-threatening because of the sudden loss of hemodynamic effects of the drug. Other serious complications include ascites and pulmonary edema. Ascites may be related to severe right heart failure but also to an increased permeability of the peritoneal membrane promoted by epoprostenol. Pulmonary edema may occur if pulmonary capillary or veins are obstructed, for example in cases of pulmonary veno-occlusive disease or pulmonary capillary hemangiomatosis, which is sometimes difficult to distinguish clinically from an IPAH (Figure 4.4). In our experience, seven patients developed fatal pulmonary edema while being treated with epoprostenol. In these patients, post mortem examination of the lungs demonstrated pulmonary veno-occlusive disease or pulmonary capillary hemangiomatosis (Humbert *et al.*, 1998; Resten *et al.*, 2002; Sitbon *et al.*, 2002).

Epoprostenol in other forms of pulmonary hypertension

In an open-label 12-week randomized trial with class III and IV PAH associated with the scleroderma spectrum of disease, treatment with continuous epoprostenol improved exercise capacity and hemodynamics (Badesch *et al.*, 2000). In addition, a number of uncontrolled studies with intravenous epoprostenol therapy also suggest improvement in patients with PAH associated with connective tissue diseases (CTD) (Humbert *et al.*, 1999; Klings *et al.*, 1999; McLaughlin *et al.*, 1999), systemic-to-pulmonary congenital cardiac shunts (McLaughlin *et al.*, 1999; Rosenzweig, Kerstein and Barst, 1999), portal hypertension (Kuo *et al.*, 1997;

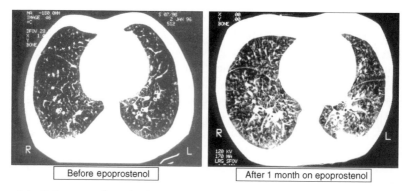

Before epoprostenol   After 1 month on epoprostenol

Figure 4.4 Pulmonary edema leading to death in a patient treated with long-term intravenous epoprostenol infusion. Post-mortem examination revealed pulmonary capillary hemangiomatosis. The diagnosis of pulmonary veno-occlusive disease or pulmonary capillary hemangiomatosis needs to be made before initiation of specific vasodilator therapy because of the risk of drug-induced severe pulmonary edema (increased driving pressure and post-capillary obstruction).

Krowka *et al.*, 1999; McLaughlin *et al.*, 1999), HIV infection (Aguilar and Farber, 2000; Nunes *et al.*, 2003), and in distal chronic thromboembolic pulmonary hypertension (Higenbottam *et al.*, 1998; Cabrol *et al.*, 2007).

Connective tissue diseases

Humbert and coworkers demonstrated the short-term efficacy of intravenous infusion of epoprostenol in 17 patients with severe PAH associated with CTD (SSc, CREST, SLE, MCTD, or Sjögren syndrome) (Humbert *et al.*, 1999). Two patients died before six weeks (from sepsis and pulmonary edema, respectively). After six weeks, exercise capacity improved in 13/15 patients (87%), with a mean increase in 6-minute walk distance of 109 m ($p = 0.01$). NYHA functional class improved in 11/15 patients (73%). Cardiac index significantly increased from 2.08 ± 0.41 to 2.65 ± 0.69 after three months on epoprostenol (Humbert *et al.*, 1999). Another study assessed the effects of continuous infusion of epoprostenol in 16 patients with severe PAH (NYHA class III or IV) associated with systemic sclerosis, mainly CREST syndrome (Klings *et al.*, 1999). During long-term treatment (0.3 to 27 months), all patients exhibited improvement in clinical status of at least one NYHA functional class. However, one patient developed right ventricular failure after six months and died, and another deteriorated after two years and died of sudden cardiac death. Persistent hemodynamic improvement was observed in four patients after one or two years of treatment (Klings *et al.*, 1999). Finally, a multicenter, randomized, open-label, controlled study compared the clinical effectiveness of 12-week epoprostenol continuous infusion with that of conventional therapy alone in 111 consecutive patients with functional class III–IV PAH associated with scleroderma spectrum of disease (Table 4.2) (Badesch *et al.*, 2000). The most frequent

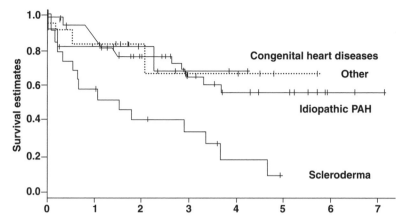

Figure 4.5 Patients with scleroderma-associated PAH have a poorer survival compared to those with idiopathic or other forms of PAH ($p = 0.002$). (Reproduced with permission from Kuhn *et al.* (2003), Outcome in 91 patients with different forms of pulmonary arterial hypertension receiving epoprostenol. *Am J Resp Crit Care Med,* 167:580–6. © American Thoracic Society.)

variants of CTD were CREST syndrome (77 patients, 69%) and diffuse scleroderma (14 patients, 13%). The 6-minute walk distance improved at week-12 in the epoprostenol group and decreased in the conventional therapy group; the treatment effect was 108 m ($p < 0.001$). Hemodynamics also improved, mainly owing to a significant increase in cardiac output. At the end of 12 weeks, 21 patients (38%) treated with epoprostenol and no patient receiving conventional therapy showed improved NYHA functional class. Only a trend toward greater improvement in the Raynaud phenomenon was seen in the epoprostenol group; 36 new digital ulcers occurred in the epoprostenol group, while 72 occurred in the conventional therapy group. Four patients died in the epoprostenol group compared with five patients in the control group. Absence of difference in survival between groups may reflect the greater complexity and multi-organ involvement in scleroderma as compared to IPAH (Badesch *et al.*, 2000). Unfortunately, it seems that epoprostenol therapy does not influence the long-term outcome of many patients with severe scleroderma-associated PAH as it appears to with IPAH (Humbert *et al.*, 1999; Kawut *et al.*, 2003; Kuhn *et al.*, 2003) (Figure 4.5).

Congenital systemic-to-pulmonary shunts

The rationale for using epoprostenol in patients with PAH related to congenital heart diseases (CHD) is based on similarity of histopathology with IPAH even if the pathogenesis might be different (Wagenvoort and Wagenvoort, 1974). Furthermore, for those patients who have had previous cardiac surgery with complete repair of their cardiac defects, post-operative physiology closely resembles IPAH (Rosenzweig,

Kerstein and Barst, 1999). Several studies showed that acute epoprostenol can provide improvement in cardiopulmonary hemodynamic in patients with PAH associated with CHD (Bush, Busst and Shinebourne, 1985; Bush *et al.*, 1987; Schranz *et al.*, 1992; Turanlahti *et al.*, 1998). Long-term effects of epoprostenol in PAH associated with CHD were reported in 1999 by Rosenzweig and coworkers (Rosenzweig, Kerstein and Barst, 1999). This study included 20 patients with PAH (17 patients in NYHA class III or IV) associated with a variety of CHD (atrial/ventricular/great vessel defects), aged from 22 months to 51 years (mean 15 years), failing to improve on conventional therapy (including surgical correction) and unresponsive to acute administration of epoprostenol. Eleven patients had had previous surgical repair at a young age, and a total of 11 patients had unoperated or residual post-operative systemic-to-pulmonary shunts at the time epoprostenol was started. At the time of the report, continuous infusion of epoprostenol had been given for 8 to 28 months in addition to conventional therapy. NYHA functional class improved in 14 patients and remained unchanged in 5 (one patient died after four months with no change). Long-term epoprostenol significantly improved mPAP (–21%), cardiac index (+69%), PVR (–52%) and mixed venous oxygen saturation. Systemic oxygen transport also improved, including those patients with residual shunts ($p < 0.001$). Finally, at the time of the report, 8/12 patients listed for LT were taken off the active transplant list because of persistent clinical and hemodynamic improvement, and one patient went from having an inoperable atrial septal defect to operable CHD.

Portopulmonary hypertension

Pulmonary arterial hypertension is a known complication of portal hypertension, with or without liver diseases. Histopathology of the pulmonary arterial lesions associated with portopulmonary hypertension (PoPH) is indistinguishable from that seen in IPAH (Krowka and Edwards, 2000). Portopulmonary hypertension usually contraindicates liver transplantation owing to high peri/post-morbidity and mortality (Krowka *et al.*, 2000).

Although randomized controlled trials have not been performed, several case series have shown substantial improvement of exercise endurance with compassionate use of epoprostenol in NYHA class III or IV PoPH patients (Kuo *et al.*, 1997; Krowka *et al.*, 1999; McLaughlin *et al.*, 1999). In a preliminary report, four patients with PoPH who received epoprostenol (10–28 ng/kg/min) over a 6–14 month period had a 29–46% decrease in mPAP and a 22–71% decrease in PVR (Kuo *et al.*, 1997). Compassionate use of epoprostenol improved NYHA functional class, exercise endurance and hemodynamics in a group of 33 patients with PAH including 7 with PoPH (McLaughlin *et al.*, 1999). In this report, patients with PoPH demonstrated better hemodynamic improvement than patients with connective-tissue diseases or congenital heart diseases. Three patients died from complications of cirrhosis (McLaughlin *et al.*, 1999). In another study, ten patients with PoPH received chronic epoprostenol infusion (6–48 ng/kg/min) over a period of between 8 days and 30 months (Krowka *et al.*, 1999). Six patients who were restudied by right heart catheterization had a $17 \pm 16\%$ (m $\pm$ SD) decrease in mPAP and a $47 \pm 12\%$ fall in PVR. Six patients died on epoprostenol after a median of 5.5 months (from complications of cirrhosis in three cases). One patient underwent liver transplantation after three months on epoprostenol (Krowka *et al.*, 1999). A retrospective chart review at two transplantation centers described long-term follow-up of 12 PoPH patients on epoprostenol (Murray *et al.*, 2002). Ten patients had a follow-up right heart catheterization after 4–28 months on epoprostenol: the mPAP decreased by 25% from 50 to 38 mm Hg and the mean PVR fell by 47% from 535 to 238 d s/cm^5. Epoprostenol was withdrawn in one patient after liver transplantation. In our center, 29 patients with severe PoPH (NYHA functional class III and IV) have been treated with long-term epoprostenol therapy for 21 ± 19 months (unpublished data). At the time of follow-up, 17 patients remained on long-term epoprostenol and 10 had died. Epoprostenol was withdrawn in two patients. One patient underwent liver transplantation and was weaned off epoprostenol. After a mean of two years on epoprostenol (mean dosage: 28 ± 8 ng/kg/min) exercise endurance and hemodynamics improved to a greater extent than in matched-IPAH patients of similar severity. In survivors, 6-minute walk distance improved by 157 $\pm$ 55 m, mPAP decreased by $25 \pm 10\%$, cardiac index increased by $43 \pm 10\%$ and PVR fell by $45 \pm 8\%$. Overall survival rates at one, two and three years were similar to those of IPAH patients on epoprostenol (78%, 72% and 59%, respectively, as compared to 85%, 70% and 63%, respectively, in IPAH).

'Tolerance' to epoprostenol therapy is similar in PoPH and in IPAH. However, it has been reported that continuous intravenous epoprostenol therapy was followed by the development of progressive splenomegaly, with worsening thrombocytopenia and leukopenia in four patients with PoPH (Findlay *et al.*, 1999). This complication may limit the usefulness of PGI$_2$ in patients with PoPH.

HIV infection

The association between PAH and HIV infection is now well recognized. In patients with PAH associated with HIV infection, lung tissue sections have revealed vascular pathology similar to that of patients with IPAH (Aguilar and Farber, 2000; Nunes *et al.*, 2003). Aguilar and Farber studied acute and long-term effects of epoprostenol in six patients with severe PAH associated with HIV infection (NYHA class III or IV). Patients were followed for 12 to 47 months (Aguilar and Farber, 2000). None responded to acute administration of i.v. adenosine or high-dose oral calcium channel blockers. However, acute administration of epoprostenol induced significant improvements in pulmonary artery pressure. Long-term epoprostenol infusion induced further sustained improvements in PAP and PVR. NYHA functional class improved in all six patients, i.e. class III or IV to class I or II (Aguilar and Farber, 2000). In a retrospective study analyzing the prognostic factors in 82 patients with PAH related to HIV infection, Nunes and coworkers described the long-term effects of epoprostenol in 20 (Nunes *et al.*, 2003). These 20 patients were followed for 6 to 47 months (mean: 17 ± 13 months). Improvement in NYHA functional class, exercise capacity (increase of 183 m in 6-minute walk distance, $p < 0.05$) and hemodynamics was observed after three months in 19/20 patients. At the last scheduled visit (mean 17 months), 12 patients were receiving epoprostenol infusion at a dose of 10 to 40 ng/kg/min (mean 22 ± 9 ng/kg/min). All exhibited sustained improvement in NYHA functional class, exercise capacity (increase of 243 m in 6-minute walked distance, $p < 0.05$), and hemodynamic. Univariate analysis showed that, in NYHA class III/IV HIV-positive PAH patients, high CD4 lymphocyte count, combination antiretroviral therapy and treatment with continuous epoprostenol infusion were all associated with improved survival (Nunes *et al.*, 2003).

Chronic thromboembolic pulmonary hypertension

Chronic thromboembolic pulmonary hypertension (CTEPH) is a well-known form of pulmonary hypertension, characterized by obstruction of the large pulmonary arteries by acute and recurrent pulmonary emboli with subsequent organization of these blood clots. Pulmonary thromboendarterectomy is the treatment of choice for patients with CTEPH; unfortunately, it cannot be performed in all CTEPH patients because of the inaccessibility of distal lesions or the presence of concomitant life-threatening diseases. In inoperable CTEPH patients, pulmonary hypertension results from organized thrombus in distal pulmonary arteries and, subsequently, pulmonary hypertensive arteriopathy develops, which is similar to that seen in PAH (Moser, 1993). In a retrospective study, Cabrol and coworkers analyzed the effects of long-term intravenous epoprostenol in 27 consecutive functional class III ($n = 20$) or IV ($n = 7$) patients with inoperable distal CTEPH (Cabrol *et al.*, 2007). After three months of epoprostenol, NYHA functional class improved by one class in 11 of 23 surviving patients, 6-minute walk distance increased by 66 m ($p < 0.0001$) and hemodynamics also improved. At the last evaluation (20 ± 8 months), functional class was improved in 9 of 18 surviving patients with sustained improvement in 6-minute walk distance (+46 m, $p = 0.03$) and hemodynamic parameters. Survival at one, two and three years was 73%, 59% and 41%, respectively (Cabrol *et al.*, 2007). Epoprostenol has also been shown to improve hemodynamics in CTEPH patients prior to pulmonary thromboendarterectomy (Nagaya *et al.*, 2003; Bresser *et al.*, 2004).

Epoprostenol in children with pulmonary arterial hypertension

Pulmonary hypertension is a rare disease in childhood. Despite an apparently greater pulmonary vasoreactivity in children compared with adults (response rate to acute vasodilator testing appears higher before the age of six years, but decreasing markedly with increasing age), raising the prospect of greater vasodilator responsiveness and better therapeutic outcomes, mean survival time on conventional therapy is indeed shorter in children than in adults (<1 year in children <16 years old versus 2 to 3 years in adults) (Barst, Maislin and Fishman, 1999).

In a retrospective study extending over 13 years and involving 77 children with IPAH aged between 7 months and 13 years, Barst and coworkers compared clinical efficacy and outcome in children receiving epoprostenol plus conventional therapy with children receiving conventional therapy alone (Barst *et al.*, 1999). The mean dose of epoprostenol increased from 4 ng/kg/min initially to 78 ng/kg/min at one year and to 122 ng/kg/min at three years. All children treated with long-term epoprostenol improved, regardless of the response with short-term vasodilator challenge. The clinical and haemodynamic improvement in 11 of 14 children listed for LT resulted in their being taken off the waiting list. Survival on epoprostenol infusion was longer than with conventional therapy alone: survival rates were 100% at one year and 94% up to four years with epoprostenol, as compared to 50% at one year, 43% at two years and 38% at three and four years on conventional therapy alone.

However, in that report, the follow-up time on epoprostenol was only 26 ± 14 months (range 10–56 months); the study was therefore extended with an additional seven years of follow-up to further define long-term outcome with epoprostenol treatment: survival rates at one, three, five and ten years were 94%, 88%, 81% and 61%, respectively; treatment success rates, for which death, transplantation and atrial septostomy were events, i.e. treatment failures, at one, three, five and ten years were 83%, 66%, 57% and 37%, respectively. Thus, it appears that treatment with continuous epoprostenol is at least as effective in children as in adults with respect to increasing survival, improving hemodynamic and relieving symptoms, although it seems to require higher doses. However, the decrease in survival and in treatment success after five years demonstrates the importance of serial re-evaluations, including the role of transplantation evaluation before treatment failure occurs (Yung *et al.*, 2004) (Figure 4.6).

The use of epoprostenol for acute vasodilator testing

The goal of acute vasodilator testing is to detect patients with PAH who are able to respond to long-term treatment with oral vasodilator, mainly calcium channel blockers (Sitbon, Humbert and Simonneau, 2002; Humbert, Sitbon and Simonneau, 2004). The most widely used drugs for vasoreactivity testing include intravenous epoprostenol (Rubin *et al.*, 1982; Simonneau *et al.*, 1986), i.v. adenosine (Morgan *et al.*, 1991; Schrader *et al.*, 1992; Nootens *et al.*, 1995), or inhaled nitric oxide (NO) (Pepke-Zaba *et al.*, 1991; Sitbon *et al.*, 1995; Jolliet *et al.*, 1997; Sitbon *et al.*, 1998; Cockrill *et al.*, 2001). Because inhaled NO does not induce systemic vasodilatation, it may be advantageous compared with epoprostenol for acute vasodilator testing in clinical practice (Sitbon *et al.*, 1995; Sitbon *et al.*, 1998).

When epoprostenol is used to test acute pulmonary vasoreactivity, acute dose ranging is started at 2–4 ng/kg/min infused peripherally, with increases by

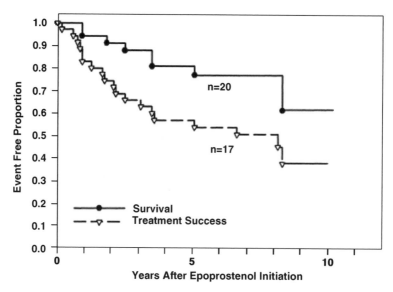

Figure 4.6 Kaplan-Meier curves for survival and treatment success in 35 children with IPAH who received epoprostenol (*n* = 35). Survival rates at one, three, five and ten years were 94%, 88%, 81% and 61%, respectively; treatment success rates at one, three, five and ten years were 83%, 66%, 57% and 37%, respectively. (Reproduced with permission from Yung *et al.*, *Circulation* 2004; 110(6):660–5).

1–2 ng/kg/min every 15 minutes or longer until dose-limiting adverse effects are experienced. The consensus definition of a favorable acute vasodilator response (at least for adult patients) is now defined as a fall in mPAP by at least 10 mm Hg to reach a value of less than 40 mm Hg, with an unchanged or increased cardiac output (Galiè *et al.*, 2004; McGoon *et al.*, 2004; Sitbon *et al.*, 2005). Patients with IPAH who meet these criteria may be treated with calcium channel blockers. However, with pediatric patients, this definition may miss an acute responder and thus the definition of an acute responder in children remains: ≥ 20% decrease in PAPm, normal or increased cardiac index and no change or a decrease in pulmonary vascular resistance/systemic vascular resistance ratio (Yung *et al.*, 2004).

Using these criteria, Barst and coworkers previously reported a five-year survival rate of 97% for IPAH acute responders treated with calcium channel blockers (Barst Maislin and Fishman, 1999); however, at an extended 10-year follow-up, the survival rate was only 81%, and treatment success (defined as freedom from death, transplantation, atrial septostomy or initiation of epoprostenol) was only 47%. In addition, a change from an acute responder to a nonresponder was a surrogate marker for treatment failure on calcium channel blockade; unfortunately, the more stringent criteria of Sitbon and coworkers for acute responders (as above) did not predict this change in children. Therefore, children with PAH who are acute responders may be treated with calcium channel blockade as first-line therapy; however, children should undergo serial acute vasodilator testing to assess the persistence of an acute response vs a change to a nonresponse. This is extremely important, particularly in light of the demonstrated efficacy of epoprostenol in nonresponders. There is no relationship between the acute and long-term effects of epoprostenol, i.e. absence of an acute response in the short term does not preclude efficacy long term (Rubin et al., 1990; McLaughlin et al., 1998), and thus acute challenge with epoprostenol is not required before initiating long-term epoprostenol infusion.

4.2 Treprostinil

The potential complications related to the central venous catheter required for intravenous infusion of epoprostenol have led to the development of treprostinil, a stable prostacyclin analogue that can be administered as a continuous subcutaneous infusion. Subcutaneous administration can be accomplished by micro-infusion pumps with small subcutaneous catheters similar to those used to administer insulin to diabetic patients. Treprostinil has a half-life of approximately 80 min when administered subcutaneously. This longer half-life reduces the potential risks associated with treatment interruption. In addition, its chemical stability permits administration at ambient temperature. Treprostinil was tested in a multicenter randomized, placebo-controlled trial involving 470 patients (all in NYHA functional classes II, III or IV) who had IPAH, PAH associated with a congenital left-to-right shunt, or associated with CTD (Table 4.4) (Simonneau, 2002).

After 12 weeks, the study showed that patients in the overall study population who received treprostinil, as compared with those who received placebo, had a modest but significant median increase of 16 m on the 6-minute walk test; patients in the IPAH group had an improvement of 19 m ($p = 0.006$). Treprostinil also improved indexes of dyspnea, signs and symptoms of pulmonary hypertension and hemodynamic measures. The greatest improvement in exercise capacity was observed in patients who could tolerate the highest doses of the drug. Local pain at the infusion site was a side effect that occurred in 85% of the patients. During the 12 week study, infusion-site pain (thought to be dose related and therefore precluding an increased dose in a substantial proportion of patients) led to discontinuation of treatment in 8%. However, subsequent data suggest that the site pain is not dose related. Despite these limitations, some patients with PAH in whom life-threatening complications developed with intravenous epoprostenol have been safely switched from i.v. epoprostenol to subcutaneous treprostinil (Vachiery et al., 2002; Rubenfire et al., 2007).

In a long-term open-label study, a sustained improvement in exercise capacity and symptoms with subcutaneous treprostinil was reported in patients with IPAH or chronic thromboembolic pulmonary hypertension, with a mean follow-up of 26 months (Lang et al., 2006). In a long-term observational study of 860 patients with PAH, the effects of subcutaneous treprostinil, followed by the addition of other PAH therapies if needed, were followed for up to four years (Barst et al., 2006). The vast majority

Table 4.4 Summary of randomized placebo-controlled, double-blind trials with nonparenteral prostanoids

	Subcutaneous Treprostinil[a]	Oral Beraprost[b]	Oral Beraprost[c]	Inhaled Iloprost[d]
Patients (n)	469	130	116	203
Duration of trial (months)	3	3	12	3
Etiology (%): Idiopathic PAH	58	48	74	54
CTD : CHD : HIV : PoPH	19 : 24 : – : –	7 : 21 : 7 : 16	10 : 16 : – : –	17 : – : – : –
CTEPH	–	–	–	28
NYHA functional class II : III : IV (%)	11 : 82 : 7	49 : 51 : 0	53 : 47 : 0	0 : 59 : 41
Placebo subtracted treatment effect:				
6-minute walk change	+16 ($p=0.006$)	+25 ($p = 0.036$)	+31 ($p = 0.098$)	+36 ($p=0.004$)
Haemodynamics (PVR)	Improved ($p=0.0001$)	Unchanged ($p=0.188$)	Unchanged ($p=0.253$)	Improved ($p<0.01$)
Clinical events[e]	Reduced	No change	No change	Reduced

Adapted from Galiè (2004).

NYHA: New York Heart Association; PAH: pulmonary arterial hypertension; CTD: connective tissue diseases; CHD: congenital heart diseases; PoPH: portopulmonary hypertension; CTEPH: chronic thromboembolic pulmonary hypertension; PVR: pulmonary vascular resistance.

[a] Simonneau et al., (2002).

[b] Galiè et al., (2002).

[c] Barst et al., (2003).

[d] Olschewski et al., (2002).

[e] Clinical events are defined as death, lung transplantation or discontinuation for clinical deterioration in the treprostinil study (Simonneau et al., 2002); death or hospitalization for worsening of symptoms related to pulmonary hypertension in EU beraprost study (Galiè et al., 2002); death, transplantation, initiation of chronic IV epoprostenol or other chronic PGI2 analogue therapy, or a >25% decrease in peak VO$_2$ during exercise from baseline in the US beraprost study (Barst et al., 2003); clinical deterioration; death; or the need for transplantation in the iloprost study (Olschewski et al., 2002).

of patients had IPAH, the remaining having PAH-associated CTD, congenital cardiac shunts, portal hypertension or HIV infection and chronic thromboembolic PH. Out of the 860 patients, 199 (23%) discontinued owing to adverse events, 136 (16%) died, 117 (14%) discontinued owing to deterioration, 29 (3%) withdrew consent and 11 (1%) underwent lung transplantation. In total, 97 patients (11%) switched from subcutaneous treprostinil to an alternative prostacyclin analogue; bosentan was added in 105 patients (12%) and sildenafil in 25 (3%). Survival rates for the whole cohort were 87% at one year and 68% at four years. In patients treated with subcutaneous treprostinil monotherapy during the observation period, survival rates were similar (88% at one year and 70% at four years). For the IPAH subset with baseline haemodynamics available ($n = 332$), survival rates were 91% at one year and 72% at four years, compared with predicted survival from the NIH Registry equation of 69% and 38%, respectively (D'Alonzo *et al.*, 1991; Barst *et al.*, 2006).

The frequency of local complications at the infusion site with the subcutaneous route has led to the study of the efficacy and safety of i.v. treprostinil, which has a potential better risk–benefit profile over intravenous epoprostenol owing to its longer half-life and stability at room temperature. The demonstration of bioequivalence between subcutaneous and i.v. treprostinil was done in healthy volunteers, with elimination half-lives of 4.6 and 4.4 h, respectively and distribution half-life of ~40 minutes (Laliberte *et al.*, 2004). In a 12-week open-label study conducted in 16 PAH patients initiating parenteral prostanoid treatment, i.e. intravenous treprostinil, the mean improvement in the 6-minute walk distance was 89 m (Tapson *et al.*, 2006). Two 12-week open-label trials have studied the feasibility of transitioning patients from intravenous epoprostenol to intravenous treprostinil (Gomberg-Maitland *et al.*, 2005; Sitbon *et al.*, 2007). In the first study, 27 of 31 patients were successfully transitioned over 24 to 48 h (4 patients transitioned back to epoprostenol) (Gomberg-Maitland *et al.*, 2005). In these 27 patients, 6-minute walk distance, Naughton–Balke treadmill test time, functional class and Borg score were maintained with intravenous treprostinil at week 12 as compared to intravenous epoprostenol before transition. However, hemodynamic measurements suggested a slight deterioration in cardiac index and PVR after 12-week intravenous treprostinil (Gomberg-Maitland *et al.*, 2005).

Similar results were observed in the second study, which investigated the feasibility of transitioning patients with PAH from intravenous epoprostenol to intravenous treprostinil using a rapid switch protocol (Sitbon *et al.*, 2007). Twelve PAH patients were enrolled in this 12-week prospective open-label study. Rapid transition to treprostinil was achieved without serious adverse events and, baseline clinical status was maintained over 12 weeks. However, the mean treprostinil dose achieved after 12 weeks was more than double the baseline epoprostenol dose (62 ± 30 vs 28 ± 14 ng/kg/min). At week 12, all patients reported less prostacyclin-related side effects with treprostinil and remained on treprostinil after study completion (Sitbon *et al.*, 2007). Long-term efficacy of intravenous treprostinil remains unknown. In addition, an increase in the number of gram-negative bloodstream infections (BSIs) among PAH patients treated with i.v. treprostinil has been raised. Recent report from the Centers for Disease Control and Prevention (CDC) indicated that the mean rates of BSI (primarily gram-negative BSI) were significantly higher for patients on treprostinil than for those on epoprostenol (Centers for Disease Control, 2007). The results do not suggest intrinsic contamination of i.v. treprostinil as a cause of the infections; the difference in rates might have been caused by differences in preparation and storage of the two agents, differences in catheter care practices, or differences in the anti-inflammatory activity of the two agents.

The stability of treprostinil offers the advantage of possible administration via an aerosol or oral route. In an experimental model, aerosolized treprostinil induced a better pulmonary vasodilator effect with less systemic vasodilatation than the same drug administered intravenously (Sandifer *et al.*, 2005). In an open-label study, a 12-week treatment with inhaled treprostinil (30–45 mg four times a day) improved 6-minute walk distance, functional class and hemodynamics in 12 patients with PAH who remained symptomatic on oral bosentan (Channick *et al.*, 2006). TRIUMPH, the subsequent 12 week randomized, multi-center, placebo controlled trial, evaluated the safety and efficacy of inhaled treprostinil as add on treatment for PAH patients who remained symptomatic on either bosentan or sildenafil. After 12 weeks, patients who received inhaled treprostinil (45 mcg inhalation four times a day), as compared with those who received placebo, had an improvement in 6-minute walk distance, i.e. 20 m increase ($p = 0.0006$) post-inhalation, and 14 m increase ($p < 0.01$) pre-inhalation. Randomized, multicenter, placebo-controlled trials are currently ongoing to determine the efficacy and safety of oral treprostinil (FREEDOM study) in patients with symptomatic PAH.

Subcutaneous treprostinil was approved as therapy for PAH in the United States in 2002 and in the European Union in 2006. Intravenous treprostinil was approved in the United States in 2004.

4.3   Iloprost

Iloprost is a chemically stable prostacyclin analogue that can be delivered through inhalation to patients with PAH (Hoeper *et al.*, 2000). The delivery system, a hand-held ultrasonic or jet nebulizer device, produces aerosol particles of appropriate size (with an optimal mass median diameter of 0.5–3.0 μm) to ensure alveolar deposition, which improves pulmonary selectivity (Gessler *et al.*, 2001). One disadvantage of iloprost is its relatively short duration of action (~1 h); because of that factor, it must be inhaled as many as 6 to 12 times a day (Hoeper *et al.*, 2000; Gessler *et al.*, 2001; Olschewski *et al.*, 2002). A 12-week randomized, multicenter, placebo-controlled trial involving 207 patients (all in NYHA functional classes III or IV) with IPAH, PAH associated with CTD, or inoperable chronic thromboembolic PH used a combined end point of 10% increase in patients' 6-minute walk test distances and an improvement in NYHA functional class (Table 4.4) (Olschewski *et al.*, 2002). Of the treated patients, 17% reached this end point, as compared with 4% of the placebo group ($p = 0.007$). The mean placebo subtracted treatment effect in the 6-minute walk test was a gain of 36 m among patients in the overall study population ($p = 0.004$) and

59 m among patients with IPAH. At 12 weeks, hemodynamic values measured after inhalation were also significantly improved in the treatment group, as compared with baseline values ($p < 0.001$), but values were largely unchanged when measured before inhalation; values both before and after inhalation were significantly worse in the placebo group than in the iloprost group. Side effects included cough and symptoms linked to systemic vasodilatation. In addition, syncope was more frequent in the iloprost group than in the placebo group (Olschewski *et al.*, 2002).

The long-term efficacy of inhaled iloprost remains to be established. In a one-year observational study of 24 patients with IPAH treated with inhaled iloprost, a significant improvement in the 6-minute walk distance was demonstrated (Hoeper *et al.*, 2000). In another observational study, 76 patient with IPAH patients treated with inhaled iloprost were prospectively followed for up to five years (Opitz *et al.*, 2005). Four endpoints were prospectively defined as: death, transplantation, switch to intravenous therapy or addition of or switch to another active oral therapy. During follow-up (535 ± 61 days), 11 patients died, 6 were transplanted, 25 were switched to intravenous prostanoids, 16 received additional or other oral therapy, and 12 patients discontinued iloprost inhalation for other reasons. Event-free survival at 3, 12, 24, 36, 48 and 60 months was 81, 53, 29, 20, 17 and 13%, respectively (Opitz *et al.*, 2005). In addition, observed survival was not statistically different than the predicted survival calculated with the NIH Registry equation. In this study, only a minority of patients (less than 20%) could be stabilized with inhaled iloprost monotherapy during a follow-up period of up to five years (Opitz *et al.*, 2005). This emphasizes the need for randomized controlled studies evaluating combination therapy with inhaled iloprost and oral agents such as endothelin-receptor antagonists or phosphodiesterase-5 inhibitors.

Iloprost can also be delivered intravenously. Continuous i.v. administration of iloprost seems to be as effective as epoprostenol in patients with PAH (Higenbottam *et al.*, 1998), even if it has only been evaluated in a small number of patients.

Inhaled iloprost was approved for class III IPAH patients in Europe in 2003 and for class III/IV PAH patients in the United States in 2004.

4.4 Beraprost

Beraprost sodium, the first biologically stable and orally active prostacyclin analogue (Okano *et al.*, 1997), is rapidly absorbed after the administration of an oral dose under fasting conditions; it reaches a peak concentration after 30 min and has an elimination half-life of 35–40 min (Galiè *et al.*, 2002). In a 12-week randomized, double-blind, placebo-controlled trial involving 130 patients (all class II or III) with PAH caused by various conditions (including IPAH, CTD, congenital left-to-right shunts, portal hypertension, and HIV infection) (Galiè *et al.*, 2002), patients in the overall study population who received beraprost (at a median dose of 80 μg, given four times a day) had a mean increase of 25 m on the 6-minute walk test, and patients with IPAH had a mean increase of 46 m ($p = 0.04$ for both comparisons) (Table 4.4). Patients with other forms of PAH had no significant changes in their exercise capacity. In the overall study population, the administration of beraprost did not significantly change hemodynamics. Side effects linked to systemic vasodilatation, mainly during the initial titration period, were frequent (Galiè *et al.*, 2002).

A 12-month randomized, double-blind, placebo-controlled trial confirmed that patients in NYHA functional class II or III who were treated with beraprost had improved scores on the 6-minute walk test at three months and six months, as compared with the placebo group (Table 4.4). However, this effect was not sustained at 9 months or 12 months, a finding that emphasizes the limitations of 3-month studies (which is the present standard for trials involving patients with PAH) (Barst *et al.*, 2003). Beraprost is an approved therapy for PAH in Korea and Japan.

4.5   Treatment selection

Intravenous epoprostenol infusion remains the treatment of choice for the most severe patients who have rapidly advanced PAH, for NYHA functional class IV patients and for those patients that have the highest risk of death (Humbert, Sitbon and Simonneau, 2004). The question of the place of other prostanoids in the therapeutic strategy of PAH is still of concern. Therapeutic guidelines suggest that inhaled iloprost and subcutaneous treprostinil may be prescribed in patients with less advanced PAH in NYHA functional class III. However, recommendations for these nonparenteral prostanoids are the same as those for oral therapies such as endothelin receptor antagonists and phosphodiesterase-5 inhibitors. Given the complexity of administering these PGI_2 analogs, the majority of clinicians prefer to use oral drugs as first-line therapy and delay introduction of prostanoids until needed based on lack of 'adequate' improvement with the oral agents alone. However, since no data are available from head-to-head comparisons of approved therapies, the choice of treatment currently is determined by clinical experience and the availability of drugs, as well as by patients' preferences (Humbert, Sitbon and Simonneau, 2004). Cost of drugs may also be taken into consideration in making treatment decisions (Table 4.5).

Table 4.5   FDA-approved prostanoids for pulmonary arterial hypertension

Drug	Route of administration	Dosage	Approximate cost of 30 days' treatment for a 70-kg patient in the US (US$)[a]
Epoprostenol (*Flolan*®)	continuous i.v. infusion	20–40 ng/kg/min	$8,000
Treprostinil (*Remodulin*®)	continuous subcutaneous or i.v. infusion	40–160 ng/kg/min	$22,000
Iloprost (*Ventavis*®)	inhaled	2.5–5 µg/inhalation, 6–9 times a day	$13,000

[a] The cost includes only the drug.

In our experience, we usually start oral therapy, e.g. ERA or PDE5 inhibitor, in most class III patients. We consider response to treatment satisfactory if the following criteria are met: NYHA class II; 6-minute walk distance >400 m; normalization of cardiac output measured by right heart catheterization; and normalization of BNP level. If these criteria are not met after three to four months on oral therapy, we add a PGI$_2$ analogue: subcutaneous treprostinil or inhaled iloprost for the less severe patients, and intravenous epoprostenol for the most severe and younger patients. What remains unknown is whether long-term benefits are greater if patients are started on i.v. epoprostenol rather than less invasive therapies, at the time of diagnosis, as opposed to deferring more invasive therapies until patients deteriorate or do not 'adequately' improve on the less invasive therapies.

4.6 Conclusions

Long-term treatment with intravenous epoprostenol improves exercise capacity, hemodynamics and survival in most patients with class III–IV IPAH, and may be currently considered as the 'gold standard' therapy for the most severe patients. In addition, epoprostenol remains the first-line treatment of choice for patients with severe unstable PAH. However, this treatment is invasive, complicated and expensive. In addition, response to long-term epoprostenol therapy may be incomplete, and adverse effects are common. Moreover, survival remains unsatisfactory (55% at five years). Randomized double-blind studies suggest that PGI$_2$ analogues (subcutaneous treprostinil, inhaled iloprost) are safe and effective, especially in IPAH. However their efficacy may be limited owing to an unfavorable pharmacokinetic profile and/or route of administration precluding the use of sufficiently high doses. Preliminary results of clinical trials evaluating combinations of prostanoids with oral drugs acting on different pathophysiologic pathways (endothelin receptor antagonists, phosphodiesterase-5 inhibitors) are promising. Further investigation is warranted.

References

Aguilar RV and Farber HW (2000) Epoprostenol (prostacyclin) therapy in HIV-associated pulmonary hypertension. *Am J Respir Crit Care Med*, **162**, 1846–50.

Badesch DB, Tapson VF, McGoon MD. *et al.* (2000) Continuous intravenous epoprostenol for pulmonary hypertension due to the scleroderma spectrum of disease. A randomized, controlled trial. *Ann Intern Med*, **132**, 425–34.

Barst RJ, Maislin G and Fishman AP (1999) Vasodilator therapy for primary pulmonary hypertension in children. *Circulation*, **99**, 1197–208.

Barst RJ, Rubin LJ, McGoon MD. *et al.* (1994) Survival in primary pulmonary hypertension with long-term continuous intravenous prostacyclin. *Ann Intern Med*, **121**, 409–15.

Barst RJ, Rubin LJ, Long WA, McGoon MD. *et al.* (1996) A comparison of continuous intravenous epoprostenol (prostacyclin) with conventional therapy for primary pulmonary hypertension.. *N Engl J Med*, **334**, 296–302.

Barst RJ, McGoon M, McLaughlin V *et al.* (2003) Beraprost therapy for pulmonary arterial hypertension. *J Am Coll Cardiol*, **41**, 2119–25.

Barst RJ, Galiè N, Naeije R. *et al.* (2006) Long-term outcome in pulmonary arterial hypertension patients treated with subcutaneous treprostinil. *Eur Respir J*, **28**, 1195–203.

Bresser P, Fedullo PF, Auger WR. *et al.* (2004) Continuous intravenous epoprostenol for chronic thromboembolic pulmonary hypertension. *Eur Respir J*, **23**, 595–600.

Bush A, Busst CM and Shinebourne EA (1985) The use of oxygen and prostacyclin as pulmonary vasodilators in congenital heart disease. *Int J Cardiol*, **9**, 267–74.

Bush A, Busst C, Knight WB and Shinebourne EA (1987) Modification of pulmonary hypertension secondary to congenital heart disease by prostacyclin therapy. *Am Rev Respir Dis*, **136**, 767–9.

Cabrol S, Souza R, Jais X. *et al.* (2007) Intravenous epoprostenol in inoperable chronic thromboembolic pulmonary hypertension. *J Heart Lung Transplant*, **26**, 357–62.

Centers for Disease Control and Prevention (CDC) (2007). Bloodstream Infections Among Patients Treated with Intravenous Epoprostenol or Intravenous Treprostinil for Pulmonary Arterial Hypertension — Seven Sites, United States, 2003–2006. *MMWR Morb Mortal Wkly Rep*, **56**, 170–2.

Channick RN, Olschewski H, Seeger W. *et al.* (2006) Safety and efficacy of inhaled treprostinil as add-on therapy to bosentan in pulmonary arterial hypertension. *J Am Coll Cardiol*, **48**, 1433–7.

Christman BW, McPherson CD, Newman JH. *et al.* (1992) An imbalance between the excretion of thromboxane and prostacyclin metabolites in pulmonary hypertension. *N Engl J Med*, **327**, 70–5.

Clapp LH, Finney P, Turcato S. *et al.* (2002) Differential effects of stable prostacyclin analogs on smooth muscle proliferation and cyclic AMP generation in human pulmonary artery. *Am J Respir Cell Mol Biol*, **26**, 194–201.

Cockrill BA, Kacmarek RM, Fifer MA. *et al.* (2001) Comparison of the effects of nitric oxide, nitroprusside, and nifedipine on hemodynamics and right ventricular contractility in patients with chronic pulmonary hypertension. *Chest*, **119**, 128–36.

Conte JV, Gaine SP, Orens JB. *et al.* (1998) The influence of continuous intravenous prostacyclin therapy for primary pulmonary hypertension on the timing and outcome of transplantation. *J Heart Lung Transplant*, **17**, 679–85.

D'Alonzo GE, Barst RJ, Ayres SM. *et al.* (1991) Survival in patients with primary pulmonary hypertension. Results from a national prospective study. *Ann Intern Med*, **115**, 343–9.

Findlay JY, Plevak DJ, Krowka MJ. *et al.* (1999) Progressive splenomegaly after epoprostenol therapy in portopulmonary hypertension. *Liver Transpl Surg*, **5**, 362–5.

Galiè N, Manes A and Branzi A (2001) Medical therapy of pulmonary hypertension. The prostacyclins. *Clin Chest Med*, **22**, 529–37.

Galiè N, Manes A and Branzi A (2002) The new clinical trials on pharmacological treatment in pulmonary arterial hypertension. *Eur Respir J*, **20**, 1037–49.

Galiè N, Humbert M, Vachiery JL. *et al.* (2002) Effects of beraprost sodium, an oral prostacyclin analogue, in patients with pulmonary arterial hypertension: a randomized, double-blind, placebo-controlled trial. *J Am Coll Cardiol*, **39**, 1496–502.

Galiè N, Torbicki A, Barst R. *et al.* (2004) Guidelines on diagnosis and treatment of pulmonary arterial hypertension. The Task Force on Diagnosis and Treatment of Pulmonary Arterial Hypertension of the European Society of Cardiology. *Eur Heart J*, **25**, 2243–78.

Geraci MW, Gao B, Shepherd DC. *et al.* (1999) Pulmonary prostacyclin synthase overexpression in transgenic mice protects against development of hypoxic pulmonary hypertension. *J Clin Invest*, **103**, 1509–15.

Gessler T, Schmehl T, Hoeper MM. *et al.* (2001) Ultrasonic versus jet nebulization of iloprost in severe pulmonary hypertension. *Eur Respir J*, **17**, 14–19.

Gomberg-Maitland M, Tapson VF, Benza RL. *et al.* (2005) Transition from intravenous epoprostenol to intravenous treprostinil in pulmonary hypertension. *Am J Respir Crit Care Med*, **172**, 1586–9.

Herner SJ and Mauro LS (1999) Epoprostenol in primary pulmonary hypertension. *Ann Pharmacother*, **33**, 340–7.

Higenbottam T, Wheeldon D, Wells F and Wallwork J (1984) Long-term treatment of primary pulmonary hypertension with continuous intravenous epoprostenol (prostacyclin). *Lancet*, **i**, 1046–7.

Higenbottam T, Butt AY, McMahon A. *et al.* (1998) Long-term intravenous prostaglandin (epoprostenol or iloprost) for treatment of severe pulmonary hypertension. *Heart*, **80**, 151–5.

Hoeper MM, Schwarze M, Ehlerding S. *et al.* (2000) Long-term treatment of pulmonary hypertension with aerolized iloprost, a prostacyclin analogue. *N Engl J Med*, **342**, 1866–70.

Humbert M, Sitbon O and Simonneau G (2004) Treatment of pulmonary arterial hypertension. *N Engl J Med*, **351**, 1425–36.

Humbert M, Sanchez O, Fartoukh M. *et al.* (1999) Short-term and long-term epoprostenol (prostacyclin) therapy in pulmonary hypertension secondary to connective tissue diseases: results of a pilot study. *Eur Respir J*, **13**, 1351–6.

Humbert M, Maitre S, Capron F. *et al.* (1998) Pulmonary edema complicating continuous intravenous prostacyclin in pulmonary capillary hemangiomatosis. *Am J Respir Crit Care Med*, **157**, 1681–5.

Jolliet P, Bulpa P, Thorens JB. *et al.* (1997) Nitric oxide and prostacyclin as test agents of vasoreactivity in severe precapillary pulmonary hypertension: predictive ability and consequences on haemodynamics and gas exchange. *Thorax*, **52**, 369–72.

Jones DK, Higenbottam TW and Wallwork J (1987) Treatment of primary pulmonary hypertension intravenous epoprostenol (prostacyclin). *Br Heart J*, **57**, 270–8.

Jones K. (1996). Prostacyclin, in *Pulmonary circulation. A handbook for clinicians*, (ed. A. J. Peacock), Chapman & Hall, pp. 115–22.

Kawut SM, Taichman DB, Archer-Chicko CL. *et al.* (2003) Hemodynamics and survival in patients with pulmonary arterial hypertension related to systemic sclerosis. *Chest*, **123**, 344–50.

Klings ES, Hill NS, Ieong MH. *et al.* (1999) Systemic sclerosis-associated pulmonary hypertension: short- and long-term effects of epoprostenol (prostacyclin). *Arthritis Rheum*, **42**, 2638–45.

Krowka MJ and Edwards WD (2000) A spectrum of pulmonary vascular pathology in portopulmonary hypertension. *Liver Transpl*, **6**, 241–2.

Krowka MJ, Frantz RP, McGoon MD. *et al.* (1999) Improvement in pulmonary hemodynamics during intravenous epoprostenol (prostacyclin): A study of 15 patients with moderate to severe portopulmonary hypertension. *Hepatology*, **30**, 641–8.

Krowka MJ, Plevak DJ, Findlay JY. *et al.* (2000) Pulmonary hemodynamics and perioperative cardiopulmonary-related mortality in patients with portopulmonary hypertension undergoing liver transplantation. *Liver Transpl*, **6**, 443–50.

Kuhn KP, Byrne DW, Arbogast PG. *et al.* (2003) Outcome in 91 consecutive patients with pulmonary arterial hypertension receiving epoprostenol. *Am J Respir Crit Care Med*, **167**, 580–6.

Kuo PC, Johnson LB, Plotkin JS. *et al.* (1997) Continuous intravenous infusion of epoprostenol for the treatment of portopulmonary hypertension. *Transplantation*, **63**, 604–6.

Laliberte K, Arneson C, Jeffs R. *et al.* (2004) Pharmacokinetics and steady-state bioequivalence of treprostinil sodium (Remodulin) administered by the intravenous and subcutaneous route to normal volunteers. *J Cardiovasc Pharmacol*, **44**, 209–14.

Lang I, Gomez-Sanchez M, Kneussl M. *et al.* (2006) Efficacy of long-term subcutaneous treprostinil sodium therapy in pulmonary hypertension. *Chest*, **129**, 1636–43.

Langleben D, Barst RJ, Badesch D. *et al.* (1999) Continuous infusion of epoprostenol improves the net balance between pulmonary endothelin-1 clearance and release in primary pulmonary hypertension. *Circulation*, **99**, 3266–71.

McGoon M, Gutterman D, Steen V. *et al.* (2004) Screening, Early Detection, and Diagnosis of Pulmonary Arterial Hypertension: ACCP Evidence-Based Clinical Practice Guidelines. *Chest*, **126**, 14S-34S.

McLaughlin VV, Shillington A and Rich S (2002) Survival in primary pulmonary hypertension: the impact of epoprostenol therapy. *Circulation*, **106**, 1477–82.

McLaughlin VV, Genthner DE, Panella MM and Rich S (1998) Reduction in pulmonary vascular resistance with long-term epoprostenol (prostacyclin) therapy in primary pulmonary hypertension. *N Engl J Med*, **338**, 273–7.

McLaughlin VV, Genthner DE, Panella MM. *et al.* (1999) Compassionate use of continuous prostacyclin in the management of secondary pulmonary hypertension: a case series. *Ann Intern Med*, **130**, 740–3.

Moncada S and Vane JR (1979) Arachidonic acid metabolites and the interactions between platelets and blood-vessel walls. *N Engl J Med*, **300**, 1142–7.

Moncada S, Gryglewski R, Bunting S and Vane JR (1976) An enzyme isolated from arteries transforms prostaglandin endoperoxides to an unstable substance that inhibits platelet aggregation. *Nature*, **263**, 663–5.

Montalescot G, Drobinski G, Meurin P. *et al.* (1998) Effects of prostacyclin on the pulmonary vascular tone and cardiac contractility of patients with pulmonary hypertension secondary to end-stage heart failure. *Am J Cardiol*, **82**, 749–55.

Morgan JM, McCormack DG, Griffiths MJD. *et al.* (1991) Adenosine as a vasodilator in primary pulmonary hypertension. *Circulation*, **84**, 1145–9.

Moser KM and Bloor CM (1993) Pulmonary vascular lesions occuring in patients with chronic major-vessel thromboembolic pulmonary hypertension. *Chest*, **103**, 685–92.

Murray ER, Merriman R, Delen FM. *et al.* (2002) Response of portopulmonary hypertension to epoprostenol therapy. *Am J Respir Crit Care Med*, **165**, A570 (abstract).

Nagaya N, Sasaki N, Ando M. *et al.* (2003) Prostacyclin therapy before pulmonary thromboendarterectomy in patients with chronic thromboembolic pulmonary hypertension. *Chest*, **123**, 338–43.

Nootens M, Schrader B, Kaufmann E. *et al.* (1995) Comparative acute effects of adenosine and prostacyclin in primary pulmonary hypertension. *Chest*, **107**, 54–7.

Nunes H, Humbert M, Sitbon O. *et al.* (2003) Prognostic Factors for Survival in Human Immunodeficiency Virus-associated Pulmonary Arterial Hypertension. *Am J Respir Crit Care Med*, **167**, 1433–9.

Okano Y, Yoshioka T, Shimouchi A. *et al.* (1997) Orally active prostacyclin analogue in primary pulmonary hypertension. *Lancet*, **349**, 1365.

Olschewski H, Simonneau G, Galiè N. *et al.* (2002) Inhaled iloprost for severe pulmonary hypertension. *N Engl J Med*, **347**, 322–9.

Opitz CF, Wensel R, Winkler J. *et al.* (2005) Clinical efficacy and survival with first-line inhaled iloprost therapy in patients with idiopathic pulmonary arterial hypertension. *Eur Heart J*, **26**, 1895–1902.

Oudiz RJ, Widlitz A, Beckmann XJ. *et al.* (2004) Micrococcus-associated central venous catheter infection in patients with pulmonary arterial hypertension. *Chest*, **126**, 90–4.

Pepke-Zaba J, Higenbottam TW, Dinh-Xuan AT. *et al.* (1991) Inhaled nitric oxide as a cause of selective pulmonary vasodilatation in pulmonary hypertension. *Lancet*, **338**, 1173–4.

Prins BA, Hu RM, Nazario B. *et al.* (1994) Prostaglandin E2 and prostacyclin inhibit the production and secretion of endothelin from cultured endothelial cells. *J Biol Chem*, **269**, 11938–44.

Resten A, Maitre S, Humbert M. *et al.* (2002) Pulmonary arterial hypertension: thin-section CT predictors of epoprostenol therapy failure. *Radiology*, **222**, 782–8.

Rich S and McLaughlin VV (1999) The effects of chronic prostacyclin therapy on cardiac output and symptoms in primary pulmonary hypertension. *J Am Coll Cardiol*, **34**, 1184–7.

Robbins IM, Christman BW, Newman JH. *et al.* (1998) A survey of diagnostic practices and the use of epoprostenol in patients with primary pulmonary hypertension. *Chest*, **114**, 1269–75.

Rosenzweig EB, Kerstein D and Barst RJ (1999) Long-term prostacyclin for pulmonary hypertension with associated congenital heart defects. *Circulation*, **99**, 1858–65.

Rubenfire M, McLaughlin VV, Allen RP. *et al.* (2007) Transition from intravenous epoprostenol to subcutaneous treprostinil in pulmonary arterial hypertension: a controlled trial. *Chest*, **132**, 764–72.

Rubin LJ, Groves BM, Reeves JT. *et al.* (1982) Prostacyclin-induced acute pulmonary vasodilation in primary pulmonary hypertension. *Circulation*, **66**, 334–8.

Rubin LJ, Mendoza J, Hood M. *et al.* (1990) Treatment of primary pulmonary hypertension with continuous intravenous prostacyclin (epoprostenol). Results of a randomized trial. *Ann Intern Med*, **112**, 485–91.

Sandifer BL, Brigham KL, Lawrence EC. *et al.* (2005) Potent effects of aerosol compared with intravenous treprostinil on the pulmonary circulation. *J Appl Physiol*, **99**, 2363–8.

Schrader BJ, Inbar S, Kaufmann L. *et al.* (1992) Comparison of the effects of adenosine and nifedipine in pulmonary hypertension. *J Am Coll Cardiol*, **19**, 1060–4.

Schranz D, Zepp F, Iversen S. *et al.* (1992) Effects of tolazoline and prostacyclin on pulmonary hypertension in infants after cardiac surgery. *Crit Care Med*, **20**, 1243–9.

Shapiro SM, Oudiz RJ, Cao T. *et al.* (1997) Primary pulmonary hypertension: improved long-term effects and survival with continuous intravenous epoprostenol infusion. *J Am Coll Cardiol*, **30**, 343–9.

Simonneau G, Hervé P, Petitpretz P. *et al.* (1986) Detection of a reversible component in primary pulmonary hypertension: value of prostacyclin acute infusion. *Am Rev Respir Dis*, **133**, A223 (Abstract).

Simonneau G, Barst RJ, Galiè N. *et al.* (2002) Continuous Subcutaneous Infusion of Treprostinil, a Prostacyclin Analogue, in Patients with Pulmonary Arterial Hypertension. A double-blind, randomized, placebo-controlled trial. *Am J Respir Crit Care Med*, **165**, 800–804.

Sitbon O, Humbert M and Simonneau, G (2002) Primary pulmonary hypertension: Current therapy. *Prog Cardiovasc Dis*, **45**, 115–28.

Sitbon O, Brenot F, Denjean A. *et al.* (1995) Inhaled nitric oxide as a screening vasodilator agent in primary pulmonary hypertension. A dose-response study and comparison with prostacyclin. *Am J Respir Crit Care Med*, **151**, 384–9.

Sitbon O, Humbert M, Jagot JL. *et al.* (1998) Inhaled nitric oxide as a screening agent for safely identifying responders to oral calcium-channel blockers in primary pulmonary hypertension. *Eur Respir J*, **12**, 265–70.

Sitbon O, Humbert M, Nunes H. *et al.* (2002a) Long-term intravenous epoprostenol infusion in primary pulmonary hypertension. Prognostic factors and survival. *J Am Coll Cardiol*, **40**, 780–8.

Sitbon O, Humbert M, Jais X. *et al.* (2005) Long-term response to calcium channel blockers in idiopathic pulmonary arterial hypertension. *Circulation*, **111**, 3105–11.

Sitbon O, Manes A, Jais X. *et al.* (2007) Rapid switch from intravenous epoprostenol to intravenous treprostinil in patients with pulmonary arterial hypertension. *J Cardiovasc Pharmacol*, **49**, 1–5.

Tahara N, Kai H, Niiyama H. *et al.* (2004) Repeated gene transfer of naked prostacyclin synthase plasmid into skeletal muscles attenuates monocrotaline-induced pulmonary hypertension and prolongs survival in rats. *Hum Gene Ther*, **15**, 1270–8.

Tapson VF, Gomberg-Maitland M, McLaughlin VV. *et al.* (2006) Safety and efficacy of IV treprostinil for pulmonary arterial hypertension: a prospective, multicenter, open-label, 12-week trial. *Chest*, **129**, 683–8.

Tuder RM, Cool CD, Geraci MW. *et al.* (1999) Prostacyclin synthase expression is decreased in lungs from patients with severe pulmonary hypertension. *Am J Respir Crit Care Med*, **159**, 1925–32.

Turanlahti MI, Laitinen PO, Sarna SJ and Pesonen E (1998) Nitric oxide, oxygen, and prostacyclin in children with pulmonary hypertension. *Heart*, **79**, 169–74.

Vachiery JL, Hill N, Zwicke D. *et al.* (2002) Transitioning from i.v. epoprostenol to subcutaneous treprostinil in pulmonary arterial hypertension. *Chest*, **121**, 1561–5.

Wagenvoort CA and Wagenvoort N (1974) Pathology of the Eisenmenger syndrome and primary pulmonary hypertension. *Adv Cardiol*, **11**, 123–30.

Yung D, Widlitz AC, Rosenzweig EB. *et al.* (2004). Outcomes in Children with Idiopathic Pulmonary Arterial Hypertension. *Circulation*, **110**, 660–5.

5 Endothelin receptor antagonists in pulmonary arterial hypertension

David B. Badesch[1] and Marc Humbert[2]

[1]*Pulmonary Hypertension Center, University of Colorado School of Medicine, Denver, USA*
[2]*Centre des Maladies Vasculaires, Université Paris-Sud, Clamart, France*

ET-1, a 21 amino acid peptide characterized in 1988, is predominantly produced by the endothelial cells and is one of the most potent vasoconstrictive agents known (Motte, McEntee and Naeije, 2006; Yanagisawa *et al.*, 1988). ET-1 is also a potent proliferative agent and is a mediator of vascular and cardiac hypertrophy and fibrosis. Endothelin-1 expression and concentration in plasma and lung tissue are elevated in patients with pulmonary arterial hypertension (PAH) (Figure 5.1) and correlations have been demonstrated between endothelin-1 plasma levels and indices of disease severity as assessed by hemodynamic parameters and exercise capacity (Figure 5.2) as well as associated with outcomes (Figure 5.3) (Montani *et al.*, 2007). This has supported the concept that endothelin receptor antagonists (ERAs) should be evaluated in patients with symptomatic PAH. The ET subtypes ETA and ETB have been identified (Plate 4) and belong to the G protein receptor superfamily. ETA receptors are expressed on smooth muscle cells and cardiac myocytes. ETB receptors are

Pulmonary Arterial Hypertension, Edited by Robyn J. Barst
© 2008 John Wiley & Sons, Ltd

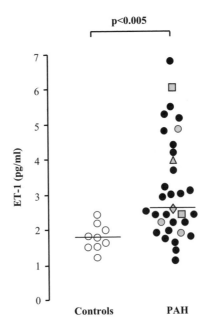

Figure 5.1   Endothelin 1 plasma concentrations in pulmonary arterial hypertension. Endothelin 1 (ET-1) plasma concentrations (pg/ml) were measured in control subjects ($n = 9$, left) and in patients with pulmonary arterial hypertension (PAH) (n = 26, right). In PAH patients, ET-1 plasma concentrations were increased in comparison to controls (p < 0.005, Mann-Whitney test). Each white circle represents measurement in controls. Each black circle represents measurement in a subject with idiopathic, familial or appetite-suppressant associated PAH. Gray shapes represent measurements in PAH associated with other conditions (square for PAH associated with sclero-derma, circle for portopulmonary hypertension, triangle for HIV-associated PAH and diamond for veno-occlusive disease). (Adapted from Montani *et al.*, 2007.)

localized predominantly on vascular endothelial cells and, to a lesser extent, on smooth muscle cells. Activation of either ETA or ETB receptors on smooth muscle cells facilitate vasoconstriction of vascular smooth muscle, stimulation of cell pro-liferation and hypertrophy of vascular smooth muscle cells. In contrast, ETB recep-tors on endothelial cells normally facilitate the release of vasodilators, e.g. nitric oxide and prostacyclin, which also exhibit antiproliferative properties (D'Orleans-Juste *et al.*, 2002; Jeffery and Wanstall, 2001; Joannides *et al.*, 1995). Furthermore, the endothelial ETB receptors are normally involved in the clearance of ET-1 from the circulatory system, particularly in the lungs and kidneys (Bohm *et al.*, 2003; Kedzierski and Yanagisawa, 2001). However, the significance of the ETB receptor on vascular smooth muscle cells in diseased states, including pulmonary hyperten-sion (PH), remains unclear. Thus although both ETA/ETB receptor antagonists and selective ETA receptor antagonists appear to be effective in the treatment of PAH, it remains unclear whether it is more advantageous to selectively block the vasocon-strictive and cell proliferative/hypertrophic effects of the ETA receptor alone while

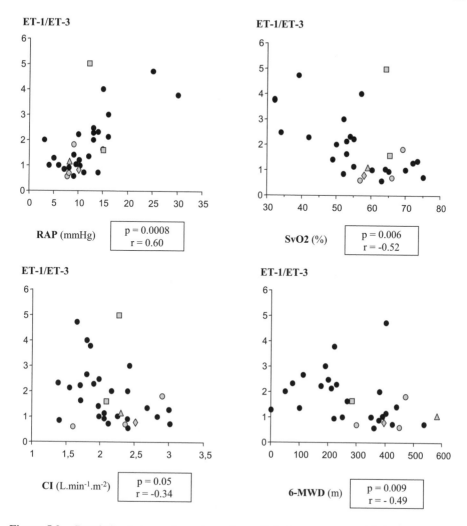

Figure 5.2 Correlation between hemodynamic or clinical parameters and ET-1/ET-3 ratio in subjects with PAH. ET-1/ET-3 ratio positively correlated with RAP ($r = 0.60$, $p < 0.001$) (top left) and negatively correlated with SvO_2 ($r = -0.52$, $p < 0.01$) (top right) and 6MWD ($r = -0.49$, $p < 0.01$) (bottom). Black circles represent measurements in subject with idiopathic, familial, or appetite suppressant-associated PAH. Gray shapes represent measurements in PAH associated with other conditions (square for PAH associated with scleroderma, circle for portopulmonary hypertension, triangle for HIV-associated PAH, and diamond for veno-occlusive disease). (Adapted from Montani *et al.*, 2007.)

maintaining the vasodilator and ET clearance functions of the ETB receptor on vascular endothelial cells or to block both the ETA and ETB receptors.

There are currently two subclasses of ERAs corresponding to non-selective ERAs (blocking both the ETA and ETB receptors), and selective ERAs targeting

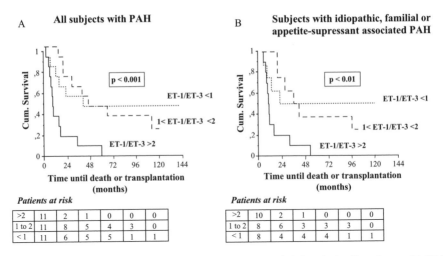

Figure 5.3 Event-free survival analysis according to ET-1/ET-3 ratio in all patients with PAH ($n = 33$). Time until death or transplantation was assessed by Kaplan-Meier analysis. Tertiles were defined as high ET-1/ET-3 ratio (> 2, $n = 11$), median ET-1/ET-3 ratio (> 1 and < 2, $n = 11$), and low ET-1/ET-3 ratio (1, $n = 11$) [$p < 0.001$ by log-rank test]. Cum = cumulative. (Adapted from Montani *et al.*, 2007.)

the ETA receptor. Bosentan (Rubin and Roux, 2002) is an orally active twice daily non-selective ERA, while sitaxsentan (Barst, 2007a) and ambrisentan (Barst 2007b) are orally active once daily ETA-selective receptor antagonists. The safety and efficacy of bosentan, sitaxsentan and ambrisentan have been evaluated in double-blind randomized clinical trials in PAH patients.

5.1 Bosentan

Bosentan was the first oral therapy approved for PAH. The pilot randomized, double-blind, placebo-controlled, multicenter trial (study 351) with bosentan was designed to assess its effects on exercise capacity and cardiopulmonary hemodynamics, as well as safety and tolerability (Channick *et al.*, 2001). Eligible patients had severe IPAH or PAH occurring in association with scleroderma (in functional classes III or IV, according to the 1998 modified New York Heart Association (NYHA) classification), despite prior treatment including vasodilators, anticoagulants, diuretics, cardiac glycosides or supplemental oxygen as clinically indicated. No class IV patients were enrolled. Patients were excluded if they were receiving chronic treatment with continuous intravenous epoprostenol. Inclusion criteria included a baseline 6-minute walking distance (6MWD) between 150 and 500 m, mean pulmonary artery pressure >25 mm Hg, mean pulmonary capillary wedge pressure <15 mm Hg, and pulmonary vascular resistance >240 dyn sec/cm^5. Thirty-two patients were randomized to receive bosentan or placebo (2:1 ratio). Patients randomized to bosentan received 62.5 mg bid for the first four weeks, followed by the target dose

(125 mg bid) unless drug-related adverse events were observed. After 12 weeks, the 6MWD increased by 70 m (from 360 ± 19 m [m $\pm$ SE] at baseline to 430 ± 14 m at week 12; $p < 0.05$) in the bosentan arm, whereas no improvement was seen with placebo (355 ± 25 m at baseline and 349 ± 44 m at week 12). The median change from baseline was +51 m with bosentan vs –6 m with placebo. The difference between treatment arms in the mean change in the 6MWD was 76 ± 31 m (mean $\pm$ SEM) in favor of bosentan (95% CI, 12–139; $p = 0.021$). Bosentan improved cardiac index, with the difference between treatment groups in the mean change at week 12 being 1.0 ± 0.2 l/min/m^2 (mean $\pm$ SEM) in favor of bosentan (95% CI, 0.6–1.4 l/min/m^2, $p < 0.001$). Bosentan decreased pulmonary vascular resistance, whereas it increased with placebo ($p < 0.0002$). Bosentan also decreased the mean pulmonary artery pressure ($p < 0.02$) and the mean right atrial pressure ($p < 0.001$), and both variables increased in the placebo group ($p < 0.005$). Functional class improved in patients treated with bosentan ($p < 0.005$). No patient received a lung transplant or died during the study. Asymptomatic increases in hepatic aminotransferases were observed in two bosentan-treated patients, but these normalized without discontinuation or change of dose.

A larger double-blind, placebo-controlled study (BREATHE-1) evaluated bosentan in 213 patients with PAH (idiopathic or associated with connective tissue disease) who were randomized to placebo, bosentan 125 or 250 mg bid for a minimum of 16 weeks (62.5 mg bid for four weeks then target dose) (Rubin *et al.*, 2002). The primary endpoint was the change in exercise capacity assessed by 6MWD, and secondary endpoints included changes in Borg dyspnea index, NYHA functional class and time to clinical worsening. Patients had symptomatic, severe PAH (NYHA functional class III–IV) despite treatment with anticoagulants, and/or vasodilators, diuretics, cardiac glycosides or supplemental oxygen as clinically indicated. Patients were randomized to receive either bosentan 62.5 mg bid for four weeks followed by the target dose (125 mg bid or 250 mg bid) or matching doses of placebo (144 patients received bosentan and 69 received placebo). After 16 weeks, bosentan improved the 6MWD by 36 m whereas deterioration (–8 m) was seen with placebo, and the difference between treatment groups in the mean change in 6MWD was 44 m in favor of bosentan (95% CI: 21 to 67 m, $p = 0.0002$; Figure 5.4). A dose response for efficacy could not be ascertained. The risk of clinical worsening was reduced by bosentan compared to placebo ($p = 0.0015$; Figure 5.5). Abnormal hepatic function (as indicated by elevated levels of alanine aminotransferase (ALT) and/or aspartate aminotransferase (AST)) occurred more frequently in the bosentan-treated patients than in the placebo-treated patients. Increases in hepatic enzymes over 3 $\times$ the upper limit of normal (ULN) occurred in 12% of the bosentan 125 mg group and in 14% of the bosentan 250 mg group; two patients (3%) in the 125 mg bid group and five (7%) in the 250 mg bid group had elevations $> 8 \times$ ULN. Hepatic function abnormalities were transient except for three patients (all in the 250 mg dosage bosentan group); these patients were withdrawn prematurely from the study. All hepatic transaminase increases have been reported to be

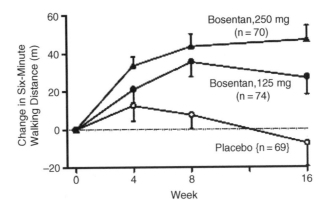

Figure 5.4 Mean (± SE) change in 6-minute walking distance from baseline to week 16 in the placebo and bosentan groups. The Mann-Whitney U test gives $p < 0.01$ for the comparison between the 125-mg dose of bosentan and placebo, and $p < 0.001$ for the comparison between the 250-mg dose and placebo. There was no significant difference between the two bosentan groups ($p = 0.18$ by the Mann-Whitney U test). (Reproduced from Rubin *et al.*, *N Engl J Med* 2002;**346**:896–903. Copyright © [2004] Massachusetts Medical Society. All rights reserved.)

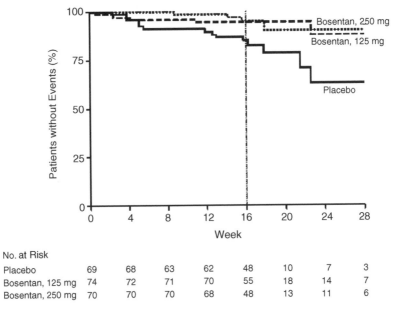

No. at Risk								
Placebo		69	68	63	62	48	10	7	3
Bosentan, 125 mg	74	72	71	70	55	18	14	7
Bosentan, 250 mg	70	70	70	68	48	13	11	6

Figure 5.5 Kaplan-Meier estimates of the proportion of patients with clinical worsening. Clinical worsening was defined by the combined end point of death, lung transplantation, hospitalization or discontinuation of the study treatment because of worsening pulmonary arterial hypertension, a need for epoprostenol therapy, or atrial septostomy. The log-rank test gives $p < 0.05$ for the comparison of the bosentan groups with the placebo group at weeks 16 and 28. There was no significant difference between the two bosentan groups at weeks 16 and 28 ($p = 0.87$). (Reproduced from Rubin *et al.*, *N Engl J Med* 2002;**346**:896–903. Copyright © [2004] Massachusetts Medical Society. All rights reserved.)

reversible with continued treatment, decrease in dose or discontinuation. Three patients died during the course of the study: two on placebo and one on bosentan.

Based on these two randomized double-blind placebo-controlled studies demonstrating improvements in exercise capacity, functional class and hemodynamic parameters, and an increase in time to clinical worsening in PAH patients, bosentan was approved for the treatment of PAH. With respect to longer term data on bosentan therapy, McLaughlin and coworkers reported that first-line therapy with bosentan monotherapy, with the addition of or transition to other therapy as needed, resulted in Kaplan–Meier survival estimates of 96% at 12 months and 89% at 24 months (McLaughlin et al., 2005). At 12 and 24 months, 85% and 70% of patients, respectively, remained alive and on bosentan monotherapy. Sitbon and coworkers compared survival in 139 functional class III IPAH treated with bosentan with historical data from 346 similar IPAH patients treated with continuous intravenous epoprostenol (Sitbon et al., 2005). Baseline characteristics suggested that the epoprostenol cohort had more severe disease. Kaplan–Meier survival estimates after one and two years were 97% and 91%, respectively, in the bosentan-treated cohort and 91% and 84%, respectively, in the epoprostenol cohort.

In a retrospective study of 86 children with IPAH and PAH associated with congenital heart disease or connective tissue disease (Rosenzweig et al., 2005), bosentan was used with or without concomitant intravenous epoprostenol or subcutaneous treprostinil. At data cutoff, 68 patients (79%) were still treated with bosentan, 13 (15%) were discontinued, and 5 (6%) had died. Median bosentan exposure was 14 months. In 90% of the patients ($n = 78$), functional class improved (46%) or was unchanged (44%) with bosentan treatment. Mean pulmonary artery pressure ($p < 0.005$) and pulmonary vascular resistance ($p < 0.01$) decreased, and Kaplan–Meier survival estimates at one and two years were 98% and 91%, respectively. Galie and coworkers evaluated bosentan therapy in a multicenter, double-blind, randomized, placebo-controlled study in patients with functional class III Eisenmenger syndrome (BREATHE-5) (Galie et al., 2006). Fifty-four patients were randomized 2:1 to bosentan vs placebo for 16 weeks. Resting systemic arterial oxygen saturation did not worsen with bosentan therapy, and compared with placebo, bosentan decreased pulmonary vascular resistance ($p < 0.05$) and mean pulmonary arterial pressure ($p < 0.05$), and increased exercise capacity ($p < 0.01$; Figure 5.6). Four patients discontinued owing to adverse events, two (5%) in the bosentan arm and two (12%) in the placebo arm. An open label multicenter study of bosentan therapy in 16 patients with HIV-associated PAH similarly demonstrated favorable effects in terms of NYHA functional class, 6MWD ($p < 0.001$), quality of life ($p < 0.001$), as well as echocardiography ($p < 0.005$) and PVR, CI and PAPm ($p < 0.005$) (Sitbon et al., 2004).

While bosentan is used relatively widely in patients with PAH, close follow-up over time of both efficacy and safety are encouraged. After approval of bosentan for treatment of PAH in the European Union, European authorities required the introduction of a post-marketing surveillance system to obtain further data on its safety

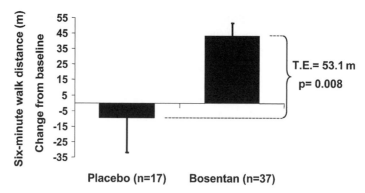

Figure 5.6 Change from baseline of 6-minute walk distance in placebo and bosentan groups. TE indicates treatment effect. (Reproduced from Galie *et al.*, *Circulation* 2006;**114**:48–54).

profile (Humbert *et al.*, 2007). For that purpose a prospective, internet-based post-marketing surveillance system was developed which solicited reports on elevated aminotransferases, medical reasons for bosentan discontinuation and other serious adverse events requiring hospitalization. Data captured included demographics, PAH etiology, baseline functional status and concomitant PAH-specific medications. Safety signals captured included death, hospitalization, serious adverse events, unexpected adverse events and elevated aminotransferases. Within 30 months, 4994 patients were included, representing 79% of patients receiving bosentan in Europe, of whom 4623 were naïve to treatment; of these 352 had elevated amino-transferases, corresponding to a crude incidence of 8% and an annualized rate of 10%. Bosentan was discontinued owing to elevated aminotransferases in 150 bosentan-naïve patients (3%) with increased hepatic transaminases reported to normalize in all patients after stopping bosentan. Safety results were consistent across subgroups and etiologies. Therefore liver function tests should be checked monthly. In addition to acute hepatotoxicity, other side effects include anemia (hematocrit may be checked every three months) and peripheral edema.

5.2 Sitaxsentan

Sitaxsentan has been studied in two randomized, double-blind, placebo-controlled trials (STRIDE-1 and STRIDE-2) (Barst *et al.*, 2004; Barst *et al.*, 2006). In STRIDE-1, 178 NYHA II, III and IV patients with either IPAH, PAH related to connective tissue disease, or PAH related to congenital systemic-to-pulmonary shunts, were equally randomized to receive placebo, sitaxsentan 100 mg or sitaxsentan 300 mg, orally once daily. Sitaxsentan improved exercise capacity assessed by 6MWD, and functional class, after 12 weeks of treatment. These benefits occurred with 100 mg and 300 mg doses, with the 6MWD placebo corrected treatment effects in the sitaxsentan groups being 35 m ($p < 0.01$) for the 100 mg dose and 33 m ($p < 0.01$) for the 300 mg dose. Functional class improved in 16/55 (29%) patients in the 100 mg group and in 19/63 (30%) patients in the 300 mg group, but only 9/60 (15%) patients in the placebo group ($p < 0.02$). Pulmonary vascular resistance decreased with sitaxsentan treatment (mean $\pm$ SD for 100 mg group: 1025 ± 694 to 805 ± 553 dyn sec/cm^5, $p < 0.001$, and 300 mg group: 946 ± 484 to 753 ± 524 dyn sec/cm^5, $p < 0.001$), and increased with placebo (911 ± 484 to 960 ± 535 dyn sec/cm^5). Cardiac index did not change after 12 weeks of placebo, but increased with sitaxsentan treatment (100 mg: 2.4 ± 0.8 to 2.7 ± 0.8 l/min/m^2, $p < 0.02$, and 300 mg: 2.3 ± 0.7 to 2.7 ± 0.9 l/min/m^2, $p < 0.001$; Figure 5.7). The incidence of liver function abnormalities, a dose-dependent ERA class effect, was lower with the 100 mg dose than with the 300 mg dose group. Elevated aminotransferase values ($> 3 \times$ normal), which reversed in all cases, occurred in 3% of the placebo group, 0% of the 100 mg group, and 10% of the 300 mg group during the 12 week study. In the 211 pilot study (sitaxsentan doses 100–500 mg bid po), elevations of hepatic transaminases $>3 \times$ upper limits of normal were seen in 7 of the 20 patients in the 12 week study; in the extension phase following the 12 week study, two cases of acute hepatitis occurred with one death; both cases occurred with the 300 mg bid dose (Barst *et al.*, 2002).

In the second randomized and controlled trial, the STRIDE-2 study (Barst, 2007), 247 PAH patients (245 were treated) with IPAH, or PAH associated with connective tissue disease or congenital heart disease were randomized to blinded placebo ($n = 62$), blinded sitaxsentan 50 mg ($n = 62$) or 100 mg ($n = 61$), or open label (6MWD, Borg dyspnea scores and NYHA functional class assessments were third-party blind) bosentan ($n = 60$). At week 18, patients treated with sitaxsentan 100 mg had an increased 6MWD compared with the placebo group (31 m, $p = 0.03$), and

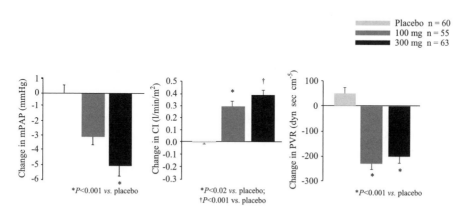

Figure 5.7 Mean ($\pm$ SE) changes in hemodynamic parameters for patients with pulmonary arterial hypertension who were treated with sitaxsentan (100 mg or 300 mg orally once daily) or placebo in STRIDE 1 (12 weeks) (Reproduced from *Barst, Expert Opin Pharmacother* 2007;**8**(1):95–109 with permission.)

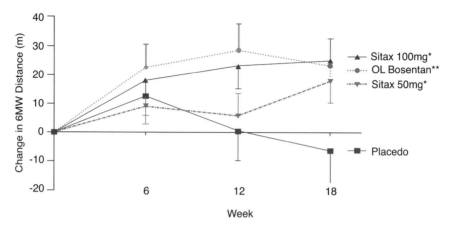

Figure 5.8 Mean (± SE) change in 6-minute walk distance from baseline to week 18 in the placebo, sitaxsentan 50-mg, sitaxsentan 100-mg, and open label bosentan groups. *$p = 0.03$ (95% confidence interval 5.37, 57.44) for comparison between the 100-mg dose of sitaxsentan and placebo, **$p = 0.05$ for open label bosentan vs placebo, and $p = 0.07$ for 50-mg sitaxsentan vs placebo. (Reproduced from *J Am Coll Cardiol*, **47**, Barst *et al.*, 2049–2056, Copyright (2006) with permission from the American College of Cardiology.)

improved functional class ($p = 0.04$). The placebo-subtracted treatment effect for sitaxsentan 50 mg was 24 m ($p = 0.07$) and for open label bosentan, 30 m ($p = 0.05$; Figure 5.8). The incidence of elevated hepatic transaminases (> 3 × the upper limit of normal) was 6% for placebo, 5% for sitaxsentan 50 mg, 3% for sitaxsentan 100 mg, and 11% for bosentan. The most frequently reported laboratory adverse event was increased international normalized ratio (INR) or prothrombin time (PT), related to sitaxsentan's inhibitory effect on the CYP2C9 P450 enzyme, the principal hepatic enzyme involved in the metabolism of warfarin. This interaction necessitates reducing the warfarin dose to achieve the desired INR, with close follow-up.

Based on these two randomized double blind placebo controlled studies demonstrating that sitaxsentan, a selective ETA receptor antagonist, when given at a dose of 100 mg/day orally has been shown to have beneficial effects on exercise capacity (i.e. 6-minute walk distance), functional class and hemodynamic parameters in PAH patients, sitaxsentan was approved for the treatment of PAH in the EU; sitaxsentan remains an investigational agent in the United States.

Because of the known association of acute hepatotoxicity with ET receptor antagonists, sitaxsentan was also evaluated as an alternative treatment option in patients discontinuing bosentan because of acute hepatotoxicity. Of 12 patients discontinuing bosentan because of acute hepatotoxicity (of whom 50% had been rechallenged with bosentan with recurrent increased hepatic transaminases) only one redeveloped elevated hepatic transaminases at 13 weeks of sitaxsentan therapy (with follow-up out to one year) (Benza *et al.*, 2007).

With respect to longer term data on sitaxsentan therapy, although efficacy is most often observed within 12 weeks of initiating ERA treatment, efficacy in some PAH subgroups such as PAH associated with congenital heart disease may not be apparent until 16–18 weeks of treatment, or longer. Long-term data over 1–2 years suggest that sitaxsentan has a durable efficacy response. At the present time, these safety and efficacy data should not be extrapolated to pediatric patients.

5.3 Ambrisentan

Ambrisentan is another oral, once-daily, ETA-selective ERA in clinical development for the treatment of PAH. A phase II dose-ranging study evaluated the efficacy and safety of four doses of ambrisentan in patients with PAH (Galie *et al.*, 2005). In this double-blind study, 64 patients with IPAH or PAH associated with connective tissue disease, anorexigen use or HIV infection were randomized to receive 1, 2.5, 5, or 10 mg once daily for 12 weeks, followed by a 12 week open label treatment period. The 6MWD (+36 m, $p < 0.0001$; Figure 5.9A) improved overall with ambrisentan, with similar increases for each dose group (range: +34 to +38 m). Other parameters, including the Borg dyspnea index, NYHA functional class, subject global assessment, mean pulmonary arterial pressure and cardiac index also improved ($p < 0.05$).

Adverse events appeared overall unrelated to dose, including the incidence of elevated serum aminotransferase concentrations $>3 \times$ the upper limit of normal (incidence of 3%). Exercise capacity continued to increase throughout the study, reaching a maximum improvement from baseline of +54m at week 12 (Figure 5.9B). Patients who completed the 24-week study were eligible to participate in a long-term, open-label extension study. Fifty-four patients continued treatment and were evaluated after one year (48 weeks) of treatment. The clinical benefits of ambrisentan were sustained over the one-year study period, including improvements in 6MWD (mean increase 55 ± 55 m, $p < 0.0001$ for all dose groups combined), Borg Dyspnea Index, and NYHA functional class.

Ambrisentan was also evaluated in two Phase III randomized, double-blind, placebo-controlled, multicenter studies (ARIES-1 and ARIES-2) (Barst, 2007b) in patients with IPAH or PAH associated with connective tissue disease, anorexigen use or HIV infection. The ARIES-1 study assessed the efficacy and safety of once-daily ambrisentan 5 or 10 mg versus placebo. A total of 202 patients were randomized to 1 of these 3 treatment groups for the 12-week study duration. Significant improvements in the placebo-corrected 6MWD change from baseline to week 12 versus placebo were seen with both dose groups (+31 m for 5 mg, $p = 0.008$; +51 m for 10 mg; $p < 0.001$). Improvements in NYHA functional class and Borg dyspnea index were also observed (Barst, 2007b). Although 6 patients in the placebo group developed clinical worsening, compared with 3 patients in each of the ambrisentan groups, this difference was not statistically significant.

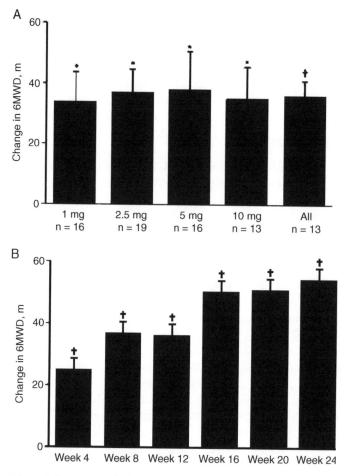

Figure 5.9 (a) Ambrisentan at all dose levels significantly increased exercise capacity as assessed by the 6-minute walk test from baseline to week 12 in patients with pulmonary arterial hypertension. (b) Improvements in 6-minute walk distance (6MWD) were maintained over 24 weeks. Data are mean ± standard error. $*p < 0.02$, $\dagger p < 0.001$ versus baseline. (Reproduced from *J Am Coll Cardiol*, **47**, Barst *et al.*, 2049–2056, Copyright (2006) with permission from the American College of Cardiology.)

In the ARIES-2 study, 192 patients with PAH were randomized to receive ambrisentan 2.5 or 5 mg or placebo once daily for 12 weeks (Barst, 2007b). Ambrisentan improved the placebo-corrected 6MWD at week 12 for patients treated with ambrisentan 2.5 mg (+32 m, $p = 0.022$) or 5 mg (+59 m, $p < 0.001$). In addition, ambrisentan delayed time to clinical worsening in each dose group versus placebo (2.5 mg: $p = 0.005$; 5 mg: $p = 0.008$). Improvements in Borg Dyspnea Index and the SF-36(r) Health Survey were also reported to be better in the ambrisentan-treated patients compared to the placebo-treated patients. Six patients died: four patients in the placebo group, two patients treated with ambrisentan 2.5 mg, and no patients who received ambrisentan 5 mg.

An integrated analysis of ARIES-1 and ARIES-2 confirmed a dose-dependent increase in 6MWD with ambrisentan treatment. All secondary efficacy endpoints demonstrated improvements for the combined ambrisentan group and in the individual 5- and 10-mg dose groups ($p < 0.05$). In addition, improvements in time to clinical worsening were seen in the combined ambrisentan group ($p = 0.0003$) and in both the 5-mg and the 10-mg dose groups individually. Based on these two double-blind randomized placebo-controlled trials demonstrating that ambrisentan improves exercise capacity, Borg dyspnea index, time to clinical worsening, NYHA functional class and quality of life compared with placebo, in conjunction with ambrisentan appearing to provide durable (at least two years) improvement in exercise capacity in a Phase II long-term extension study, ambrisentan was approved for the treatment of PAH.

An open label Phase II study of ambrisentan was performed to evaluate the risk of LFT abnormalities in patients with PAH who had previously discontinued bosentan and/or sitaxsentan because of liver toxicity. Thirty-six patients were evaluated, 86% of whom had discontinued bosentan, 6% had discontinued sitaxsentan, and 8% had discontinued both. The median duration of treatment with ERA prior to discontinuation was nine weeks. None of the 36 patients enrolled in the study had a recurrence of LFT abnormalities that resulted in discontinuation of ambrisentan during the initial 12-week evaluation period. One patient experienced a transient increase in hepatic aminotransferase$>3 \times$ upper limit of normal (ULN) that resulted in dose reduction. No further elevations$>3 \times$ ULN have been observed with ambrisentan exposure of more than one year (Barst, 2007b).

5.4 Safety and tolerability with endothelin receptor antagonists

These three ERAs were all generally safe and well tolerated in all of the PAH clinical studies. The most frequently reported adverse events with ERAs were peripheral edema, nasal congestion, upper respiratory tract infection, headache, flushing and nausea and did not appear to be dose related.

Liver abnormalities have been associated with ERAs as a class, and to date necessitate monthly liver function testing (LFT). In the 16-week BREATHE-1 study with bosentan, 12% of patients developed hepatic aminotransferase concentrations $>3 \times$ ULN and 3% developed hepatic aminotransferase concentrations$>8 \times$ ULN in the 125-mg target dose group (Rubin et al., 2002). In the 18-week STRIDE-2 study with sitaxsentan, the incidence of hepatic aminotransferases $>3 \times$ ULN was 3% for sitaxsentan 100 mg (Barst et al., 2006). The incidence of acute hepatotoxicity $>3 \times$ ULN in the ambrisentan clinical trials was 2% during the Phase II, 24-week study. At the start of the long-term extension study (i.e. after 24 weeks of ambrisentan treatment), 48% of patients were receiving the maximal dose of ambrisentan (10 mg); no additional elevations of ALT and/or AST $>3 \times$ ULN were observed after one year follow-up (Galie *et al.*, 2005). In the pivotal 12-week ARIES-1 and ARIES-2 studies, no patients treated with ambrisentan developed hepatic aminotransferases $>3 \times$ ULN (Barst, 2007b).

Decreases in hemoglobin concentration have also been recognized as a class effect associated with ERAs, with an average decrease from baseline to week 12 of -0.8 g/dl without further decreases thereafter for all three of the ERAs studied to date. Sitaxsentan signifcantly decreases warfarin metabolism and thus requires reducing the warfarin dose to achieve the desired INR, with close follow-up. Ambrisentan does not appear to affect the metabolism of warfarin. (Kenyon and Nappi, 2003; Dingemanse and van Giersbergen, 2004; Barst *et al.*, 2006).

ET-1 is expressed in tissues during embryogenesis (including in the mouse brachial epithelium, optic vesicle and endothelial cells of large blood vessels), and abnormal craniofacial, great vessel, heart, thyroid and thymus development occurs in ET-1 deficient mice. Thus, although the effects of ERAs on human development are unknown, teratogenic risks of ERAs as a class have to be presumed. It should be noted that bosentan and sitaxsentan may reduce the effects of hormonal contraception and it is recommended to add a second method of contraception in bosentan or sitaxsentan-treated women. In males, there is also a concern that the ERAs as a class may cause testicular atrophy and male infertility. Younger males who may consider conceiving in the future should be informed of this possibility prior to taking an ERA.

5.5 Conclusions

Three ERAs (bosentan, sitaxsentan, and ambrisentan) have been evaluated in randomized, controlled clinical trials in patients with symptomatic PAH. It remains unclear whether a selective ETA receptor antagonist or an ETA/ETB receptor antagonist will prove to be more efficacious in the treatment of PAH. In addition, whether various PAH subgroups such as PAH associated with connective tissue disease or associated with congenital heart disease may respond more or less favorably with a selective ETA receptor antagonist than an ETA/ETB receptor antagonist is also unknown. Furthermore, whether an ERA should be first-line monotherapy, i.e. as opposed to a PDE5 inhibitor or a prostacyclin analogue, is also unclear. Whether there is an additive or synergistic effect of an ERA with a prostanoid (e.g. epoprostenol, iloprost or treprostinil) and/or a PDE-5 inhibitor (e.g. sildenafil or tadalafil) is yet to be determined. As observed in many chronic diseases, e.g. diabetes, congestive heart failure and asthma, combination therapy (an area of active investigation and optimism) may further improve the overall efficacy for treating patients with PAH, but further data from controlled studies is needed.

References

Abraham DJ., Vancheeswaran R., Dashwood MR. *et al.* (1997) Increased levels of endothelin-1 and differential endothelin type A and B receptor expression in scleroderma-associated fibrotic lung disease. *Am J Pathol*; **151**(3):831–841.

Barst RJ. (2007a) Sitaxsentan: a Selective Endothelin-A Receptor Antagonist, for the Treatment of Pulmonary Arterial Hypertension. *Expert Opin Pharmacother*; 8(1):95–109.

Barst RJ. (2007b) A Review of Pulmonary Arterial Hypertension: Role of Ambrisentan. *Vasc Health Risk Man*; **3**(1):11–22.

Barst RJ., Rich S., Widlitz A. *et al.* (2002) Clinical efficacy of sitaxsentan, an endothelin-A receptor antagonist, in patients with pulmonary arterial hypertension: open-label pilot study. *Chest*; **121**:1860–1868.

Barst RJ., Langleben D., Frost A. *et al.* (2004) Sitaxsentan therapy for pulmonary arterial hypertension. *Am J Respir Crit Care Med*; **169**:441–447.

Barst RJ., Langleben D., Badesch D. *et al.* (2006) Treatment of pulmonary arterial hypertension with the selective endothelin-A receptor antagonist sitaxsentan. *J Am Coll Cardiol*; **47**:2049–2056.

Bauer M., Wilkens H., Langer F. *et al.* (2002) Selective upregulation of endothelin B receptor gene expression in severe pulmonary hypertension. *Circulation*; **105**(9):1034–1036.

Benza RL., Mehta S., Keogh A. *et al.* (2007) Treatment for Patients with Pulmonary Arterial Hypertension Discontinuing Bosentan. *J Heart Lung Transplant*; **26**:63–69.

Bohm F., Pernow J., Lindstrom J., Ahlborg G. (2003) ET_A receptors mediate vasoconstriction, whereas ET_B receptors clear endothelin-1 in the splanchnic and renal circulation of healthy men. *Clin Sci (Lond)*; **104**(2):143–151.

Channick RN., Simonneau G., Sitbon O. *et al.* (2001) Effects of the dual endothelin-receptor antagonist bosentan in patients with pulmonary hypertension: a randomised placebo-controlled study. *Lancet*; **358**:1119–1123.

Dingemanse J., van Giersbergen PL. (2004) Clinical pharmacology of bosentan, a dual endothelin receptor antagonist. *Clin Pharmacokinet*; **43**:1089–1115.

D'Orleans-Juste P., Labonte J., Bkaily G. *et al.* (2002) Function of the endothelin(B) receptor in cardiovascular physiology and pathophysiology. *Pharmacol Ther*; **95**(3):221–238.

Dupuis J., Jasmin JF., Prie S., Cernacek P. (2000) Importance of local production of endothelin-1 and of the ET(B)Receptor in the regulation of pulmonary vascular tone. *Pulm Pharmacol Ther*;13(3):135–140.

Galie N., Badesch D., Oudiz R. *et al.* (2005) Ambrisentan therapy for pulmonary arterial hypertension. *J Am Coll Cardiol*; **46**:529–535.

Galie N., Beghetti M., Gatzoulis MA. *et al.* (2006) Bosentan therapy in patients with Eisenmenger syndrome: a multicenter, double-blind, randomized, placebo-controlled study. *Circulation*; **114**:48–54.

Humbert M., Seagal ES., Kiely DG. *et al.* (2007) Results of European post-marketing surveillance of bosentan in pulmonary hypertension. *Eur Resp J*; **30**(2):338–344.

Jeffery TK., Wanstall JC. (2001) Pulmonary vascular remodeling: a target for therapeutic intervention in pulmonary hypertension. *Pharmacol Ther*; **92**(1):1–20.

Joannides R., Haefeli WE., Linder L. *et al.* (1995) Nitric oxide is responsible for flow-dependent dilatation of human peripheral conduit arteries in vivo. *Circulation*; **91**(5):1314–1319.

Kedzierski RM., Yanagisawa M. (2001) Endothelin system: the double-edged sword in health and disease. *Annu Rev Pharmacol Toxicol*; **41**:851–876.

Kenyon KW., Nappi JM. (2003) Bosentan for the treatment of pulmonary arterial hypertension. *Ann Pharmacother*; **37**:1055–1062.

McCulloch KM., MacLean MR. (1995) EndothelinB receptor-mediated contraction of human and rat pulmonary resistance arteries and the effect of pulmonary hypertension on endothelin responses in the rat. *J Cardiovasc Pharmacol*; **26** Suppl 3:S169–176.

McCulloch KM., Docherty C., MacLean MR. (1998) Endothelin receptors mediating contraction of rat and human pulmonary resistance arteries: effect of chronic hypoxia in the rat. *Br J Pharmacol*; **123**(8):1621–1630.

McLaughlin VV., Sitbon O., Badesch DB. *et al.* (2005) Survival with first-line bosentan in patients with primary pulmonary hypertension. *Eur Respir J*; **25**:244–249.

Montani D., Souza R., Binkert C. *et al.* (2007) Endothelin-1/endothelin-3 ratio: a potential prognostic factor of pulmonary arterial hypertension. *Chest*; **131**:101–108.

Motte S., McEntee K., Naeije R. (2006) Endothelin receptor antagonists. *Pharmacol Ther*; **100**:386–414.

Rosenzweig EB., Ivy DD., Widlitz A. *et al.* (2005) Effects of long-term bosentan in children with pulmonary arterial hypertension. *J Am Coll Cardiol*; **46**:697–704.

Rubin LJ., Roux S. (2002) Bosentan: a dual endothelin receptor antagonist. *Expert Opin Investig Drugs*; **11**(7):991–1002.

Rubin LJ., Badesch DB., Barst RJ. *et al.* (2002) Bosentan therapy for pulmonary arterial hypertension. *N Engl J Med*; **346**:896–903.

Sitbon O., Gressin V., Speich R. *et al.* (2004) Bosentan for the treatment of human immunodeficiency virus-associated pulmonary arterial hypertension. *Am J Respir Crit Care Med*; **170**: 1212–1217.

Sitbon O., McLaughlin VV., Badesch DB. *et al.* (2005) Survival in patients with class III idiopathic pulmonary arterial hypertension treated with first line oral bosentan compared with an historical cohort of patients started on intravenous epoprostenol. *Thorax*; **60**:1025–1030.

Yanagisawa M., Kurihara H., Kimura S. *et al.* (1988) A novel potent vasoconstrictor peptide produced by vascular endothelial cells. *Nature*; **332**(6163):411–415.

6 Phosphodiesterase-5 inhibitors in pulmonary arterial hypertension

Hossein A. Ghofrani, Werner Seeger and Friedrich Grimminger

Department of Internal Medicine, University Hospital Giessen and Marburg GmbH, Giessen, Germany

6.1 The origins of phosphodiesterase-5 inhibitor development

Nitrate drugs are an exogenous source of nitric oxide (NO), a labile gas that can diffuse across cell membranes into vascular smooth muscle cells where it stimulates the action of soluble guanylate cyclase to convert guanosine triphosphate (GTP) to cyclic guanosine monophosphate (cGMP) (Moncada, Palmer and Higgs, 1991). The formation of cGMP initiates a cascade of reactions that decreases intracellular calcium levels, thereby promoting vascular smooth muscle relaxation (Pfeifer *et al.*, 1999; Lucas *et al.*, 2000). Thus nitrates act as mixed dilators of arteries and veins. The resulting decrease in peripheral vascular resistance and cardiac preload, coupled with improved perfusion of ischemic myocardium, led to its clinical development for angina. However, the therapeutic potential of nitrates is limited by the rapid induction of tachyphylaxis with prolonged administration (Parker and Parker, 1998). Although the precise mechanism of tolerance to nitrates is not clear,

Table 6.1 PDE Nomenclature and families

PDE Family	Subfamily (number of splice variants)	Substrate
1	A (4), B (1), C (5)	cAMP/cGMP
2	A (3)	cAMP/cGMP
3	A (1), B (1)	cAMP/cGMP
4	A (8), B (3), C (4), D (5)	cAMP
5	A (3)	cGMP
6	A (1), B (1), C (1)	cGMP
7	A (3), B (1)	cAMP
8	A (5), B (1)	cAMP
9	A (6)	cGMP
10	A (2)	cAMP/cGMP
11	A (4)	cAMP/cGMP

PDE: phosphodiesterase; cAMP: cyclic adenosine monophosphate; cGMP: cyclic guanosine monophosphate.

treatment that does not directly increase NO levels might circumvent this problem. Thus, it was hypothesized that a downstream target in the NO/cGMP pathway could be modulated. Cyclic nucleotides (cAMP and cGMP) are degraded by intracellular phosphodiesterases (PDEs) (Plate 4). To date, eleven PDE subtypes have been recognized. PDE3 and PDE4 catalyze the breakdown of cAMP, while PDE1 and PDE2 catalyze the breakdown of both cAMP and cGMP. The fifth member of this group, PDE5, catalyzes the breakdown of cGMP (Tables 6.1 and 6.2). PDE5 is present in the smooth muscle of the systemic vasculature and in platelets. Studies by Corbin and coworkers demonstrated that the regulatory domain in the amino-terminal portion of PDE5 contains the phosphorylation site (Ser-92), the two allosteric cGMP-binding sites *a* and *b*, and at least a portion of the dimerization domain. The catalytic domain in the carboxyl-terminal portion of the protein contains the two Zn^{2+}-binding motifs A and B, and a cGMP substrate-binding site (Plate 5) (Corbin and Francis, 1999).

The introduction of sildenafil to the market revolutionized the treatment of erectile dysfunction (ED), and within a few weeks of approval, over one million patients in the US had received prescriptions for sildenafil. The first-line treatment of ED began to move from specialists such as urologists and psychiatrists to a general practice setting and in 1998, case reports of myocardial infarction (MI), stroke and sudden death were reported in patients taking sildenafil for ED. However, subsequent clinical trials and epidemiological studies have not demonstrated that sildenafil provokes MI or stroke when used in accordance with the prescribing instructions (Herrmann *et al.*, 2000; Arruda-Olsen *et al.*, 2002; DeBusk *et al.*, 2004; Wysowski, Farinas and Swartz, 2002; Boshier, Wilton and Shakir, 2004). Indeed there are now multiple scientific papers suggesting a potential utility of sildenafil

Table 6.2 Physiological and/or functional roles of PDEs

PDE family	Role(s)	Evidence[a]
1	Vascular smooth muscle proliferation; Ca^{2+} modulation of olfaction	Broad distribution, but highest levels in proliferatingvascular smooth muscle cells, testes, heart, and neural tissues (e.g., olfactory epithelial cells); binding and inactivation by Ca^{2+}/calmodulin
2	Regulation of Ca^{2+} channels, olfaction, platelet aggregation, and aldosterone secretion	Broad distribution, but highest levels in brain and adrenal cortex[b]
3	Cardiac contractility, insulin secretion, and lipolysis	Broad distribution, but particular abundance in adipose tissue, liver, cardiac muscle, vascular smooth muscle, and platelets; inhibited by drugs with cardiotonic, vasodilatory, thrombolytic, and antiplatelet aggregation properties; stimulated by insulin, leptin, and insulin-like growth factor
4	Immunological and inflammatory signaling processes; smooth muscle tone; depression	Broad distribution, highest levels in neural and endocrine tissue; inflammatory cells thought to participate in the pathogenesis of inflammatory diseases (i.e., asthma and chronic obstructive pulmonary disease), preferentially express PDE4
5	Penile erection; smooth muscle tone of vasculature, airways, and gastrointestinal tract	Abundant distribution in smooth muscle; clinical efficacy of the PDE5-specific inhibitor, sildenafil, for treatment of erectile dysfunction
6	Vision	Distribution in rod and cone photoreceptor cells; some visual defects related to PDE6 mutations
7	T-lymphocyte activation and proliferation; skeletal muscle metabolism	Distribution is predominantly in T-lymphocytes (PDE7A1); PDE7 mRNA is abundant in skeletal muscle tissue, T-lymphocytes, and B-lymphocytes, but protein and activity are readily measurable only in T-lymphocytes
8	T-cell activation	PDE8A mRNA widely expressed (highest in testis); PDE8B is unique to thyroid gland
9	Possibly maintains basal intracellular cGMP levels or natriuresis and vascular tone	mRNA widely expressed, particularly in spleen, intestine, kidney, heart, and brain
10	Unknown	Human PDE10 widely distributed
11	Sperm capacitation; other functions unknown	mRNA occurs at highest levels in skeletal muscle, prostate, kidney, liver, pituitary and salivary glands, and testis; protein localised to vascular smooth muscle cells, cardiac myocytes, corpus cavernosum of the penis, prostate, and skeletal muscle

PDE: phosphodiesterase; cGMP: cyclic guanosine monophosphate.
[a]Francis, Turko and Corbin, 2001; Fawcett *et al.*, 2000; Beavo, 1995; Dousa, 1999; Hayashi *et al.*, 1998; Soderling, Bayuga and Beavo (1998).
[b]Yang *et al.*, 1994.
[c]Pyne and Furman, 2003.
[d]Glavas *et al.*, 2001.
Adapted from Ghofreni *et al.*, 2006

in protecting the ischemic myocardium and in treating stroke (Fox *et al.*, 2003; Halcox *et al.*, 2002; Bocchi *et al.*, 2002; Mahmud, Hennessy and Feely, 2001; Katz *et al.*, 2000; Desouza *et al.*, 2002; Ockaili *et al.*, 2002; Zhang *et al.*, 2002).

Since 2000, there have been occasional case reports (Egan and Pomeranz, 2000; Cunningham and Smith, 2001; Pomeranz *et al.*, 2002; Pomeranz and Bhavsar, 2005) of non-anterior ischemic optic neuropathy (NAION) in patients taking sildenafil. Although NAION is the most common acute optic neuropathy in people over 50 years of age, it is a relatively rare event, causing partial visual loss in one eye, and is associated with various risk factors including cardiovascular disease and a small cup : disk ratio. In a published review of clinical trial data (Gorkin *et al.*, 2006), Gorkin and coworkers estimated an incidence of 2.8 cases of NAION per 100,000 patient-years of sildenafil exposure, which is similar to estimates reported in men aged > 50 years in the general US population (2.5–11.8 cases per 100,000) (Hattenhauer *et al.*, 2006; Johnson and Arnold, 1994). Recently, the original authors of many of the case reports published a further review (Fraunfelder, Pomeranz and Egan, 2006) and concluded that most of the case reports of NAION may be an expected coincidence, as sildenafil is frequently used by patients who are older, vasculopathic and already at risk of NAION, and conclude that the only patients who should avoid PDE5 inhibitors for visual reasons are those who have previously suffered NAION in one eye.

6.2 Pulmonary hypertension as a new indication for phosphodiesterase-5 inhibitor treatment

After the approval of sildenafil for the treatment of ED, thoughts started to turn to other potential indications. Sanchez and coworkers observed up-regulation of phosphodiesterase (PDE5) gene expression in pulmonary hypertensive lungs (Sanchez *et al.*, 1998). Furthermore, it was observed that zaprinast (M&B 22948), E4021 and dipyridamole (a relatively non-selective PDE inhibitor with PDE5-inhibitory activity) appeared to play a role in ameliorating the increased pulmonary arterial pressure (PAP) in experimental pulmonary hypertension (PH) models (Ziegler *et al.*, 1998; Ichinose *et al.*, 1998; Ichinose *et al.*, 1995; Nagamine, Hill and Pearl, 2000; Thusu *et al.*, 1995). With the availability of the more potent and selective PDE5 inhibitor, sildenafil, a series of preclinical and clinical investigations were conducted to investigate its potential role as a therapeutic agent in pulmonary vascular diseases. The first placebo-controlled study (Pfizer study 1024) evaluated the dose–response of intravenous sildenafil. This study, conducted between 1998 and 2000, showed that sildenafil selectively reduced pulmonary artery pressure (PAP) and pulmonary vascular resistance (PVR) in more than 80 patients with pulmonary arterial hypertension (PAH), pulmonary venous hypertension and/or hypoxic PH. It was also observed that the effect reached a plateau at a plasma concentration of ~100 ng/ml of sildenafil. During this period, interest in the role of sildenafil in PH gained significant momentum.

6.3 Role of phosphodiesterase-5 in the pulmonary vasculature

Nitric oxide is constitutively produced in the lung by NO synthases (NOS). The main cellular sources of lung NO production are the vascular endothelium and the airway epithelium (Bohle *et al.*, 2000; German *et al.*, 2000). Adaptation of the perfusion distribution to well-ventilated areas of the lung (ventilation/perfusion (V/Q) matching) is regulated primarily by local NO production (Ide *et al.*, 1999; Grimminger *et al.*, 1995), since the most prominent stimulus for local NO production in the lung is alveolar distension during inspiration (Grimminger *et al.*, 1995; Ghofrani *et al.*, 2004a; Weissmann *et al.*, 2000; Schulz *et al.*, 2000; Spriestersbach *et al.*, 1995). Thus, local NO release results in redirection of blood flow to well-ventilated areas of the lung (V/Q matching) (Plate 6). NOS is regulated at the transcriptional and post-translational levels (Michelakis, 2003). The most important cyclic GMP degrading phosphodiesterase – PDE-5 – is abundantly expressed in lung tissue (Ahn *et al.*, 1991; Fink *et al.*, 1999; Giordano *et al.*, 2001; Wharton *et al.*, 2005). When compared with the expression of PDE5 in other tissues such as the myocardium, the expression and activity of PDE5 is considerably higher in lung tissue (Corbin *et al.*, 2005). PDE5 is thus an ideal target for treatment of pulmonary vascular disorders, including PAH, and PH associated with underlying lung disorders. Moreover, sildenafil is the first oral drug with the potential to augment NO-related vasodilatation in regions of perfusion demand and, in the case of the lung, prevent wasted perfusion (venous admixture) and wasted ventilation (dead space ventilation).

In 1991, Haynes and coworkers demonstrated that the PDE5 inhibitor zaprinast decreased the vasoconstrictor response of isolated rat lungs to acute alveolar hypoxia (Haynes *et al.*, 1991). Zaprinast was also shown to induce selective pulmonary vasodilatation when compared to its effects on the systemic circulation in intact anesthetized newborn lambs exposed to acute hypoxia (Braner *et al.*, 1993), and in chronically hypoxic rats (Cohen *et al.*, 1996). However, in the latter study, the PDE5 inhibitor E4021 turned out to be more selective for the pulmonary vascular bed, without any dilating effects in the systemic circulation. Inhibition of hypoxic pulmonary vasoconstriction (HPV) was also achieved in isolated rabbit lungs by zaprinast (Weissmann *et al.*, 2000). Investigations with the PDE5 inhibitor sildenafil in isolated perfused rodent lungs demonstrated a marked inhibition of HPV (Zhao *et al.*, 2001; Zhao *et al.*, 2003), thereby confirming that PDE5 inhibitors act as potent pulmonary vasodilators. Oral treatment of chronically hypoxic mice with sildenafil prevented the development of PH (Zhao *et al.*, 2001). In these studies, Zhao and coworkers also demonstrated that it was not only NO derived from endothelial nitric oxide synthase (eNOS) that contributed to these effects of the PDE5 inhibitor (Zhao *et al.*, 2001). These observations are consistent with their more recent study demonstrating that in natriuretic peptide (NPR-A) knockout mice, sildenafil decreased the PH and right ventricular hypertrophy, suggesting that the natriuretic peptide pathway may play a major role in the effects of sildenafil (Zhao *et al.*, 2003). While all of the above investigations initiated the sildenafil treatment at the onset of hypoxia, Sebkhi and coworkers demonstrated that starting sildenafil after established hypoxic PH also reduced pulmonary artery pressure and pulmonary vascular muscularization in lungs from chronically hypoxic rats (Sebkhi *et al.*, 2003). These investigations therefore demonstrated that PDE5 inhibition appears to have remodeling effects, with selective effects on the pulmonary vascular resistance. Thus, the selective pulmonary effects of PDE5 inhibitors appear attributable to a high level of PDE5 in the pulmonary circulation compared with the systemic circulation (Ahn *et al.*, 1991, Giordano *et al.*, 2001; Corbin *et al.*, 2005; Hanson *et al.*, 2003), and that NO production in the lung is high, akin to the situation in the corpus cavernosum (Grimminger *et al.*, 1995; Spriestersbach *et al.*, 1995; Nangle, Cotter and Cameron, 2003; Bloch *et al.*, 1998). Itoh and others recently reported that sildenafil alone, and in combination with the prostacyclin analogue beraprost, decreased right ventricular systolic pressure (RVSP), right heart hypertrophy and pulmonary vascular medial wall thickness in the MCT-induced rat PH model (Itoh *et al.*, 2004). The beneficial effects of sildenafil after the development of PH yielded similar results (Schermuly *et al.*, 2004), i.e. sildenafil reduced pulmonary artery pressure and vascular muscularization in the MCT-PH model rat lungs, and reduced the expression of matrix metalloproteinases (MMP) 2 and 9 after development of PH. In addition, the degree of fully muscularized small (< 50 μm) pulmonary arteries was decreased.

6.4 Clinical experience with sildenafil for the treatment of chronic pulmonary hypertension

The vasodilatory effects of inhaled NO appear to be restricted to the pulmonary vasculature. Nitric oxide, with its very short half-life, i.e. ~20 s, is used as a screening agent for acute pulmonary vasoreactivity (Sitbon *et al.*, 1998), and is effective in improving gas exchange in selected patients with adult respiratory distress syndrome (ARDS) (Rossaint *et al.*, 1993). Weaning from chronic NO treatment in patients with ARDS has been facilitated by oral sildenafil (Atz and Wessel 1999). The first case report of an adult patient with PAH treated chronically with high doses of oral sildenafil indicated that this approach could be effective (Prasad, Wilkinson and Gatzoulis, 2000). An early report using oral sildenafil in a child with severe PH also appeared efficacious, raising interest not only within the medical community but also in the media (Abrams, Schulze-Neick and Magee, 2000; Patole and Travadi, 2002; Oliver and Webb, 2002). Sildenafil is frequently given if a patient cannot be easily weaned off inhaled NO, e.g. after 'corrective' open heart surgery in children with systemic-to-pulmonary shunts. The sildenafil is then weaned or continued based on whether the patient has persistent PH post-operatively.

Trials addressing the characterization of the acute effects of sildenafil on pulmonary and systemic hemodynamics in a larger number of patients with PAH showed that sildenafil effectively reduces pulmonary vascular resistance in a dose-dependent manner (Ghofrani *et al.*, 2002a). Notably, the vasodilator effects are predominantly restricted to the pulmonary circulation and appear to be greater than the effects seen with inhaled NO. In combination with inhaled iloprost, augmentation of the pulmonary vasodilator effect of each single agent was observed (Ghofrani *et al.*, 2002a; Wilkens *et al.*, 2001). Long-term oral sildenafil treatment in PAH patients has been investigated in a number of single-center studies, all suggesting its high efficacy and safety (Kothari and Duggal, 2002; Sastry *et al.*, 2002; Sastry *et al.*, 2004).

Interestingly, sildenafil appears to be effective also for treating patients with PH with etiologies other than idiopathic PAH. In patients with human immunodeficiency virus (HIV)-related PH, sildenafil was similarly effective in reducing pulmonary vascular resistance as it was in idiopathic PAH (Schumacher *et al.*, 2001; Carlsen, Kjeldsen and Gerstoft, 2002). Recent data also suggest that long-term oral sildenafil treatment in patients with inoperable chronic thromboembolic PH is beneficial (Ghofrani *et al.*, 2003a; Reichenberger *et al.*, 2007).

6.5 Pivotal trial and approval of sildenafil for the treatment of pulmonary arterial hypertension (SUPER-1 study)

Based on studies between 1998 and 2001 suggesting the efficacy of sildenafil for the treatment of PAH, a large randomized, double-blind, placebo-controlled international trial was carried out to confirm that treatment with sildenafil is safe and efficacious for the treatment of PAH. The SUPER-1 (Sildenafil Use in Pulmonary HypERtension) study (started in 2002) included 278 patients with symptomatic PAH treated either with placebo or sildenafil (20, 40, or 80 mg) orally three times daily (TID) for 12 weeks. The primary end-point – as in many previous PAH trials – was the change from baseline to week 12 in the 6-minute walk distance (6MWD). Sildenafil, in all three applied doses, improved exercise capacity (~45–50 m; placebo corrected value), functional class and hemodynamics, as compared to placebo-treated patients, and was well tolerated (Galie *et al.*, 2005). In addition, patients completing the double-blind phase were eligible to enter a long-term extension trial, conducted over a two-year period with 80 mg sildenafil TID. The increase in the 6MWD achieved after three months in the placebo-controlled phase was maintained after one year of therapy in the patients who continued on sildenafil, as were the improvements in functional class, both indicative of maintenance of the effect; however, these long-term data were uncontrolled and observational; in addition, patients could have had additional PAH therapies added at the discretion of the investigator.

Based on the favorable effects of this new oral treatment, sildenafil was approved by the FDA and the EMEA in 2005 for the treatment of patients with symptomatic PAH. Both agencies approved only the 20 mg TID dose, as a non-significant dose–effect relationship between 20 and 80 mg TID was observed with regard to the primary endpoint of the study, the change in 6MWD over 12 weeks of treatment, in the overall patient population. However, there were significant dose responses demonstrated in some of the secondary endpoints, e.g. mean pulmonary arterial pressure (mPAP) and PVR in the overall population, as well as in some subgroup analyses, e.g. idiopathic PAH, with respect to improvement in 6MWD. Moreover, in the majority of prior short- and long-term studies, daily doses of 100 up to 300 mg were investigated and reported to be efficacious and well tolerated (Ghofrani *et al.*, 2002; Wilkens *et al.*, 2001; Kothari and Duggal, 2002; Sastry *et al.*, 2004; Michelakis *et al.*, 2003). Thus, future studies are warranted addressing the long-term efficacy of 20 mg TID, higher doses, or perhaps lower doses, of sildenafil for the treatment of PAH. However, the duration of action of sildenafil reported from some clinical and experimental settings may not be accurately reflected by plasma levels and the applied dosage (Moncada *et al.*, 2004). One possible explanation is that intracellular rebinding of sildenafil to the catalytic site of PDE5 could occur repeatedly and may retard clearance of the inhibitor from the cells; it has also been shown that the affinity of sildenafil to PDE5 increases after intracellular phosphorylation of the enzyme (Mullershausen *et al.*, 2003). This led to the hypothesis that sildenafil may saturate the PDE5 enzyme intracellularly with higher affinity than previously estimated. However, whether the conformational changes of the PDE5 and the slow dissociation rate of sildenafil from the enzyme reflect dose effects remains speculative (Francis *et al.*, 1998; Gopal, Francis and Corbin, 2001; Corbin and Francis, 2002; Huai *et al.*, 2004).

6.6   Other phosphodiesterase-5 inhibitors

In a comparative clinical trial, 60 consecutive PAH patients (NYHA classification II–IV) undergoing right heart catheterization for acute pulmonary vasoreactivity testing received initial short-term NO inhalation and were subsequently assigned to oral intake of 50 mg sildenafil ($n = 19$), 10 mg ($n = 7$) or 20 mg ($n = 9$) vardenafil, or 20 mg ($n = 9$), 40 mg ($n = 8$) or 60 mg ($n = 8$) tadalafil (Ghofrani *et al.*, 2004b) (Figure 6.1). Hemodynamics and gas exchange responses were assessed over a subsequent 120 min observation period. All three PDE-5 inhibitors caused significant pulmonary vasorelaxation, accompanied by an increase in cardiac output, with maximum effects obtained after 40–45 min (vardenafil), 60 min (sildenafil) and 75–90 min (tadalafil). Sildenafil and tadalafil, but not vardenafil, caused a significant reduction of the pulmonary-to-systemic vascular resistance ratio. Significant improvement in systemic arterial oxygenation, corresponding to that observed during NO inhalation, was noted only with sildenafil. Thus, the three PDE-5 inhibitors (Table 6.3) appeared to differ in kinetics of pulmonary vasorelaxation (most rapid effect by vardenafil), selectivity for the pulmonary circulation (sildenafil and tadalafil, but not vardenafil) and impact on systemic arterial oxygenation (improvement only after sildenafil). Tadalafil has also been shown to be safe and efficacious for the treatment of symptomatic pulmonary arterial hypertension as monotherapy

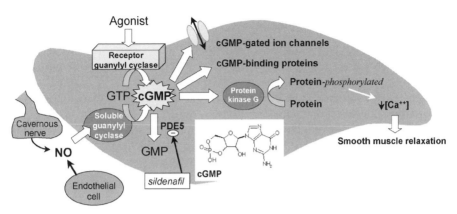

Figure 6.1 Comparison of the structure of the selective PDE5 inhibitors, sildenafil, tadalafil and vardenafil with that of the native substrate cGMP. (Adapted from Ghofrani, Osterloh and Grimminger, 2006.)

and as add on therapy to bosentan in the randomized, double-blind, placebo-controlled PHIRST trial (**P**ulmonary arterial **H**ypertens**I**on and **R**espon**S**e to **T**adalafil). Compared with placebo treated patients, patients treated with tadalafil had increased exercise capacity, improved hemodynamics, and less clinical worsening.

Table 6.3 PDE inhibition and selectivity

Compound	Geometric mean IC_{50} values (µM) (fold selectivity versus PDE5 in parentheses)					
	PDE1	PDE2	PDE3	PDE4	PDE5	PDE6 (rod)
Sildenafil	0.281 (80)	>30 (>8570)	16.2 (4630)	7.68 (2190)	0.00350	0.037 (11)
Tadalafil	>30 (>4450)	>100 (>14,800)	>100 (>14,800)	>100 (>14,800)	0.00674	1.26 (187)
Vardenafil	0.070 (500)	6.20 (44,290)	>1.0 (>7140)	6.10 (43,570)	0.00014	0.0035 (25)
	PDE6 (cone)	PDE7A	PDE8A	PDE9A	PDE10A	PDE11A
Sildenafil	0.034 (10)	21.3 (6090)	29.8 (8510)	2.61 (750)	9.80 (2800)	2.73 (780)
Tadalafil	1.30 (193)	>100 (>14,800)	>100 (>14,800)	>100 (>14,800)	>100 (>14,800)	0.037 (5)
Vardenafil	0.0006 (4)	>30 (>214,000)	>30 (>214,000)	0.581 (4150)	3.0 (21,200)	0.162 (1160)

IC_{50}s were determined using either native enzyme purified from human tissue (PDE1, heart; PDEs 2, 3, and 5, corpus cavernosum; PDE4, skeletal muscle; PDE6, retina) or using recombinant human enzymes expressed in $Sf9$ cells (PDEs 7–11) and purified by anion-exchange chromatography. PDE: phosphodiesterase; IC_{50}: drug concentration necessary to inhibit 50% of enzyme activity. Adapted from Gbekor et al., 2002.

6.7 Combination therapy

As in many other progressive diseases, patients with PAH may experience clinical and hemodynamic deterioration despite ongoing initial effective monotherapy with the currently available disease-specific PAH drugs (i.e. PDE5i, prostanoids, endothelin receptor antagonists). It may thus be reasonable to consider combination therapy from another complementary group of drugs. However, because of unknown risks, costs, drug interactions, etc., combination therapy is not generally recommended until randomized, controlled trial data is available that demonstrates safety and efficacy with the various possible combinations and in the various PAH subgroups.

Experience to date with combination of phosphodiesterase-5 inhibitors and prostanoids

The combination of prostanoids and sildenafil has potential as synergistic treatment for PAH. The combination of sildenafil plus inhaled iloprost has to date been studied in three small trials. During a randomized, controlled acute trial, 30 patients (17 PAH, 13 chronic thromboembolic PH) in NYHA functional class III–IV were given either sildenafil in one of two doses (12.5 mg or 50 mg) or sildenafil plus inhaled iloprost (Ghofrani $et\ al.$, 2002). Before randomization, the pulmonary hemodynamic effects of NO alone and of inhaled iloprost alone were tested. Inhaled iloprost showed a greater and longer-lasting effect than did NO (60–90 min vs 5 min). The efficacy of sildenafil was dose-dependent. The best results were obtained with high-dose sildenafil (50 mg) plus inhaled iloprost. Using this combination, the PVR decreased ~50% with a concomitant ~50% increase in cardiac index, with maintenance of effect for more than 3 h. Another pilot study involving five idiopathic PAH patients reported similar results. Inhaled iloprost decreased mPAP more than sildenafil (reduction by 9.4 vs 6.4 mm Hg; $p < 0.05$). Receiving a combination of the two drugs led to a greater decrease in mPAP than with inhaled iloprost alone (13.8 vs 9.4 mm Hg; $p < 0.009$). Systemic blood pressure remained unaffected (Wilkens $et\ al.$, 2001).

The third trial was a long-term observational study examining the effects of adding sildenafil in 14 patients whose condition deteriorated during the course of long-term treatment with inhaled iloprost after an initial improvement (Ghofrani $et\ al.$, 2003b). Before the start of iloprost monotherapy, the patients had an average 6MWD of 217 m. With inhaled iloprost, the distance walked initially improved to 305 m before deteriorating over the course of 18 months to 256 m. At this point sildenafil was added, leading to an improvement in the 6MWD to 346 m. The combination therapy thus resulted in a walk distance (346 m) that was above the distance attained with the initial monotherapy (305 m) – even though more than 18 months had passed. The effect of the combination was

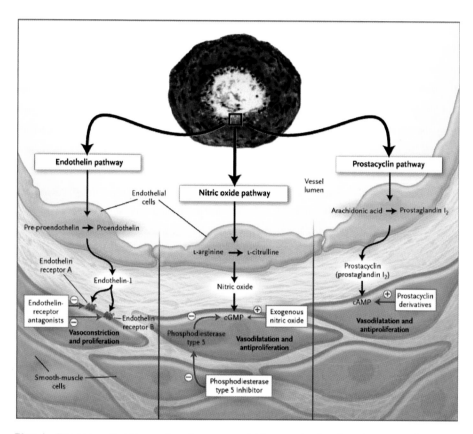

Plate 1 Targeted medical therapy for pulmonary arterial hypertension based on the prostacyclin pathway, the nitric oxide pathway and the endothelin pathway. Reproduced with permission from Humbert *et al.*, *N. Engl. J. Med.* 2004; 351:1425. Copyright © [2004] Massachusetts Medical Society. All rights reserved.

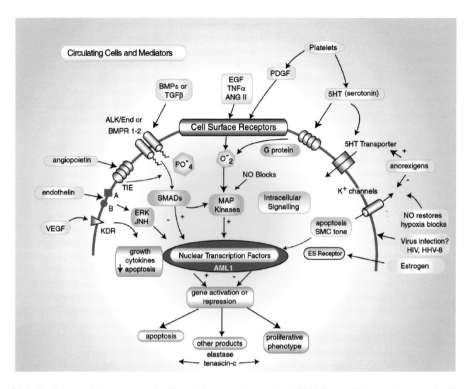

Plate 2 Some cellular processes implicated in the pathogenesis of PAH. Extracellular mediators and cells (platelets) are highlighted in yellow, cell surface receptors and ion channels in purple, intracellular signaling in blue, and nuclear responses in green. See text for detailed descriptions of pathogenic mechanisms and interactions among the many pathways that span the extracellular, membrane, cytosolic, and nuclear domains. VEGF indicates vascular endothelial growth factor; its receptor is KDR. Intracellular transduction of this pathway is poorly understood. Endothelin is vasoactive and a mitogen, acting through Ca2+ channels and ERK/Jun kinases. TIE is the angiopoietin receptor, a system found to be upregulated in pulmonary vascular disease. Alk1 and BMPR1–2 are receptors of the TGF-ß superfamily, and BMP indicates bone morphogenetic protein. Alk1 mutations cause hereditary hemorrhagic telangiectasia and some cases of PPH. Epidermal growth factor (EGF), tumor necrosis factor (TNF)- , angiotensin II (ANGII), and platelet-derived growth factor (PDGF) are all proliferative stimuli that act through tyrosine kinase receptors and are partially transduced by intracellular oxidant species. In the intracellular domain, SMADs are regulatory proteins that activate nuclear transcription factors and interact with MAP kinases. AML1 is a nuclear transcription factor of potential importance. Elastase, downstream of AML1, has been implicated in vascular disease in experimental animals. Viral proteins are found in vascular lesions in the lungs of patients with PAH, raising the possibility that they participate in its pathogenesis. Reproduced with permission from Newman *et al.*, *Circulation* 2004; 109:2947–2952.

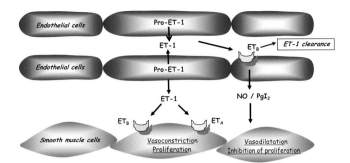

Plate 3 Endothelin 1 pathways in the pulmonary circulation. Pulmonary artery endothelial cells (blue) produce endothelin-1 (ET-1) from its precursor pro-endothelin 1. Released ET-1 binds to endothelin receptors A and/or B on pulmonary artery smooth muscle cells (red) promoting vasoconstriction and smooth muscle cell growth. When interacting with endothelin receptors B on endothelial cells, ET-1 stimulates the generation of local mediators of vascular tone, such as nitric oxide and prostaglansin I2. These factors modulate the effects of ET-1 in the cardiovascular system through their opposing vasorelaxant action. Endothelin B receptors on endothelial cells also contribute to the clearance of circulating ET-1.

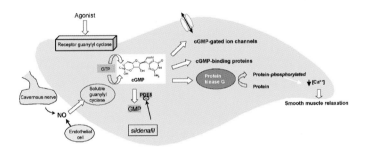

Plate 4 The NO/cGMP signaling pathway, showing stimuli promoting the synthesis of cGMP, downstream intracellular signaling targets modulated by cGMP, and the role of PDEs in cGMP breakdown. This pathway mediates relaxation of vascular smooth muscle and penile erection (upon sexual stimulation) and pulmonary vasodilatation (continuously). Smooth muscle relaxation is in part mediated via protein kinase G (PKG) activation, potassium channel opening and decreases in intracellular calcium levels (Michelakis, 2003). PDE5 is the target for sildenafil, and other PDE5 inhibitors in the treatment of chronic vascular disorders. NO, nitric oxide; PDE, phosphodiesterase; cGMP, cyclic guanosine monophosphate; GMP, guanosine monophosphate; GTP, guanosine triphosphate. Adapted from Ghofrani, Osterloh and Grimminger, 2006.

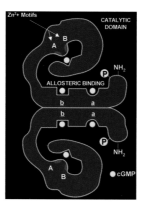

Plate 5 Working model of PDE5. The regulatory domain in the amino-terminal portion contains a phosphorylation site and two allosteric cGMP-binding sites, a and b, that are theorized to be involved in a cGMP negative-feedback loop. The catalytic domain in the carboxyl-terminal portion contains two Zn2+-binding motifs, A and B, and a cGMP-binding substrate site. cGMP, cyclic guanosine monophosphate; PDE5, phosphodiesterase type 5. Reproduced with permission from Corbin and Francis, 1999.

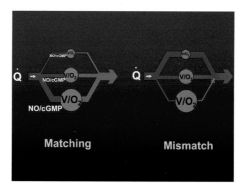

Plate 6 Adaptation of blood flow to ventilation in the pulmonary circulation. Blood flow (Q) in the pulmonary circulation is ideally directed to well-ventilated areas (symbolized by big V (ventilation) and O_2 (oxygenation) in the largest alveolus (light blue circle at bottom of figure)) to ensure optimal gas exchange ('matching'), whereas only a small amount of blood flows through areas of minimal or no ventilation, respectively (midsize and small alveolus, respectively) (left panel). Lung vessel dilatation is mainly regulated by the compartmentalized production of NO and subsequent intracellular cGMP formation, where alveolar distension and oxygenation represent the most potent stimuli for this local NO release. Alternatively, less NO/cGMP is produced in non-ventilated areas of the lung, resulting in hypoxic vasoconstriction (the so called von Euler–Liljestrand mechanism). During application of non-selective vasodilators and/or under disease conditions (e.g. chronic obstructive lung disease or lung fibrosis, or during sepsis and acute respiratory distress syndrome), vasodilatation is induced in poorly- or non-ventilated areas of the lung resulting in venous admixture and worsening of gas-exchange ('mismatch', right panel). Sildenafil appears to preferentially dilate pulmonary vessels in well-ventilated areas of the lung, thereby both reducing overall pulmonary vascular resistance and improving overall oxygenation ('re-matching' drug) (Ghofrani et al., 2002b; Ghofrani et al., 2004c)

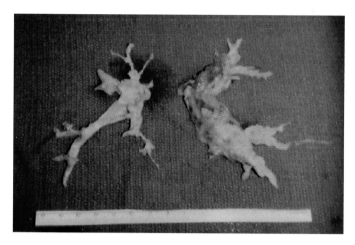

Plate 7 Specimens dissected from right and left pulmonary arteries during pulmonary endarterectomy (PEA) in a patient with CTEPH.

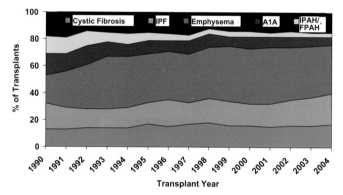

Plate 8 Indications for adult lung transplantation by year. IPF: idiopathic pulmonary fibrosis; A1A: alpha-1 antitrypsin deficiency; IPAH: idiopathic or familial pulmonary arterial hypertension. (Data from ISHLT Registry 2006)

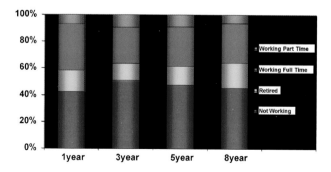

Plate 9 Employment status of surviving adult lung recipients. (Data from ISHLT Registry: April 1994–June 2005.)

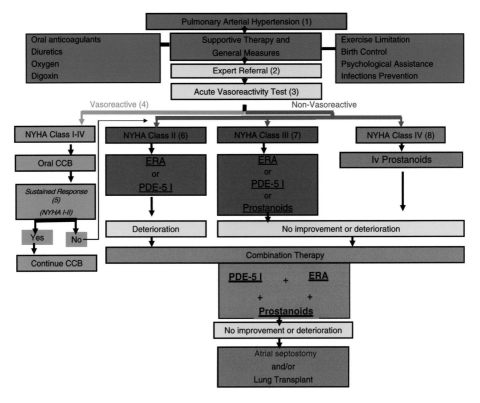

Plate 10 Pulmonary arterial hypertension treatment algorithm.

(1) Different treatments have been evaluated mainly in sporadic idiopathic pulmonary arterial hypertension patients (IPAH), and in PAH associated with scleroderma or to anorexigen use. Extrapolation of these recommendations to the other PAH subgroups should be done with caution.

(2) Owing to the complexity of the acute vasoreactivity tests, and of the treatment options available, it is strongly recommended that consideration be given to referral of patients with PAH to a specialized center.

(3) Acute vasoreactivity test should be performed in all patients with PAH even if the greater incidence of positive response is achieved in patients with IPAH and PAH associated to anorexigen use.

(4) A positive acute response to vasodilators is defined as a fall in mean pulmonary artery pressure of at least 10 mm Hg to less than or equal to 40 mm Hg, with an increase or no change in cardiac output during acute challenge with inhaled NO, IV epoprostenol, or IV adenosine.

(5) Sustained response to calcium channel blockers (CCB) is defined as patients being in NYHA functional class I or II with near-normal hemodynamics after several months of treatment.

(6) In patients in NYHA functional class II, first line therapy may include phosphodiesterase-5 inhibitors or oral endothelin receptor antagonists

(7) In patients in NYHA functional class III, first line therapy may include phosphodiesterase-5 inhibitors, oral endothelin receptor antagonists, chronic IV epoprostenol or prostanoid analogues.

(8) Most experts consider that NYHA functional class IV patients (regardless of response with acute vasore-activity testing) should be treated with IV prostanoids (survival improvement, worldwide experience and rapidity of action).

CCB: calcium channel blockers; ERA: endothelin receptor antagonists; IV: continuous intravenous; PDE5 I: phosphodiesterase-5 inhibitors; BAS: balloon atrial septostomy.

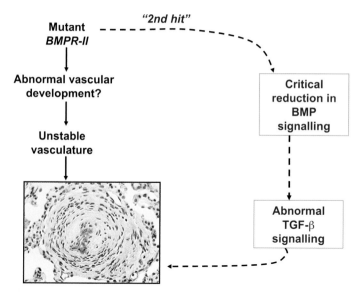

Plate 11 Potential role of BMPR2 mutations in PAH. (Personal communication Nicholas Morrell, MD.)

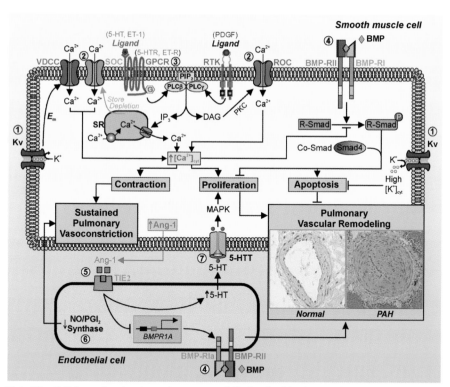

Plate 12 Cellular and molecular pathways potentially involved in the transformation of the normal to the hypertensive pulmonary vessel phenotype. These processes involve both endothelial and smooth muscle cell-dependent pathways, as well as interactions between the two cell types. According to this model, vasoconstriction, proliferation and altered apoptosis are involved, to varying degrees, in the pathologic transformation from normal to disease state

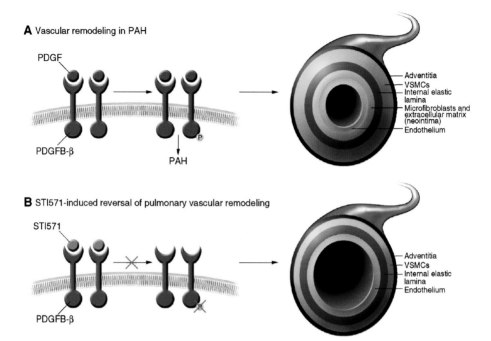

A Vascular remodeling in PAH

PDGF

PDGFB-β

PAH

Adventitia
VSMCs
Internal elastic lamina
Microfibroblasts and extracellular matrix (neointima)
Endothelium

B STI571-induced reversal of pulmonary vascular remodeling

STI571

PDGFB-β

Adventitia
VSMCs
Internal elastic lamina
Endothelium

Plate 13 Schematic representation of pulmonary vascular remodeling in the small pulmonary arteries in PAH. (A) PDGF receptor (PDGFR) expression and phosphorylation (P) in pulmonary arteries are increased in PAH, which activates downstream signaling pathways that promote the abnormal proliferation and migration of vascular smooth muscle cells, as well as the formation of a layer of microfibroblasts and extracellular matrix (termed the neointima) between the internal elastic lamina and the endothelium. These changes underlie the structural and functional abnormalities in the vessel wall that lead to pulmonary vascular disease. (B) Schermuly and coworkers demonstrated that administration of the PDGF receptor antagonist STI571, i.e. imatinib mesylate, induces a reversal of the pulmonary vascular remodeling in two different animal models of pulmonary hypertension. STI571 prevents phosphorylation of the PDGF receptor and consequently suppresses activation of downstream signaling pathways associated with PAH. Reproduced from Barst RJ (2005) PDGF Signaling in pulmonary arterial hypertension. *J Clin Invest* **115**:2691–2694.

retained throughout the 12-month observation period (349 m at the end of the trial; $p = 0.002$).

The PACES-1 trial

The addition of sildenafil to long-term intravenous epoprostenol (EPO) treatment was investigated in the PACES-1 (**P**ulmonary **A**rterial hypertension **C**ombination study of **E**poprostenol and **S**ildenafil) trial (Simonneau *et al.*, 2007). In this 16-week international, double-blind, placebo-controlled, parallel group study, 267 patients with PAH on stable dose EPO were randomized to sildenafil or placebo. Patients randomized to sildenafil received 20 mg orally TID, uptitrated to 40 mg and to 80 mg TID, as tolerated, at four-week intervals. The primary endpoint was change from baseline in exercise capacity measured by the 6MWD. Secondary endpoints included change from baseline in mPAP, time to clinical worsening, and Borg dyspnea score. There was a treatment-adjusted increase of 26.0 m ($p < 0.001$) in 6MWD with subjects in the sildenafil-EPO group. The combination therapy also decreased mPAP to a greater extent than EPO alone (−3.9 mm Hg, $p < 0.0001$). Time to clinical worsening was also longer in patients on combination therapy compared with EPO monotherapy ($p < 0.012$). No patients died when treated with combination therapy compared with seven deaths in the EPO alone group. Thus, sildenafil-EPO combination therapy was more effective than EPO alone in improving exercise capacity, mPAP and time to clinical worsening over 16 weeks.

Combination of phosphodiesterase-5 inhibitors and endothelin receptor antagonists

The first open label study adding sildenafil to the endothelin receptor antagonist bosentan after transient improvement with bosentan demonstrated an increase in exercise capacity with the addition of sildenafil (Hoeper *et al.*, 2004). The 6MWD at baseline was 346 ± 66 m and improved to 403 ± 80 m three months after starting bosentan treatment. However, this effect was not sustained and, after 11 ± 5 months, the walk distance had declined to 277 ± 80 m. At this point, sildenafil was added to bosentan. Three months later, the 6MWD had increased to 392 ± 61 m and the patients remained stable throughout the median follow-up of 9 months (range 6–12 months); increases in maximum oxygen uptake during cardiopulmonary exercise testing were consistent with the improvements observed in 6MWD. The combination of bosentan and sildenafil appeared well tolerated. These preliminary data suggest that combining bosentan and sildenafil may be safe and effective in patients with idiopathic PAH, and support further investigation.

6.8   Potential new indications for phosphodiesterase-5 inhibitors outside pulmonary arterial hypertension

Raynaud's phenomenon and digital ulcers in connective tissue diseases (CTD)

Patients with PAH often complain about intermittent, temperature-dependent peripheral vasospasms resulting in perfusion deficiencies in their fingers and toes, i.e. Raynaud's phenomenon, even in the absence of a defined CTD (Celoria, Friedell and Sommers, 1960; Smith and Kroop, 1957; D'Alonzo *et al.*, 1991). When treated with vasodilators, these symptoms may improve in parallel with, but also independent of, improvements in hemodynamics. Raynaud's phenomenon and digital ulcers are of even higher prevalence and clinically more important in patients with systemic sclerosis, limited sclerosis or systemic lupus erythematosus (SLE) (Kallenberg, 1995). Treatment currently includes calcium channel blockers, infused prostanoids, and alpha-2 blockade (Pope *et al.*, 2000; Belch and Ho, 1996; Boin and Wigley, 2005).

However, the clinical efficacy of these therapies is often modest at best. A growing number of uncontrolled trials suggest efficacy with sildenafil for the treatment of digital ulcerations and Raynaud's phenomenon in patients with scleroderma with or without PH (Kamata *et al.*, 2005; Gore and Silver, 2005; Rosenkranz *et al.*, 2003; Lichtenstein, 2003). In a pilot randomized, controlled trial, Fries and coworkers investigated the effects of sildenafil (50 mg bid) on symptoms and capillary perfusion in patients with Raynaud's phenomenon (Fries *et al.*, 2005); only patients who showed insufficient improvement when previously treated with other vasodilators were studied. In contrast to the effects of placebo, chronic sildenafil treatment for four weeks reduced the frequency and duration of Raynaud attacks and lowered the Raynaud's condition score. Moreover, capillary blood flow velocity increased in all patients, and the capillary flow velocity of all patients more than quadrupled after sildenafil treatment (Fries *et al.*, 2005). Interestingly, while sildenafil had clear effects in the diseased vascular areas, significant reductions in systemic blood pressure were not reported. This is consistent with the notion of selectivity of sildenafil for certain vascular beds (e.g. pulmonary circulation, corpus cavernosum) and indicates that PDE5 may be differentially expressed in the affected vasculature of digital ulcers as opposed to non-affected regions of the systemic circulation (Maurice *et al.*, 2003). Taken together, there is rationale to further evaluate sildenafil as treatment for Raynaud's phenomenon and digital ulcerations.

Pulmonary hypertension associated with ventilatory disorders

When PH is associated with interstitial lung disease, systemic administration of vasodilators increases blood flow to low- or non-ventilated areas of the lung by interfering with the physiological hypoxic vasoconstrictor mechanism. This worsens pre-existent V/Q mismatch and increases shunt flow (Agusti and Rodriguez-Roisin, 1993). The decrease in systemic arterial oxygenation and wasting of the small ventilatory reserve of these patients are important negative consequences of this effect. Oral sildenafil, however, has been shown to cause pulmonary vasodilatation in patients with lung fibrosis and PH, with an overall vasodilatory potency corresponding to that of intravenous prostacyclin. In contrast to an infused prostanoid, selectivity for well-ventilated lung areas was demonstrated with sildenafil, resulting in improvement, rather than deterioration, in gas exchange (Ghofrani *et al.*, 2002b). PH impairs right ventricular performance due to increased right heart afterload. However, it is still unclear to what extent exercise capacity is limited by this mechanism.

In a recent investigation, this issue was addressed under conditions of acute hypoxia at sea level, and with prolonged hypoxia at the altitude of Mount Everest Base Camp (Ghofrani *et al.*, 2004c). These investigations were performed in healthy volunteers to exclude other confounding factors that might have added to the limitation of exercise capacity in patients with chronic hypoxia (e.g. muscle wasting, chronic immobilization, etc.). Both acute and prolonged hypoxia induced significant PH in the study subjects. As expected, exercise capacity was reduced as a consequence of severe hypoxemia and significant PH. Sildenafil reduced PH under resting conditions as well as during exercise. An interesting finding was that the reversal of PH resulted in an immediate improvement in exercise capacity, regardless of improvements in systemic arterial oxygenation. Further studies investigating the effects of acute and chronic sildenafil administration in hypoxic PH confirmed the anti-pulmonary hypertensive potential, and the beneficial effects of sildenafil on exercise performance, under these conditions (Richalet *et al.*, 2005; Hsu *et al.*, 2006). The results of these studies stimulated further investigations addressing the therapeutic potential of sildenafil in patients with chronic hypoxic PH as it occurs in various chronic diseases (e.g. chronic obstructive lung disease (COPD), interstitial lung disease, and obstructive sleep apnea, etc.) (Naeije, 2005; Higenbottam, 2005; Voelkel and Cool, 2003; Barbera, Peinado and Santos, 2003). In fact, there is work that supports the possibility of effective treatment of PH in patients with advanced COPD (Alp *et al.*, 2005). Based on the significant impact of COPD on public health, further studies in this field are warranted.

Sildenafil in heart failure

Chronic heart load leads to ventricular hypertrophy as an initial process of adaptation and may ultimately result in ventricular dilatation and failure if not treated (Jessup and Brozena, 1995). Although cardiac hypertrophy applies to disorders that lead to both left ventricular and to right ventricular loading, there are important differences with respect to the reversibility of muscular hypertrophy of the two ventricles. While the right ventricle – even at advanced stages of dilatation and decompensation – can virtually normalize structure and function once the load is reduced effectively, left ventricular hypertrophy is only partly reversible once a certain degree of hypertrophy has been exceeded (Anversa *et al.*, 1995; Anversa *et al.*, 1992). In chronic PH, right ventricular dysfunction is the most common cause of death; however, effective reduction of PVR, e.g. after lung transplantation, can reverse right ventricular hypertrophy in addition to PAP and PVR (Kasimir *et al.*, 2004). Wilkins and coworkers suggest that treatment of PAH with sildenafil not only improves functional capacity, but also reduces right ventricular mass in these patients, as assessed by magnetic resonance imaging (Wilkins *et al.*, 2005). To date, reduction of right ventricular hypertrophy in patients with chronic PH has been attributed to treatment-related reductions in right ventricular load (Kentera and Susic, 1980; Rich and Brundage, 1987; Pelouch *et al.*, 1997; O'Blenes *et al.*, 2001). However, the observations of Wilkins and others raise the possibility of a direct anti-hypertrophic effect of sildenafil on cardiomyocytes (Takimoto *et al.*, 2005). In another study, Takimoto and others reported that sildenafil reduced ventricular hypertrophy and improved myocardial function in a mouse model of chronic left ventricular pressure load (induced by transaortic constriction) in a protein kinase G-1-dependent manner (Takimoto *et al.*, 2005). In addition, cGMP levels were shown to inversely correlate with the cardiac hypertrophy in an isoproterenol-induced cardiac hypertrophy model in rats (Hassan and Ketat, 2005).

However, the potential benefit of sildenafil in chronic heart failure may result from a variety of actions in addition to its effect on ventricular hypertrophy. Multiple investigations have indicated that sildenafil should be cautiously administered only to selected patients with left heart failure (Katz *et al.*, 2005; Lepore *et al.*, 2005; Hirata *et al.*, 2005; Freitas *et al.*, 2006; Fisher *et al.*, 2005; Webster *et al.*, 2004; Alaeddini *et al.*, 2004; Guazzi *et al.*, 2004; Mickley and Poulsen, 2004; Mikhail, 2004). Endothelial function (the ability of arterioles to increase regional blood flow in response to appropriate stimuli such as ischemia) is limited in chronic congestive heart failure, and in an elegant study, Katz and coworkers showed that sildenafil could improve endothelial function in such patients (Katz *et al.*, 2005). Further studies investigating the long-term effects of PDE5 inhibitors in patients with these diseases appear warranted. In addition, by virtue of its effects on vasodilatation, arterial stiffness and wave reflection, sildenafil may reduce aortic pressure and augmentation index, and thus could have a role in systemic hypertension (Mahmud, Hennessy and Feely, 2001).

6.9 Conclusions

PDE5 inhibitors, e.g. sildenafil, were initially developed for the treatment of systemic hypertension and angina. However, sildenafil subsequently evolved into a novel treatment for erectile dysfunction. Sildenafil was then further developed as an oral treatment for PAH, and also appears effective in treating Raynaud's phenomenon associated with systemic sclerosis and digital ulceration. The PDE5 inhibitor tadalafil is also being developed as an oral treatment for PAH. In later investigative studies, PDE5 inhibitors also appear to have promise in the treatment of respiratory disorders with ventilation/perfusion mismatch, congestive cardiac failure, systemic hypertension and even stroke. Although these findings might appear quite disparate and unrelated, in fact all of the above disorders are characterized by regional deficiencies in blood supply. The successful application of PDE5 inhibitors (as opposed to non-selective vasodilators) to treat these conditions can be understood in terms of the ability of these drugs to reverse endothelial dysfunction, and to selectively improve regional blood flow in areas of greatest need. Many patients with erectile dysfunction or PAH are now benefiting from the advances in our understanding of vascular biology and pathophysiology, and the advent of selective inhibitors of PDE5. In addition, sildenafil and other PDE5 inhibitors may have increased efficacy when used in combination with other disease-specific targeted PAH drugs, e.g. endothelin receptor antagonists and/or prostanoids. It is hoped that the clinical potential of these mechanisms to treat other serious medical conditions such as those described above will soon be realized, so that more patients may benefit from these breakthroughs in science, technology and medicine.

References

Abrams, D., Schulze-Neick, I. and Magee, A.G. (2000) Sildenafil as a selective pulmonary vasodilator in childhood primary pulmonary hypertension. *Heart* **84**, E4.

Agusti, A.G. and Rodriguez-Roisin, R. (1993) Effect of pulmonary hypertension on gas exchange. *Eur. Respir. J.* **6**, 1371–1377.

Ahn, H.S. *et al.* (1991) Ca/CaM-stimulated and cGMP-specific phosphodiesterases in vascular and non-vascular tissues. *Adv. Exp. Med. Biol.* **308**, 191–197.

Alaeddini, J. *et al.* (2004) Efficacy and safety of sildenafil in the evaluation of pulmonary hypertension in severe heart failure. *Am. J. Cardiol.* **94**, 1475–1477.

Alp, S., Skrygan, M., Schmidt, W.E. and Bastian, A. (2005) Sildenafil improves hemodynamic parameters in COPD-an investigation of six patients. *Pulm. Pharmacol. Ther.* **19**, 386–390.

Anversa, P., Capasso, J.M., Olivetti, G. and Sonnenblick, E.H. (1992) Cellular basis of ventricular remodeling in hypertensive cardiomyopathy. *Am. J. Hypertens.* **5**, 758–770.

Anversa, P. *et al.* (1995) Ischemic cardiomyopathy: myocyte cell loss, myocyte cellular hypertrophy and myocyte cellular hyperplasia. *Ann. N.Y. Acad. Sci.* **752**, 47–64.

Arruda-Olson, A.M. *et al.* (2002) Cardiovascular effects of sildenafil during exercise in men with known or probable coronary artery disease: a randomized crossover trial. *JAMA* **287**, 719–725.

Atz, A.M. and Wessel, D.L. (1999) Sildenafil ameliorates effects of inhaled nitric oxide withdrawal. *Anesthesiology* **91**, 307–310.

Barbera, J.A., Peinado, V.I. and Santos, S. (2003) Pulmonary hypertension in chronic obstructive pulmonary disease. *Eur. Respir. J.* **21**, 892–905.

Beavo, J.A. (1995) Cyclic nucleotide phosphodiesterases: functional implications of multiple isoforms. *Physiol. Rev.* **75**, 725–748.

Belch, J.J. and Ho, M. (1996) Pharmacotherapy of Raynaud's phenomenon. *Drugs* **52**, 682–695.

Bloch, W. *et al.* (1998) Evidence for the involvement of endothelial nitric oxide synthase from smooth muscle cells in the erectile function of the human corpus cavernosum. *Urol. Res.* **26**, 129–135.

Bocchi, E.A. *et al.*(2002) Sildenafil effects on exercise, neurohormonal activation and erectile dysfunction in congestive heart failure: a double-blind, placebo-controlled, randomized study followed by a prospective treatment for erectile dysfunction. *Circulation* **106**, 1097–1103.

Bohle, R.M. *et al.* (2000) Cell type-specific mRNA quantitation in non-neoplastic tissues after laser-assisted cell picking. *Pathobiology* **68**, 191–195.

Boin, F. and Wigley, F.M. (2005) Understanding, assessing and treating Raynaud's phenomenon. *Curr. Opin. Rheumatol.* **17**, 752–760.

Boshier, A., Wilton, L.V. and Shakir, S.A. (2004) Evaluation of the safety of sildenafil for male erectile dysfunction: experience gained in general practice use in England in 1999. *BJU. Int.* **93**, 796–801.

Braner, D.A., Fineman, J.R., Chang, R. and Soifer, S.J. (1993) M&B 22948, a cGMP phosphodiesterase inhibitor, is a pulmonary vasodilator in lambs. *Am. J. Physiol.* **264**, H252-H258.

Carlsen, J., Kjeldsen, K. and Gerstoft, J. (2002) Sildenafil as a successful treatment of otherwise fatal HIV-related pulmonary hypertension. *AIDS* **16**, 1568–1569.

Celoria, G.C., Friedell, G.H. and Sommers, S.C. (1960) Raynaud's disease and primary pulmonary hypertension. *Circulation* **22**, 1055–1059.

Cohen, A.H. *et al.* (1996) Inhibition of cyclic 3'-5'-guanosine monophosphate-specific phosphodiesterase selectively vasodilates the pulmonary circulation in chronically hypoxic rats. *J. Clin. Invest.* **97**, 172–179.

Corbin, J.D. and Francis, S.H. (1999) Cyclic GMP phosphodiesterase-5: target of sildenafil. *J. Biol. Chem.* **274**, 13729–13732.

Corbin, J.D. and Francis, S.H. (2002) Pharmacology of phosphodiesterase-5 inhibitors. *Int. J. Clin. Pract.* **56**, 453–459.

Corbin, J.D., Beasley, A., Blount, M.A. and Francis, S.H. (2005) High lung PDE5: A strong basis for treating pulmonary hypertension with PDE5 inhibitors. *Biochem. Biophys. Res. Commun.* **334**, 930–938.

Cunningham, A.V. and Smith, K.H. (2001) Anterior ischemic optic neuropathy associated with viagra. *J. Neuroophthalmol.* **21**, 22–25.

D'Alonzo, G.E. *et al.* (1991) Survival in patients with primary pulmonary hypertension. Results from a national prospective registry. *Ann. Intern. Med.* **115**, 343–349.

DeBusk, R.F. *et al.* (2004) Efficacy and safety of sildenafil citrate in men with erectile dysfunction and stable coronary artery disease. *Am. J. Cardiol.* **93**, 147–153.

Desouza, C. *et al.* (2002) Acute and prolonged effects of sildenafil on brachial artery flow-mediated dilatation in type 2 diabetes. *Diabetes Care* **25**, 1336–1339.

Dousa, T.P. (1999) Cyclic-3',5'-nucleotide phosphodiesterase isozymes in cell biology and pathophysiology of the kidney. *Kidney Int.* **55**, 29–62.

Egan, R. and Pomeranz, H. (2000) Sildenafil (Viagra) associated anterior ischemic optic neuropathy. *Arch. Ophthalmol.* **118**, 291–292.

Fawcett, L. *et al.* (2000) Molecular cloning and characterization of a distinct human phosphodiesterase gene family: PDE11A. *Proc. Natl. Acad. Sci. USA* **97**, 3702–3707.

Fink, T.L. *et al.* (1999) Expression of an active, monomeric catalytic domain of the cGMP-binding cGMP-specific phosphodiesterase (PDE5). *J. Biol. Chem.* **274**, 34613–34620.

Fisher, P.W. *et al.* (2005) Phosphodiesterase-5 inhibition with sildenafil attenuates cardiomyocyte apoptosis and left ventricular dysfunction in a chronic model of doxorubicin cardiotoxicity. *Circulation* **111**, 1601–1610.

Fox, K.M. *et al.* (2003) Sildenafil citrate does not reduce exercise tolerance in men with erectile dysfunction and chronic stable angina. *Eur. Heart J.* **24**, 2206–2212.

Francis, S.H., Turko, I.V. and Corbin, J.D. (2001) Cyclic nucleotide phosphodiesterases: relating structure and function. *Prog. Nucleic Acid Res. Mol. Biol.* **65**, 1–52.

Francis, S.H. *et al.* (1998) Ligand-induced conformational changes in cyclic nucleotide phosphodiesterases and cyclic nucleotide-dependent protein kinases. *Methods* **14**, 81–92.

Fraunfelder, F.W., Pomeranz, H.D. and Egan, R.A. (2006) Nonarteritic anterior ischemic optic neuropathy and sildenafil. *Arch. Ophthalmol.* **124**, 733–734.

Freitas, D. *et al.* (2006) Sildenafil improves quality of life in men with heart failure and erectile dysfunction. *Int. J. Impot. Res.* **18**, 210–212.

Fries, R., Shariat, K., von Wilmowsky, H. and Bohm, M. (2005) Sildenafil in the treatment of Raynaud's phenomenon resistant to vasodilatory therapy. *Circulation* **112**, 2980–2985.

Galie, N. *et al.* (2005) Sildenafil citrate therapy for pulmonary arterial hypertension. *N. Engl. J. Med.* **353**, 2148–2157.

Gbekor, E. *et al.* (2002) Phosphodiesterase 5 inhibitor profiles against all human phosphodiesterase families: Implications for use as pharmacological tools. *J. Urol.* **167**, 246.

German, Z. *et al.* (2000) Molecular basis of cell-specific endothelial nitric-oxide synthase expression in airway epithelium. *J. Biol. Chem.* **275**, 8183–8189.

Ghofrani, H.A., Osterloh, I.H. and Grimminger, F. (2006) Sildenafil: from angina to erectile dysfunction to pulmonary hypertension and beyond. *Nat. Rev. Drug Disc.* **5**, 689–702.

Ghofrani, H.A. *et al.* (2002a) Combination therapy with oral sildenafil and inhaled iloprost for severe pulmonary hypertension. *Ann. Intern. Med.* **136**, 515–522.

Ghofrani, H.A. *et al.* (2002b) Sildenafil for treatment of lung fibrosis and pulmonary hypertension: a randomised controlled trial. *Lancet* **360**, 895–900.

Ghofrani, H.A. *et al.* (2003a) Sildenafil for long-term treatment of nonoperable chronic thromboembolic pulmonary hypertension. *Am. J. Respir. Crit. Care Med.* **167**, 1139–1141.

Ghofrani, H.A. *et al.* (2003b) Oral sildenafil as long-term adjunct therapy to inhaled iloprost in severe pulmonary arterial hypertension. *J. Am. Coll. Cardiol.* **42**, 158–164.

Ghofrani, H.A. *et al.* (2004a) Nitric oxide pathway and phosphodiesterase inhibitors in pulmonary arterial hypertension. *J. Am. Coll. Cardiol.* **43**, 68S-72S.

Ghofrani, H.A. *et al.* (2004b) Differences in hemodynamic and oxygenation responses to three different phosphodiesterase-5 inhibitors in patients with pulmonary arterial hypertension: a randomized prospective study. *J. Am. Coll. Cardiol.* **44**, 1488–1496.

Ghofrani, H.A. *et al.* (2004c) Sildenafil increased exercise capacity during hypoxia at low altitudes and at Mount Everest base camp: a randomized, double-blind, placebo-controlled crossover trial. *Ann. Intern. Med.* **141**, 169–177.

Giordano, D *et al.* (2001) Expression of cGMP-binding cGMP-specific phosphodiesterase (PDE5) in mouse tissues and cell lines using an antibody against the enzyme amino-terminal domain. *Biochim. Biophys. Acta* **1539**, 16–27.

Glavas, N.A. *et al.* (2001) T cell activation up-regulates cyclic nucleotide phosphodiesterases 8A1 and 7A3. *Proc. Natl. Acad. Sci. USA* **98**, 6319–6324.

Gopal, V.K., Francis, S.H. and Corbin, J.D. (2001) Allosteric sites of phosphodiesterase-5 (PDE5). A potential role in negative feedback regulation of cGMP signaling in corpus cavernosum. *Eur. J. Biochem.* **268**, 3304–3312.

Gore, J. and Silver, R. (2005) Oral sildenafil for the treatment of Raynaud's phenomenon and digital ulcers secondary to systemic sclerosis. *Ann. Rheum. Dis.* **64**, 1387.

Gorkin, L., Hvidsten, K., Sobel, R.E. and Siegel, R. (2006) Sildenafil citrate use and the incidence of nonarteritic anterior ischemic optic neuropathy. *Int. J. Clin. Pract.* **60**, 500–503.

Grimminger, F. *et al.* (1995) Nitric oxide generation and hypoxic vasoconstriction in buffer-perfused rabbit lungs. *J. Appl. Physiol.* **78**, 1509–1515.

Guazzi, M. *et al.* (2004) The effects of phosphodiesterase-5 inhibition with sildenafil on pulmonary hemodynamics and diffusion capacity, exercise ventilatory efficiency and oxygen uptake kinetics in chronic heart failure. *J. Am. Coll. Cardiol.* **44**, 2339–2348.

Halcox, J.P. *et al.*(2002) The effect of sildenafil on human vascular function, platelet activation and myocardial ischemia. *J. Am. Coll. Cardiol.* **40**, 1232–1240.

Hanson, K.A. *et al.* (1998) Chronic pulmonary hypertension increases fetal lung cGMP phosphodiesterase activity. *Am. J. Physiol.* **275**, L931-L941.

Hassan, M.A. and Ketat, A.F. (2005) Sildenafil citrate increases myocardial cGMP content in rat heart, decreases its hypertrophic response to isoproterenol and decreases myocardial leak of creatine kinase and troponin T. *BMC. Pharmacol.* **5**, 10.

Hattenhauer, M.G. *et al.* (1997) Incidence of nonarteritic anterior ischemic optic neuropathy. *Am. J. Ophthalmol.* **123**, 103–107.

Hayashi, M. *et al.* (1998) Molecular cloning and characterization of human PDE8B, a novel thyroid-specific isozyme of 3',5'-cyclic nucleotide phosphodiesterase. *Biochem. Biophys. Res. Commun.* **250**, 751–756.

Haynes, J., Jr., Kithas, P.A., Taylor, A.E. and Strada, S.J. (1991) Selective inhibition of cGMP-inhibitable cAMP phosphodiesterase decreases pulmonary vasoreactivity. *Am. J. Physiol.* **261**, H487-H492.

Herrmann, H.C., Chang, G., Klugherz, B.D. and Mahoney, P.D. (2000) Hemodynamic effects of sildenafil in men with severe coronary artery disease. *N. Engl. J. Med.* **342**, 1622–1626.

Higenbottam, T. (2005) Pulmonary hypertension and chronic obstructive pulmonary disease: a case for treatment. *Proc. Am. Thorac. Soc.* **2**, 12–19.

Hirata, K., Adji, A., Vlachopoulos, C. and O'Rourke, M.F. (2005) Effect of Sildenafil on Cardiac Performance in Patients With Heart Failure. *Am. J. Cardiol.* **96**, 1436–1440.

Hoeper, M.M. *et al.* (2004) Combination therapy with bosentan and sildenafil in idiopathic pulmonary arterial hypertension. *Eur. Respir. J.* **24**, 1007–1010.

Hsu, A.R. *et al.* (2006) Sildenafil improves cardiac output and exercise performance during acute hypoxia, but not normoxia. *J. Appl. Physiol.* **100**, 2031–2040.

Huai, Q. *et al.* (2004) Crystal structures of phosphodiesterases 4 and 5 in complex with inhibitor 3-isobutyl-1-methylxanthine suggest a conformation determinant of inhibitor selectivity. *J. Biol. Chem.* **279**, 13095–13101.

Ichinose, F., Adrie, C., Hurford, W.E. and Zapol, W.M. (1995) Prolonged pulmonary vasodilator action of inhaled nitric oxide by Zaprinast in awake lambs. *J. Appl. Physiol* **78**, 1288–1295.

Ichinose, F. *et al.* (1998) Selective pulmonary vasodilation induced by aerosolized zaprinast. *Anesthesiology* **88**, 410–416.

Ide, H. *et al.* (1999) Regulation of pulmonary circulation by alveolar oxygen tension via airway nitric oxide. *J. Appl. Physiol* **87**, 1629–1636.

Itoh, T. *et al.* (2004) A combination of oral sildenafil and beraprost ameliorates pulmonary hypertension in rats. *Am. J. Respir. Crit. Care Med.* **169**, 34–38.

Jessup, M. and Brozena, S. (1995) Heart failure. *N. Engl. J. Med.* **348**, 2007–2018.

Johnson, L.N. and Arnold, A.C. (1994) Incidence of nonarteritic and arteritic anterior ischemic optic neuropathy. Population-based study in the state of Missouri and Los Angeles County, California. *J. Neuroophthalmol.* **14**, 38–44.

Kallenberg, C.G. (1995) Overlapping syndromes, undifferentiated connective tissue disease and other fibrosing conditions. *Curr. Opin. Rheumatol.* **7**, 568–573.

Kamata, Y., Kamimura, T., Iwamoto, M. and Minota, S. (2005) Comparable effects of sildenafil citrate and alprostadil on severe Raynaud's phenomenon in a patient with systemic sclerosis. *Clin. Exp. Dermatol.* **30**, 451.

Kasimir, M.T. *et al.* (2004) Reverse cardiac remodelling in patients with primary pulmonary hypertension after isolated lung transplantation. *Eur. J. Cardiothorac. Surg.* **26**, 776–781.

Katz, S.D. *et al.*(2000) Acute type 5 phosphodiesterase inhibition with sildenafil enhances flow-mediated vasodilation in patients with chronic heart failure. *J. Am. Coll. Cardiol.* **36**, 845–851.

Katz, S.D. *et al.* (2005) Efficacy and safety of sildenafil citrate in men with erectile dysfunction and chronic heart failure. *Am. J. Cardiol.* **95**, 36–42.

Kentera, D. and Susic, D. (1980) Dynamics of regression of right ventricular hypertrophy in rats with hypoxic pulmonary hypertension. *Respiration* **39**, 272–275.

Kothari, S.S. and Duggal, B. (2002) Chronic oral sildenafil therapy in severe pulmonary artery hypertension. *Indian Heart J.* **54**, 404–409.

Lepore, J.J. *et al.* (2005) Hemodynamic effects of sildenafil in patients with congestive heart failure and pulmonary hypertension: combined administration with inhaled nitric oxide. *Chest* **127**, 1647–1653.

Lichtenstein, J.R. (2003) Use of sildenafil citrate in Raynaud's phenomenon: comment on the article by Thompson et al. *Arthritis Rheum.* **48**, 282–283.

Lucas, K.A. *et al.* (2000) Guanylyl cyclases and signaling by cyclic GMP. *Pharmacol. Rev.* **52**, 375–414.

Mahmud, A., Hennessy, M. and Feely, J. (2001) Effect of sildenafil on blood pressure and arterial wave reflection in treated hypertensive men. *J. Hum. Hypertens.* **15**, 707–713.

Maurice, D.H. *et al.* (2003) Cyclic nucleotide phosphodiesterase activity, expression and targeting in cells of the cardiovascular system. *Mol. Pharmacol.* **64**, 533–546.

Michelakis, E.D. (2003) The role of the NO axis and its therapeutic implications in pulmonary arterial hypertension. *Heart Fail. Rev.* **8**, 5–21.

Michelakis, E.D. *et al.* (2003) Long-term treatment with oral sildenafil is safe and improves functional capacity and hemodynamics in patients with pulmonary arterial hypertension. *Circulation* **108**, 2066–2069.

Mickley, H. and Poulsen, T.S. (2004) Use of sildenafil is safe in men with congestive heart failure. *Arch. Intern. Med.* **164**, 2068.

Mikhail, N. (2004) Efficacy and safety of sildenafil in patients with congestive heart failure. *Arch. Intern. Med.* **164**, 2067–2068.

Moncada, S., Palmer, R.M. and Higgs, E.A. (1991) Nitric oxide: physiology, pathophysiology and pharmacology. *Pharmacol. Rev.* **43**, 109–142.

Moncada, I. *et al.* (2004) Efficacy of sildenafil citrate at 12 hours after dosing: re-exploring the therapeutic window. *Eur. Urol.* **46**, 357–360.

Mullershausen, F. *et al.* (2003) Direct activation of PDE5 by cGMP: long-term effects within NO/cGMP signaling. *J. Cell Biol.* **160**, 719–727.

Naeije, R. (2005) Pulmonary hypertension and right heart failure in chronic obstructive pulmonary disease. *Proc. Am. Thorac. Soc.* **2**, 20–22.

Nagamine, J., Hill, L.L. and Pearl, R.G. (2000) Combined therapy with zaprinast and inhaled nitric oxide abolishes hypoxic pulmonary hypertension. *Crit. Care Med.* **28**, 2420–2424.

Nangle, M.R., Cotter, M.A. and Cameron, N.E. (2003) An in vitro study of corpus cavernosum and aorta from mice lacking the inducible nitric oxide synthase gene. *Nitric Oxide* **9**, 194–200.

O'Blenes, S.B. *et al.* (2001) Hemodynamic unloading leads to regression of pulmonary vascular disease in rats. *J. Thorac. Cardiovasc. Surg.* **121**, 279–289.

Ockaili, R., Salloum, F., Hawkins, J. and Kukreja, R.C. (2002) Sildenafil (Viagra) induces powerful cardioprotective effect via opening of mitochondrial K(ATP) channels in rabbits. *Am. J.
Physiol. Heart Circ. Physiol* **283**, H1263-H1269.

Oliver, J. and Webb, D.J. (2002) Sildenafil for "blue babies". Such unlicensed drug use might be
justified as last resort. *Brit. Med. J.* **325**, 1174.

Parker, J.D. and Parker, J.O. (1998) Nitrate therapy for stable angina pectoris. *N. Engl. J. Med.* **338**,
520–531.

Patole, S. and Travadi, J. (2002) Sildenafil for "blue babies". Ethics, conscience and science have
to be balanced against limited resources. *Brit. Med. J.* **325**, 1174.

Pelouch, V. *et al.* (1997) Regression of chronic hypoxia-induced pulmonary hypertension, right ventricular hypertrophy and fibrosis: effect of enalapril. *Cardiovasc. Drugs Ther.* **11**, 177–185.

Pfeifer, A. *et al.* (1999) Structure and function of cGMP-dependent protein kinases. *Rev. Physiol.
Biochem. Pharmacol.* **135**, 105–149.

Pomeranz, H.D. and Bhavsar, A.R. (2005) Nonarteritic ischemic optic neuropathy developing soon
after use of sildenafil (viagra): a report of seven new cases. *J. Neuroophthalmol.* **25**, 9–13.

Pomeranz, H.D., Smith, K.H., Hart, W.M., Jr. and Egan, R.A. (2002) Sildenafil-associated nonarteritic anterior ischemic optic neuropathy. *Ophthalmology* **109**, 584–587.

Pope, J. *et al.* (2000) Iloprost and cisaprost for Raynaud's phenomenon in progressive systemic
sclerosis. *Cochrane. Database. Syst. Rev.*CD000953.

Prasad, S., Wilkinson, J. and Gatzoulis, M.A. (2000) Sildenafil in primary pulmonary hypertension.
N. Engl. J. Med. **343**, 1342.

Pyne, N.J. and Furman, B.L. (2003) Cyclic nucleotide phosphodiesterases in pancreatic islets.
Diabetologia **46**, 1179–1189.

Reichenberger, F. *et al.* (2007) Long-term treatment with sildenafil in chronic thromboembolic pulmonary hypertension. *Eur. Respir. J.* **30**, 922–927.

Rich, S. and Brundage, B.H. (1987) High-dose calcium channel-blocking therapy for primary pulmonary hypertension: evidence for long-term reduction in pulmonary arterial pressure and
regression of right ventricular hypertrophy. *Circulation* **76**, 135–141.

Richalet, J.P. *et al.* (2005) Sildenafil inhibits altitude-induced hypoxemia and pulmonary hypertension. *Am. J. Respir. Crit. Care Med.* **171**, 275–281.

Rosenkranz, S. *et al.* (2003) Sildenafil improved pulmonary hypertension and peripheral blood flow
in a patient with scleroderma-associated lung fibrosis and the raynaud phenomenon. *Ann. Intern.
Med.* **139**, 871–873.

Rossaint, R. *et al.* (1993) Inhaled nitric oxide for the adult respiratory distress syndrome. *N. Engl.
J. Med.* **328**, 399–405.

Sanchez, L.S. *et al.* (1998) Cyclic-GMP-binding, cyclic-GMP-specific phosphodiesterase (PDE5)
gene expression is regulated during rat pulmonary development. *Pediatr. Res.* **43**, 163–168.

Sastry, B.K., Narasimhan, C., Reddy, N.K. and Raju, B.S. (2004) Clinical efficacy of sildenafil in
primary pulmonary hypertension: a randomized, placebo-controlled, double-blind, crossover
study. *J. Am. Coll. Cardiol.* **43**, 1149–1153.

Sastry, B.K. *et al.* (2002) A study of clinical efficacy of sildenafil in patients with primary pulmonary hypertension. *Indian Heart J.* **54**, 410–414.

Schermuly, R.T. *et al.* (2004) Chronic sildenafil treatment inhibits monocrotaline-induced pulmonary hypertension in rats. *Am. J. Respir. Crit. Care Med.* **169**, 39–45.

Schulz, R. *et al.* (2000) Decreased plasma levels of nitric oxide derivatives in obstructive sleep
apnoea: response to CPAP therapy. *Thorax* **55**, 1046–1051.

Schumacher, Y.O., Zdebik, A., Huonker, M. and Kreisel, W. (2001) Sildenafil in HIV-related pulmonary hypertension. *AIDS* **15**, 1747–1748.

Sebkhi, A. *et al.* (2003) Phosphodiesterase type 5 as a target for the treatment of hypoxia-induced pulmonary hypertension. *Circulation* **107**, 3230–3235.

Simonneau, G. *et al.* (2008) Safety and Efficacy of Sildenafil-Epoprostenol Combination Therapy in Patients with Pulmonary Arterial Hypertension (PAH). *Annals of Internal Medicine* 2008 (in press).

Sitbon, O. *et al.* (1998) Inhaled nitric oxide as a screening agent for safely identifying responders to oral calcium-channel blockers in primary pulmonary hypertension [see comments]. *Eur. Respir. J.* **12**, 265–270.

Smith, W.M. and Kroop, I.G. (1957) Raynaud's disease in primary pulmonary hypertension. *J. Am. Med. Assoc.* **165**, 1245–1248.

Soderling, S.H., Bayuga, S.J. and Beavo, J.A. (1998) Cloning and characterization of a cAMP-specific cyclic nucleotide phosphodiesterase. *Proc. Natl. Acad. Sci. USA* **95**, 8991–8996.

Spriestersbach, R. *et al.* (1995) On-line measurement of nitric oxide generation in buffer-perfused rabbit lungs. *J. Appl. Physiol.* **78**, 1502–1508.

Takimoto, E. *et al.* (2005) Chronic inhibition of cyclic GMP phosphodiesterase 5A prevents and reverses cardiac hypertrophy. *Nat. Med.* **11**, 214–222.

Thusu, K.G., Morin, F.C., III, Russell, J.A. and Steinhorn, R.H. (1995) The cGMP phosphodiesterase inhibitor zaprinast enhances the effect of nitric oxide. *Am. J. Respir. Crit. Care Med.* **152**, 1605–1610.

Voelkel, N.F. and Cool, C.D. (2003) Pulmonary vascular involvement in chronic obstructive pulmonary disease. *Eur. Respir. J. Suppl* **46**, 28s-32s.

Webster, L.J., Michelakis, E.D., Davis, T. and Archer, S.L. (2004) Use of sildenafil for safe improvement of erectile function and quality of life in men with New York Heart Association classes II and III congestive heart failure: a prospective, placebo-controlled, double-blind crossover trial. *Arch. Intern. Med.* **164**, 514–520.

Weissmann, N. *et al.* (2000) Nitric oxide (NO)-dependent but not NO-independent guanylate cyclase activation attenuates hypoxic vasoconstriction in rabbit lungs. *Am. J. Respir. Cell Mol. Biol.* **23**, 222–227.

Wharton, J. *et al.* (2005) Antiproliferative effects of phosphodiesterase type 5 inhibition in human pulmonary artery cells. *Am. J. Respir. Crit. Care Med.* **172**, 105–113.

Wilkens, H. *et al.* (2001) Effect of inhaled iloprost plus oral sildenafil in patients with primary pulmonary hypertension. *Circulation* **104**, 1218–1222.

Wilkins, M.R. *et al.* (2005) Sildenafil versus Endothelin Receptor Antagonist for Pulmonary Hypertension (SERAPH) Study. *Am. J. Respir. Crit. Care Med.* **171**, 1292–1297.

Wysowski, D.K., Farinas, E. and Swartz, L. (2002) Comparison of reported and expected deaths in sildenafil (Viagra) users. *Am. J. Cardiol.* **89**, 1331–1334.

Yang, Q. *et al.* (1994) A novel cyclic GMP stimulated phosphodiesterase from rat brain. *Biochem. Biophys. Res. Commun.* **205**, 1850–1858.

Zhang, R. *et al.*(2002) Sildenafil (Viagra) induces neurogenesis and promotes functional recovery after stroke in rats. *Stroke* **33**, 2675–2680.

Zhao, L. *et al.* (2001) Sildenafil inhibits hypoxia-induced pulmonary hypertension. *Circulation* **104**, 424–428.

Zhao, L. *et al.* (2003) M.R. Beneficial effects of phosphodiesterase 5 inhibition in pulmonary hypertension are influenced by natriuretic Peptide activity. *Circulation* **107**, 234–237.

Ziegler, J.W. *et al.* (1998) Effects of dipyridamole and inhaled nitric oxide in pediatric patients with pulmonary hypertension. *Am. J. Respir. Crit Care Med.* **158**, 1388–1395.

7 Combination therapy for pulmonary arterial hypertension

Anne Keogh[1] and Marius Hoeper[2]

[1]*University of NSW, Randwick, Australia*
[2]*Department of Respiratory Medicine and Critical Care Medicine,*
Hannover Medical School, Hannover, Germany

7.1 Background

Why do pulmonary arterial hypertension patients need combination
therapy? – rationale

Many patients, but not all, respond symptomatically to monotherapy with oral, inhaled, subcutaneous (SC) or intravenous (IV) therapies. A minority of patients may even achieve normal or near-normal hemodynamics, symptoms and functional class on monotherapy. A substantial subgroup, however, do not and in those patients combination treatment may be beneficial. In addition, the initial response to monotherapy is not always sustained. It is speculated that combination therapy may be more efficacious than monotherapy (Benza *et al.*, 2007).

In systemic hypertension, left ventricular failure and other comparable conditions, combined use of agents targeting multiple pathways has proven more efficacious than monotherapy thereby serving as a conceptual model for the treatment of PAH. Although survival in PAH has improved with current treatment modalities, it is still far from ideal.

Pulmonary Arterial Hypertension, Edited by Robyn J. Barst
© 2008 John Wiley & Sons, Ltd

Synthesis statement

Concomitant combination therapy has not been adequately studied. The single small trial of epoprostenol initiation with add on bosentan 48 hours later showed only trends without significant benefits.

In contrast, sequential add on therapy has achieved successful endpoints for a wide range of combinations, e.g. bosentan add iloprost, epoprostenol add sildenafil, bosentan add sildenafil, beraprost or iloprost add bosentan, treprostinil add bosentan, and iloprost add sildenafil.

Efficacy limitations on monotherapy

Monotherapy with either oral, inhaled and intravenous agents has in general terms, improved 12–18-week endpoints modestly: 6-minute walk distance (6MWD) increases by 30–50 m above baseline, 20% to 40% of patients improve by 1 to 2 functional classes and clinical worsening (death, transplantation, atrial septostomy or addition of intravenous agents) is reduced. In terms of hemodynamics, mean pulmonary artery pressure (mPAP) is reduced by between 2% and 6%, cardiac output increased by 20–30%, and pulmonary vascular resistance reduced by approximately 20%.

Maintenance monotherapy

The success of maintenance with monotherapy varies with agent and the treatment group. The percentage of patients stable and remaining on bosentan monotherapy is 85% at one year (McLaughlin *et al.*, 2003) and 57% at three years (Provencher *et al.*, 2005), for sildenafil monotherapy 85% at 12 months (Galie *et al.*, 2005), for epoprostenol 85% at 12 months (Sitbon *et al.*, 2002), for treprostinil 85% at 12 months (McLaughlin *et al.*, 2003) and 42–77% for inhaled iloprost at 12 months (Opitz *et al.*, 2005; Hoeper *et al.*, 2005a) whilst for beraprost, efficacy tends to be lost after six months, perhaps because patients cannot always tolerate an optimal dosage (Barst *et al.*, 2003a).

Therapeutic benefits in some cases of idiopathic pulmonary arterial hypertension (IPAH) and the majority of cases of pulmonary arterial hypertension (PAH) associated with other conditions such as connective tissue diseases (CTDs) commonly diminish over time.

Treatment goals

Various target treatment goals may be set. Examples are normalization of pulmonary artery pressure, or of exercise pulmonary artery pressure, brain natriuretic peptide (BNP) or pro N-terminal BNP (pro NT-BNP) or improvement on echocardiography of pericardial effusion, right atrial area, right ventricular ejection fraction, right ventricular ejection time (Tei index), mitral valve early filling and left ventricular

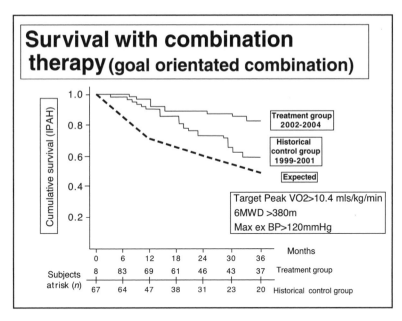

Figure 7.1 Survival with goal orientated combination therapy. Where target goal was not met, an ordered sequence of drugs PDE5 was purposed. (Reproduced with permission from Hoeper *et al.*, (2005), *Eur Respir J* **26**:858–63. ©European Respiratory Society Journals Ltd.)

end-diastolic dimension. For 6MWD, > 325 m vs < 325 m or > 380 m vs < 380 m, depending upon the study, is a cut point, defining prognosis.

The best treatment goals are simply normalization of every parameter and to enable the diagnosis of PAH to be consistent with a normal life expectancy.

One approach already tested is goal-oriented treatment with combination therapy to achieve the following targets: A 6MWD of > 380 m, VO_2 max > 10.4 mls/kg/min, a systolic blood pressure at exercise > 120 mm Hg and for patients to be in at least NYHA Class II (Hoeper *et al.*, 2005a) (Figure 7.1). A large analysis of survival, utilizing this goal-oriented approach to combination therapy was undertaken in 123 pulmonary arterial hypertension patients. The treatment group (2002–2004) was managed with combination therapy, when mandated by VO_2 max < 10.4 mls/kg/min, 6MWD < 380 m or maximal exercise systolic blood pressure < 120 mm Hg. The predefined order of treatment was bosentan, then add sildenafil, then add inhaled iloprost. Compared with a historic control group and compared with expected survival by the National Institute of Health (NIH) survival equation derived from the NIH primary pulmonary arterial hypertension (PPH) Registry in the 1980s, survival was markedly improved by the targeted approach, with over 80% three-year survival. The use of combination treatment also significantly diminished the combined endpoint of death, transplantation and initiation of intravenous prostanoid treatment (Hoeper *et al.*, 2005a).

7.2   Combination therapy to date

Combination therapy to date has involved the combination of two drugs from three classes: prostanoids, endothelin receptor antagonists and phosphodiesterase 5 inhibitors (Table 7.1). Their differing modes of action may be complementary. The specific mechanisms are covered in Chapters 4, 5 and 6.

Beyond simple additive effects, some combinations may have a synergistic action, e.g. there is evidence that ET-1 suppresses nitric oxide (NO) production, primarily through the ET_A receptor. Endothelin receptor antagonists (ETRAs) are thus expected to enhance NO generation in PAH. Addition of a PDE5 inhibitor could augment the effects of the increased NO production. Increased cGMP via PDE5 inhibition is associated with inhibition of PDE3 and, consequently, reduced catabolism of cAMP. Moreover, there is evidence that cAMP favorably affects NO function. Therefore, the combination of a PDE5 inhibitor and an ETRA may be synergistic.

Similarly the combination of sildenafil with inhaled iloprost, which acts more locally and less systemically, also may be synergistic, echoing the effects seen in acute challenge with these two agents (Ghofrani et al., 2002).

The evidence in combination therapy

Combination therapy can be started concurrently (with the drugs started within a day or so of each other) or sequentially. Two main outcomes to be borne in mind are the safety of the combination and their combined efficacy.

Concurrent/simultaneous trials

BREATHE-2 – Randomized, placebo-controlled trial: epoprostenol add bosentan

In the BREATHE-2 trial, 33 patients (mean age 46 years) with WHO Class III (76%) or IV (24%) IPAH or PAH related to CTD were started on epoprostenol IV for two days starting at 2 ng/kg/min and uptitrated to 14 ng/kg/min. Patients were randomized (2:1 ratio) at day 2 to either epoprostenol with added placebo ($n = 11$), or epoprostenol with added bosentan ($n = 22$). The primary endpoint at 16 weeks was change in total pulmonary resistance (TPR) (Humbert et al., 2004). Although TPR decreased with epoprostenol/bosentan by 41% (from 1697 ± 142 to 1016 ± 78 dyn s/cm^5) vs 23% with epoprostenol/placebo (1628 ± 154 to 1242 ± 153 dyn s/cm^5), the difference was not significant ($p = 0.08$). The change in 6MWD was also not significant (combination +68 m vs baseline, epoprostenol alone +74 m vs baseline) nor were the changes in Borg dyspnea score, functional class, clinical worsening, death or other hemodynamic parameters. However, limitations of the study were small sample size and suboptimal dose of epoprostenol. An unexpected

Table 7.1 Combination therapy trials reported

Trial	Year	n	Design	Condition, FC	Design	Agents	Duration (weeks)	Endpoint	
BREATHE-2	2004	33	R,P-C	Adult IPAH, CTD, III, IV	Simultaneous	IV Epoprostenol + bosentan vs epoprostenol + placebo	16	Total pulmonary resistance	No significant difference
STEP-1	2006	67	R,P-C	Adult IPAH, CTD, III, IV	Sequential	Bosentan, add inhaled iloprost or placebo	12	6MWD +26m $p=0.051$	FC $p = 0.0023$, developed clinical deterioration $p=0.02$, PAPm $p <0.001$ PVR $p \leq 0.001$
PACES-1	2006	264	R,P-C	Adult IPAH, CTD, III, IV	Sequential	IV Epoprostenol add sildenafil or placebo	16	6MWD +26m ($p < 0.001$)	Developed clinical deterioration $p < 0.012$ PAPm $p < 0.0001$
COMBI-1	2006	40	R,P-C, O/L	Adult IPAH	Sequential	Bosentan, add inhaled iloprost or bosentan alone	12	6MWD	Futility analysis premature discontinuation
Hoeper	2004	9	Open Label	Adult IPAH, III	Sequential	Bosentan add sildenafil	52	6MWD + 115m	Peak VO_2 +33%
Hoeper	2003	20	Open Label	Adult IPAH, III	Sequential	Beraprost or inhaled iloprost, add bosentan	12	6MWD + 58m	Peak VO_2 +25%
Benza	2004	19	Open Label	Adult IPAH, CTD, IV	Sequential	SC treprostinil, add bosentan	78	6MWD + 67m	PAPm RAPm improved FC $p = 0.002$
Kotlyar	2006	107	Open Label	IPAH, CTD, CTEPH, miscellaneous	Sequential	Drug one add drug two	24	6MWD +41m $p<0.001$	FC improved $p < 0.05$ Echo RVSP reduced by 10 mm Hg $p < 0.05$

(Continued)

Table 7.1 *(Continued)*

Trial	Year	n	Design	Condition, FC	Design	Agents	Duration (weeks)	Endpoint	
Ghofrani	2003	14	Open Label	IPAH, CTD	Sequential	Inhaled iloprost add sildenafil	12	6MWD +90m p=0.002	Improved FC, PVRI, mPAP
Ruiz	2006	20	Open Label	IPAH, HIV toxic oil, III, IV	Sequential	IV epoprostenol or SC treprostinil or iloprost, add sildenafil	104	6MWD +105m p=0.04	Improved RV function and FC
Diaz	2005	12	Open Label	Adult, IPAH, SLE, RA, CTD, miscellaneous, III, IV	Sequential	Epoprostenol or SC treprostinil add bosentan	34	6MWD + 44m	FC improved in 75%, RV score improved in 50%
Seyfarth	2005	16	Open Label	Adult, IPAH, miscellaneous	Sequential	Beraprost or iloprost (inhaled or IV) add bosentan	54	6MWD +43m p<0.001	Improved Tei index, FC improved in 56%
BREATHE-3	2005	86	Open Label	Pediatric, IPAH, CHD, I-IV	Simultaneous	Treprostinil or epoprostenol add bosentan	14	Hemodynamics, FC, safety	FC improved or stable in 90% PA red p = 0.005 PVR fell p = 0.01
Rozenzweig	2005	86	Open Label	Pediatric, IPAH. CHD, I-IV	Simultaneous	SC treprostinil or IV epoprostenol add bosentan	14	Hemodynamics, FC, study	FC improved or stable in 90% PAPM red p = 0.005 PVR p=0.01
Ivy	2004	8	Open Label	Pediatric, sequential	Sequential	IV epoprostenol add bosentan	52	FC, hemodynamics	Reduced epoprostenol dosage and side effects

CHD: congenital heart disease; CTD: connective tissue disease; FC: functional class; IPAH: idiopathic pulmonary arterial hypertension; P-C: placebo controlled; R: randomized; SC: subcutaneous; RA: rheumatoid arthritis.

finding (not significant), was a trend to reduction in prostacyclin side effects with combination – similar to results seen in children. On bosentan–epoprostenol 59% of patients experienced jaw pain vs 91% of those randomized to placebo–epoprostenol. Abnormal hepatic function was less frequent in the bosentan–epoprostenol group (9% vs 18%). On the other hand, lower limb edema was three times more frequent (27% vs 9%) and diarrhea more than twice as frequent (55% vs 27%) in patients treated with the combination regimen.

Summary note: Starting bosentan two days after starting epoprostenol showed non-significant trends to improvement over 16 weeks in TPR, but not 6MWD or clinical parameters. Study design may have limited conclusions.

Sequential trials

STEP-1 – Randomized, controlled trial: bosentan add inhaled iloprost

The STEP-1 phase II trial was the iloprost inhalation solution Safety and pilot efficacy Trial in combination with bosentan for Evaluation in PAH (Figure 7.2). Fifteen USA sites enrolled a total of 67 patients with IPAH or PAH CTD in Class III (94%) or IV (6%) (McLaughlin *et al.*, 2006). Patients were required to have been stable on bosentan for > 16 weeks but with 6MWD still limited to 100–425 m (mean 338 m). Randomization was double-blind, placebo-controlled to bosentan and inhaled iloprost (six times daily) or to bosentan with inhaled placebo (six times daily). The change in 6MWD at week 12 vs baseline (measured immediately

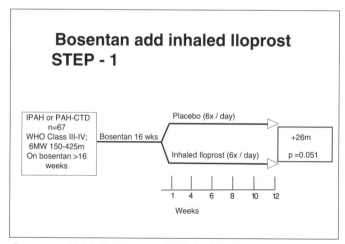

Figure 7.2 Bosentan add inhaled iloprost STEP-1 trial. (Reproduced with permission from McLaughlin *et al.* (2006). Randomized study of adding inhaled iloprost to existing bosentan in pulmonary arterial hypertension. *Am J Resp Crit Care Med*, **174**:1257–63. ©American Thoracic Society.)

after inhalation) on bosentan/iloprost was +30 m vs bosentan/placebo +4 m, for a placebo-corrected improvement of +26 m ($p = 0.051$). Compared with bosentan/placebo, combination therapy resulted in increased functional class in 34% vs 6% ($p = 0.0023$), no clinical deterioration on iloprost combination (vs 15% on placebo, $p = 0.0219$), mPAP reduced by 8 mm Hg ($p = 0.001$) and pulmonary vascular resistance (PVR) reduced by 54 dyn s/cm^5 ($p = 0.0007$). Dyspnea also improved with the addition of iloprost, defined by a reduction in Borg dyspnea scale from baseline ($p = 0.03$). The number of significant adverse events and syncope was similar, and no patients in either group died or demonstrated elevated hepatic transaminases. Compliance with inhalations in each arm was high at 90% (McLaughlin *et al.*, 2006).

Summary note: Patients stable on bosentan but still Class III or IV had modest improvements over 12 weeks in 6MWD, functional class and hemodynamics with the addition of inhaled iloprost.

COMBI – Randomized, open, controlled trial: bosentan add inhaled iloprost

Like STEP-1, the COMBI trial evaluated the safety and efficacy of adding inhaled iloprost in IPAH patients who were stable on bosentan treatment (Hoeper *et al.*, 2006). This trial, however, was terminated prematurely after a futility analysis predicted failure with respect to the primary endpoint. Thus, only 40 patients were enrolled and there were no differences in the outcome measures, i.e. 6MWD, maximum oxygen uptake, quality of life or functional class.

Summary note: Viewed together with the results from STEP-1, the advantage of adding inhaled iloprost to bosentan has not been convincingly demonstrated and requires further study.

PACES-1 randomized, placebo-controlled trial: epoprostenol add sildenafil

The PACES-1 trial randomized 267 patients with Class III to IV disease, IPAH, CTD related or post repair CHD, who were already on epoprostenol continuous IV infusion, to either added sildenafil or added placebo (Figure 7.3). The placebo-corrected 6MWD treatment effect at week 16 vs baseline was +26 m ($p < 0.001$). The combination therapy also decreased mPAP to a greater extent than epoprostenol monotherapy ($p < 0.0001$). Time to clinical worsening was significantly longer in patients on combination therapy compared with epoprostenol monotherapy ($p = 0.012$). Side effects were similar for both treatment groups. (Simonneau *et al.*, 2008)

Summary note: Patients stable on IV epoprostenol but still limited, i.e. 6MWD < 450 m, improved over 16 weeks in 6MWD, hemodynamics and clinical worsening with the addition of sildenafil.

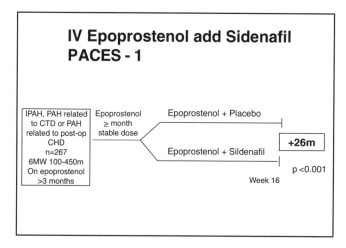

IV Epoprostenol add Sidenafil PACES - 1

IPAH, PAH related to CTD or PAH related to post-op CHD n=267 6MW 100-450m On epoprostenol >3 months	Epoprostenol ≥ month stable dose	Epoprostenol + Placebo / Epoprostenol + Sildenafil

+26m

p <0.001

Week 16

Figure 7.3 Epoprostenol add sildenafil. PACES-1 trial. (Simonneau 2008 *Ann Int Med* (in press)).

Bosentan add sildenafil – open label

In a European trial treating patients with IPAH, sildenafil was added when the clinical benefits of bosentan had declined in nine patients, (functional Class III 89%; mean age 39 ± 9 years) (Figure 7.4). Mean RA pressure was 9 ± 5 mm Hg, mPAP 62 ± 12 mm Hg and CI 1.6 ± 0.3 l/min/m² consistent with advanced disease. Bosentan was started at a dose of 62.5 mg po bid and increased to 125 mg po bid after four weeks. Sildenafil was then added at a dose of 25 mg three or four times daily and increased to a total daily dose of 150 mg in patients with suboptimal responses to sildenafil, based on predefined 6MWT and cardiopulmonary exercise testing cutpoints (Hoeper *et al.*, 2004).

The baseline 6MWD distance was 346 ± 66 m, which improved by 57 m, to 403 ± 80 m (16%; $p = 0.0003$) on bosentan. By 11 ± 5 months of bosentan monotherapy, the mean 6MWD had declined 31%, to 277 ± 80 m and was below baseline. Three months after adjunctive sildenafil however, 6MWD rose by 115 m (42%; $p = 0.007$), to 392 ± 61 m. This effect was sustained with follow-up of up to 12 months.

Consistent with these findings, cardiopulmonary exercise testing demonstrated an increase in peak oxygen uptake by 24% after three months of bosentan treatment, then fell to near baseline levels at treatment month 11. However, three months after addition of sildenafil, peak oxygen uptake rose 33%, to a higher level than during bosentan monotherapy.

Combination therapy was well tolerated. All patients reported transient mild flushing and headache with initiation of sildenafil. There was no syncope, liver function test abnormalities, deaths or serious adverse events ascribed to combination treatment.

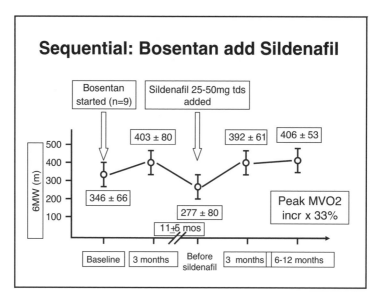

Figure 7.4 Sequential bosentan add sildenafil. (Reproduced with permission from Hoeper *et al.*, (2004), *Eur Respir J* **24**:1007–10. ©European Respiratory Society Journals Ltd.)

Summary note: Sildenafil appeared to serve as a safe and effective rescue agent in the face of waning clinical response to bosentan.

Beraprost or iloprost add bosentan – open label

In an open label experience, patients on at least three months of oral beraprost (n = 11) or inhaled iloprost (n = 9) had bosentan added (Hoeper *et al.*, 2003). All 20 patients had IPAH, mean age 46 years, female (70%) and functional Class III (85%).

Bosentan add-on therapy appeared to be efficacious for up to six months. The 6MWD increased 64, m from prostanoids baseline, to three months after adding bosentan, and rose a further 15m after six months on combination. Cardiopulmonary exercise testing showed a range of significant benefits with combination therapy at three months compared with prostanoids baseline, including a 25% increase in VO_2 max from 11.0 mls/kg/min at baseline to 13.8 mls/kg/min at three months (p = 0.001) and a 15% improvement in anaerobic threshold (from 10.2 to 11.7 mls/kg/min; p = 0.007).

Treatment was well tolerated in all patients, with no symptomatic systemic hypotension or syncope. Mild leg edema reversed spontaneously and only mild anemia was noted in half the patients. Liver function test abnormalities in two patients resolved despite continued bosentan dosing (Hoeper *et al.*, 2003).

Summary note: Although limitations were lack of randomization without a placebo control, this study suggests possible benefits of adding bosentan to beraprost or iloprost therapy.

Treprostinil add bosentan – open label

In a study at the University of Alabama, Birmingham, bosentan was added in 19 patients with PAH (9 IPAH, 10 CTD PAH) already receiving SC treprostinil monotherapy who remained NYHA Class III after a year of therapy ($n = 12$) or who had intolerable site pain ($n = 7$) (Benza *et al.*, 2004). Patients included 13 women and 6 men with mean age 49 ± 15 years. The mean duration of treprostinil was 770 ± 307 days at a dose of 38 ± 18 ng/kg/min at the time of initiation of bosentan.

In this study, the last observation on combination therapy (18 ± 4 months) was compared to pre-treprostinil and to pre-bosentan values. There were serial improvements in mPAP (60 ± 4, 56 ± 4, 47 ± 3 mm Hg), and mean right atrial pressure (7 ± 1, 10 ± 2, 5 ± 7 mm Hg), as well as an incremental improvement in the 6MWD (307 m ± 14, 333 m ± 18, 374 m ± 25) and Borg dyspnea scale (4.3 ± 0.6, 3.6 ± 0.5, 2.9 ± 0.4). However, these differences were only statistically significant after the addition of bosentan. Symptomatically, before the addition of treprostinil, 18 patients were NYHA Class III–IV (94%). After the addition of treprostinil, 57% remained Class III and 43% were Class II ($p = 0.007$). At the last observation on combined therapy, 74% were NYHA Classes I or II and 16% NYHA Class III ($p = 0.002$ vs pre-treprostinil) (Benza *et al.*, 2004).

Summary note: The addition of bosentan to continuous SC treprostinil in patients with moderate/severe PAH improved hemodynamic status, exercise capacity and functional class.

Inhaled iloprost add sildenafil – open label

A German group suggests that sildenafil is also a viable rescue agent in the presence of waning clinical effects of inhaled iloprost in patients with severe PAH (Ghofrani *et al.*, 2002; Ghofrani *et al.*, 2003) (Figure 7.5). Among 73 patients who were being treated with inhaled iloprost (mean of nine inhalations daily), 14 (19%) experienced clinical worsening on treatment. These 14 patients were assigned to open label sildenafil uptitrated to a total daily target dose of 75–150 mg (three split doses). The mean age was 58 years, 64% had IPAH and 36% had PAH associated with CTD. Monthly follow-up visits were conducted and outcomes measured quarterly through to treatment month 12. Disease was advanced with baseline mPAP 58.4 ± 2.4 mm Hg, cardiac index 2.0 ± 0.2 l/min/m^2, PVR index of 2312 ± 271 dyn s m^2/cm^5, and 6MWD distance 217 m.

Initiation of inhaled iloprost increased 6MWD by 88 m (41%) within the first three months. However, much of this initial increment was lost on continued iloprost monotherapy, with 6MWD declining toward baseline (256 m) at treatment month 18 ± 4. Adjunctive sildenafil reversed this decline, augmenting 6MWD to 346 m (35% rise; $p = 0.002$ vs pre-sildenafil) after three months of combination treatment, with this benefit persisting at 12 month follow-up.

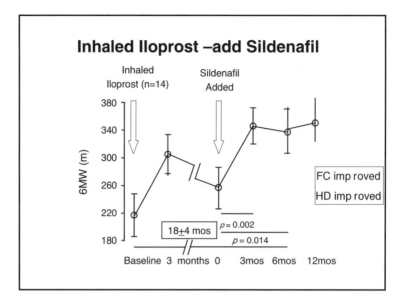

Figure 7.5   Inhaled iloprost add sildenafil (Reproduced from *J Am Coll Cardiol*, **42**(1), Ghofrani *et al.*, 158–64, Copyright (2003) with permission from the American College of Cardiology.)

Consistent with these effects, improvements in functional class and cardiopulmonary hemodynamics (cardiac index, PVR index, mPAP) were also noted. Combination therapy appeared to be well tolerated, with no sildenafil-related serious untoward effects over six months. No patients had syncope or dizziness. Two patients died of pneumonia.

Summary note: When the effect of iloprost is waning in IPAH or PAH associated with CTD, the addition of sildenafil may provide rescue.

Long-term prostanoids add sildenafil

Twenty patients had received prostanoids (7 epoprostenol, 22 ± 6 ng/kg/min, 8 treprostinil 32 ± 6 ng/kg/min and 5 iloprost 140 ± 22 ng/kg/min) for a mean of 19 months (6–34 months) (Ruiz *et al.*, 2006). All were Class III or IV or had syncope with 6MWD 350 ± 121 m. Etiology was IPAH in 13, toxic oil PAH in 6 and HIV-related PAH in 1.

Twelve months after adding sildenafil, improvements were noted in Class (baseline 3.0 ± 0.5, to 2.1 ± 0.8, $p < 0.001$), 6MWD (baseline 351 ± 121 to 430 ± 86, $p < 0.02$), RV diastolic diameter (50 ± 8 to 43 ± 8 mm, $p = 0.002$), and RA area (baseline 21 ± 6 to 18 ± 6, $p = 0.06$).

The majority were followed up to 24 months with further improvements seen in 6MWD with sustained benefit in functional class, although there was no further evidence of RV reverse remodeling.

Summary note: This study provides further evidence that the addition of sildenafil to various prostanoids appears safe and efficacious in patients with advanced PAH.

Australian national experience of sequential combination therapy

In an attempt to capture data about open label double drug usage, a large retrospective collaborative review in Australia followed patients started on one drug, followed by the addition of a second PAH-specific agent (Kotlyar *et al.*, 2006) (Figure 7.6). The study group comprised 107 patients, mean age 51 ± 18 years (range 14–87), who had been on monotherapy for a mean of 18 ± 12 months (range 0.1–56 months) and who were either deteriorating or who were showing evidence of persistent PAH clinically, hemodynamically or by echocardiography. The underlying diagnosis was IPAH 51%, CTD 35%, chronic thromboembolic 6%, arteriovenous malformation 2% and CHO 5%.

Combination therapy varied. In order of frequency, first drug was bosentan (66%), sildenafil (22%), ambrisentan (6%) and sitaxsentan (6%). In order of frequency, the second drug added was sildenafil (68%), inhaled iloprost (17%), bosentan (12%) and ambrisentan (3%). Data was combined for the purpose of analysis.

At initiation of first drug, 6MWD was 313 ± 110 m and increased to 386 ± 98 m after three months, but declined to 316 ± 117 m by 18 ± 12 months of monotherapy. The addition of the second agent increased 6MWD after three months to 357 ±

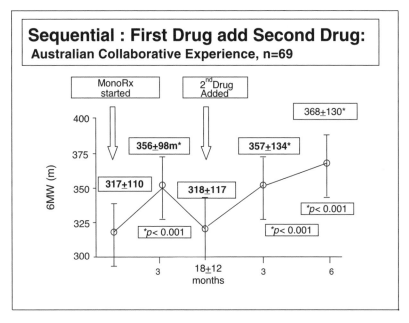

Figure 7.6 Sequential: First drug add second drug: Australian collaborative experience (Reproduced from Kotlyar *et al.*, 2006, *Heart, Lung and Circulation* 15S:S78. Courtesy of Elsevier.)

134 m ($p < 0.001$) and after six months of combination 368 ± 130 m ($p < 0.001$). Functional class improved from 3.1 ± 0.7 at start of combination to 2.4 ± 0.7 ($p < 0.05$) at three months and the echocardiographic estimate of RV systolic pressure fell from 84 ± 18 to 74 ± 14 ($p < 0.05$) at three months of combination. All combinations were well tolerated. Eighteen-month survival from start of combination was 93% in IPAH and 79% for scleroderma-related disease. Follow-up is ongoing.

Summary note: While retrospective, this review captures the broadening range of practice in combination therapy, with improvement in 6MWD across combinations, and reinforces the ability of add-on therapy to retrieve a deteriorating situation in some patients.

Pediatric

Treprostinil or epoprostenol add bosentan – sequential open label

In a small open label study, 19 children with PAH were treated with bosentan with a target total daily dose of (split dosage) 62.5 mg for children 10–20 kg weight, 125 mg for 20–40 kg weight and 250 mg for > 40 kg weight. During the first four weeks of bosentan therapy, half the target dose was administered each day, with the dose increased to target if treatment was well tolerated. Pharmacokinetic and hemodynamic parameters were obtained at baseline and after 12 weeks of bosentan treatment.

Bosentan produced hemodynamic improvement and was well tolerated. The mean change from baseline in mPAP was –8 mm Hg (95% CI, –12.2 to –3.7 mm Hg) and that in PVR index was –300 dyn sec m^2/cm^5 (95% CI, –576 to –24 dyne sec m^2/cm^5). The exposure to bosentan was 43%, 67% and 75%, respectively, of the exposure seen in adult patients, for patients with body weights of 10–20 kg, 20–40 kg and > 40 kg. These pharmacokinetic data suggested that these children might have received suboptimal doses of bosentan. Based on these data, a follow-up study was carried out to determine bosentan dose selection that would result in similar exposure to bosentan for children with PAH to that for adults with PAH. However, a follow-up study did not demonstrate any significant difference in pharmacokinetic data in children receiving 4 mg/kg/dose orally twice daily versus 2mg/kg/dose orally twice daily.

In a retrospective study, 86 children with PAH commenced bosentan with or without concurrent SC treprostinil or IV epoprostenol. Bosentan dosing was 62.5 mg twice daily for children 10–20 kg weight, 125 mg twice daily for 20–40 kg and 250 mg twice daily for > 40 kg weight. Treprostinil or epoprostenol dose adjustments were discretionary (Rosenzweig et al., 2005). Bosentan improved functional class in 46% of patients but FC war unchanged in 44%. Kaplan–Meier survival was 91% by two years. Bosentan treatment also lowered both mPAP (from 64 mm Hg to 57 mm Hg; $p = 0.005$) and PVRI (from 20 U m^2 to 15 U m^2, $p = 0.01$), and was well tolerated. Peripheral edema was observed in 8% and systemic hypotension in 3%. Fatigue led to discontinuation in 2%, 9 and 11 months after the initiation of bosentan treatment, and systemic arterial oxygen desaturation resulted in discontinuation in 2%, 5 and 7 months after the initiation of bosentan; both patients had unrepaired congenital heart disease. Both of these adverse events reversed following bosentan discontinuation.

Summary note: This retrospective study showed that bosentan appears safe and efficacious for children with PAH, both as monotherapy and as and adjunct to prostanoid treatment.

Epoprostenol add bosentan

In a further pediatric study, addition of bosentan enabled reduction in IV epoprostenol dosage, with decreases in prostanoid side effects without apparent hemodynamic or clinical compromise (Ivy *et al.*, 2004). Curiously the improvements in WHO functional class and hemodynamics were more pronounced for the children who started bosentan without concomitant prostanoid therapy than for those treated with combined bosentan and prostanoids. This may have been be explained by the difference that the patients who needed prostanoid treatment before bosentan initiation had more advanced disease at bosentan initiation.

Summary note: This study showed that select children with PAH may be transitioned from intravenous epoprostenol to oral therapies. It needs to be noted, however, that such an approach carries substantial risks and requires close long-term surveillance.

Pharmacokinetics

A concern with combination therapy is drug interactions.

An example is in a bosentan–sildenafil regimen, i.e. both components are CYP3A4 substrates (Barst *et al.*, 2003b). Sildenafil at steady state dosage (80 mg three times daily) led to a 50% increase in the systemic exposure (AUC) of bosentan and a 42% increase in the maximum concentration (C_{max}) of bosentan when administered at 125 mg twice daily (Paul *et al.*, 2005). In addition, because bosentan induces CYP3A4, bosentan reduced sildenafil plasma levels by 60% – possibly reducing the efficacy of sildenafil (Paul *et al.*, 2005). The clinical relevance of these interactions is unclear and, in practice to date, this combination has not led to dose adjustment of either drug.

The TRAX non-interventional, prospective web-based database evaluating long-term safety of bosentan, demonstrated no increased risk of liver toxicity in patients taking bosentan plus sildenafil compared to bosentan alone (Hoeper 2005b).

The potential for interactions may be diminished when sildenafil is administered with the selective endothelin antagonists sitaxsentan (a CYP2C9 substrate and weak inhibitor of CYP3A4/5) or ambrisentan. Sildenafil has been shown to have no effect on sitaxsentan plasma concentrations. Sitaxsentan caused only a minor pharmacokinetic interaction with sildenafil (increase in C_{max} 18% and AUC 28%) (Coyne, *et al.*, 2005). Ambrisentan has no relevant interactions with cytochrome P450 isoenzymes (Rubin, *et al.*, 2005).

Other considerations are interactions with other commonly prescribed concomitant medications. Bosentan induces CYP3A4 isoenzymes and reduces circulating levels of simvastatin and glyburide (Dingemanse, *et al.*, 2003; van Giersberger *et al.*, 2002). Sitaxsentan inhibits CYP2C9 P450 enzymes and increases circulating levels of warfarin, resulting in a 40–50% lower dosage requirement of warfarin with increased monitoring as appropriate when sitaxsentan and warfarin are combined (Barst *et al.*, 2002). The prostacyclin analogues treprostinil and iloprost are metabolized by side-chain oxidation and are not CYP enzyme substrates, reducing the chance of interaction with PDE5 inhibitors or ERAs.

Sildenafil (50 mg three times a day) and atorvastatin (20 mg daily) were added to bosentan (125 mg two times a day) (12-week randomized trial), in 23 patients with PAH. Two patients discontinued early owing to side effects but no liver toxicity was seen (Gomberg-Maitland *et al.*, 2005).

New pathophysiological targets for future combination therapy

Future candidates for consideration with combination therapy include: vasointestinal peptide (VIP), the PDGF antagonist imatinib (tyrosine kinase pathway), adrenomedullin, serotonin transport inhibitors such as fluoxetine, potassium channel openers such as anandamide, elastase inhibitors, autologous gene therapy inducing eNOS or BMPR receptor delivery, endothelial progenitor cells, and perhaps antiproliferative agents such as mTOR inhibitors. Type 1, 3 and 4 phosphodiesterase inhibitors and cGMP augmenting agents are also under development.

7.3 Conclusions

To date, information on combination therapy with disease-specific targeted PAH agents comes from a limited number of patients in several randomized, placebo-controlled trials, and from patients in single center or national open label uncontrolled studies. Moreover, truly long-term data are completely absent. The vast global experience of open label combination therapy remains unreported. Nevertheless, combination therapy to date of drugs from different classes appears safe, with clinical efficacy observed with most combinations. However, combination therapy does not yet have a firm place in evidence-based PAH treatment algorithms (Badesch *et al.*, 2004).

Data on simultaneous initiation of therapies is limited to epoprostenol with added bosentan in a small number of patients, which suggested safety of the combination but only trends toward efficacy.

In contrast, data with sequential therapy, in the face of waning efficacy with monotherapy, has been evaluated more fully with promising results. This is true not just of 6MWD but of other symptoms (when measured) such as hemodynamics, echocardiographic and peak oxygen utilization. The benefits of sequential therapy appear consistent between randomized, placebo-controlled trials and open label reports. The response to the second agent in open label reports appears to be at least as good if not better than the initial response to the first agent.

All combinations to date appear to be safe and well tolerated without excess adverse events or deaths. Nevertheless, combinations of drugs require heightened levels of monitoring for side effects and potential drug interactions.

The new scientific trend in monotherapy is not only to determine the effective dose of agent but to determine the minimum dose and duration of monotherapy which is effective with minimal toxicity. The same question remains to be explored and is just as important in the context of combination therapy.

The appropriate time at which to introduce a second agent is unclear. The time to optimal response with monotherapy appears to be 12 weeks for epoprostenol and sildenafil, and perhaps 16 weeks for ERAs although these data are led in essence by the clinical trial designs used for registration purposes. Responses to a second agent in deteriorating monotherapy groups are evident. However, although pre-emptive combination therapy introduced earlier in the course of PAH may prove to be more efficacious in preventing continued pulmonary vascular remodeling, deterioration and in targeting the goal of cure, data is currently not available.

Whether attempts at withdrawal of initial therapy are warranted after a period of combined therapy is an important question for the future. Perceived ineffective therapy may actually be stabilizing disease, and withdrawal may be potentially detrimental; however, again, data are lacking. For this reason, additions, or withdrawals or transitioning in the era of combination therapy should be done vigilantly and with clear cut and predetermined endpoints.

More information is needed for the less responsive scleroderma PAH patients and other rarer subgroups of PAH. Similarly, information regarding the appropriate hierarchy of drugs is also needed.

In conclusion, for patients with suboptimal improvement in endpoints (functional class, 6MWD distance, BNP levels or hemodynamics) or with waning clinical responses with monotherapy, and/or severe PAH persisting or progressing despite monotherapy, sequential combination regimens targeted to more than one pathobiologic disease mechanism may offer clinical benefit.

As is true with monotherapy, the cost of combination therapies, and hence equitable access, will be a major consideration.

However, few patients, even on combination therapy, return to a normal life, and it remains uncertain if combinations of current therapies will ever 'cure' PAH.

Acknowledgement

Our gratitude to Cathy Borg, Australia, for her careful preparation of this manuscript.

References

Badesch D., Abman S., Ahern G. *et al.* (2004) Medical therapy for pulmonary arterial hypertension: ACCP evidence-based clinical practice guidelines. *Chest* **126**:35S–62S.

Barst R., Rich S., Widlitz A., Horn E. *et al.* (2002) Clinical efficacy of sitaxsentan, an endothelin-A receptor antagonist, in patients with pulmonary arterial hypertension: open-label pilot study. *Chest* **121**:1860–68.

Barst R., McGoon M., McLaughlin V. *et al.* (2003a) Beraprost therapy for pulmonary arterial hypertension. *JACC* **41**:2119–25.

Barst RJ., Ivy D., Dingemanse J. *et al.* (2003b) Single- and Multiple-Dose Pharmacokinetics of Bosentan in Pediatric Patients with Pulmonary Arterial Hypertension. *Clin Pharmacol Ther* **73**:372–382.

Benza R., Rayburn B., Tallaj J. *et al.* (2004) Efficacy of a combination of oral bosentan and continuous subcutaneous infusion of treprostinil in pulmonary arterial hypertension. Proceedings of the American Thoracic Society 100th International Conference, May 21–26 2004, Orlando, FL. *Am J Resp Crit Care Med* **169**(7):A174.

Benza R., Park M., Keogh A., Girgis R. (2007) Management of pulmonary arterial hypertension with a focus on combination therapies. *Transplant* **26**:437–46.

Coyne T., Garces P., Kramer W. (2005) No clinical interaction between sitaxsentan and sildenafil. Proceedings of the American Thoracic Society 101st International Conference, San Diego, CA.

Diaz E., Bair N., Banjac S., Jennings C. (2005) Addition of bosentan to epoprostenol in patients with pulmonary arterial hypertension. Proceedings of the American Thoracic Society 101st International Conference, San Diego, CA.

Dingemanse J., Schaarschmidt D., van Giersbergen P. (2003) Investigation of the mutual pharmacokinetic interactions between bosentan, a dual endothelin receptor antagonist, and simvastatin. *Clin Pharmacokinet* **42**(3):293–301.

Galie N., Ghofrani H., Torbicki A. *et al.* (2005) Sildenafil citrate therapy for pulmonary arterial hypertension (SUPER-1 study). *N Engl J Med* **353**:2148–57.

Ghofrani H., Wiedemann R., Rose F. *et al.* (2002) Combination therapy with oral sildenafil and inhaled iloprost for severe pulmonary hypertension. Ann Intern Med **136**(7):515–22.

Ghofrani HA., Rose F., Schermuly RT. *et al.* (2003) Oral sildenafil as long-term adjunct therapy to inhaled iloprost in severe pulmonary arterial hypertension. *J Am Coll Cardiol* **42**(1):158–64.

Gomberg-Maitland M., McLaughlin V., Gulati M., Rich S. (2005) Efficacy and safety of sildenafil and atorvastatin added to bosentan on therapy for pulmonary arterial hypertension. Proceedings of the American Thoracic Society 101st International Conference, San Diego, CA.

Hoeper MM., Taha N., Bekjarova A. *et al.* (2003) Bosentan treatment in patients with primary pulmonary hypertension receiving nonparenteral prostanoids. *Eur Respir J* **22**(2):330–4.

Hoeper MM., Faulenbach C., Golpon H. *et al.* (2004) Combination therapy with bosentan and sildenafil in idiopathic pulmonary arterial hypertension. *Eur Respir* **24**(6):1007–10.

Hoeper M., Markevych I., Spiekerkoetter E. *et al.* (2005a) Goal oriented treatment and combination therapy for pulmonary arterial hypertension. *Eur Respir J* **26**(5):858–63.

Hoeper M., Kiely D., Carlsen J. *et al.* (2005b) Safety profile of pulmonary arterial hypertension patients treated with bosentan and sildenafil. Results from the European Surveillance Program. ATS San Diego.

Hoeper M., Leuchte H., Halank M. *et al.* (2006) Combining inhaled iloprost with bosentan in patients with idiopathic pulmonary arterial hypertension. *Eur Respir* **28**:691–4.

Humbert M., Barst RJ., Robbins IM. *et al.* (2004) Combination of bosentan with epoprostenol in pulmonary arterial hypertension. BREATHE-2 *Eur Respir J* **24**(3):353–9.

Ivy DD., Doran A., Claussen L. *et al.* (2004) Weaning and discontinuation of epoprostenol in children with idiopathic pulmonary arterial hypertension receiving concomitant bosentan. *Am J Cardiol* **93**(7):943–6.

Kotlyar E., Keogh A., Macdonald P. *et al.* (2006) Dual therapy for pulmonary arterial hypertension *Heart Lung Circ* **15S**:S78.

McLaughlin V., Gaine S., Barst R. *et al.* (2003) Efficacy and safety of treprostinil: an epoprostenol analog for primary pulmonary hypertension. *J Cardiovasc Pharmacol* **41**(2):293–9.

McLaughlin V., Oudiz R., Frost A. *et al.* (2006) Randomized study of adding inhaled iloprost to existing bosentan in pulmonary arterial hypertension. *Am J Respir Crit Care Med* **174**:1257–63.

Morice AH., Mulrennan S., Clark A (2005) Combination therapy with bosentan and phosphodi-esterase-5 inhibitor in pulmonary arterial hypertension. *Eur Respir J* **26**(1):180;author reply 180–1.

Opitz C., Wensel R., Winkler J. *et al.* (2005) Clinical efficacy and survival with first-line inhaled iloprost therapy in patients with idiopathic pulmonary arterial hypertension. Sep;**26**(18):1895–902.

Paul GA., Gibbs JS., Boobis AR. *et al.* (2005) Bosentan decreases the plasma concentration of sildenafil when coprescribed in pulmonary hypertension. *Br J Clin Pharmacol* **60**(1):107–112.

Provencher S., Sitbon O., Humbert M. *et al.* (2005) Predictors of long term efficacy of bosentan in idiopathic pulmonary arterial hypertension. Proc of Amer Thoracic Soc 101st International Conference, San Diego, CA.

Rosenzweig EB., Dunbar D., Widlitz A. *et al.* (2005) Effects of long term bosentan in children with pulmonary arterial hypertension. *J Am Coll Cardiol* **46**(4):697–704.

Rubin L., Dufton C., Gerber M. (2005) Ambrisentan for pulmonary arterial hypertension. *Future Cardiol* **1**(4):425–432.

Ruiz MJ., Escribano P., Delgardo J. *et al.* (2006) Efficacy of sildenafil as a rescue therapy for patients with severe pulmonary arterial pulmonary hypertension and given long term treatment with prostanoids: a 2 year experience. *J Heart Lung Transplant* **25**:1353–7.

Seyfarth H., Panky H., Hamnerschmidt S. *et al.* (2005) Bosentan improves exercise tolerance and TEI index in patients with pulmonary hypertension and prostanoid therapy. *Chest* **128**:709–13.

Simonneau G., Rubin LJ., Galie N. *et al.* (2008) For the Pulmonary Arterial Hypertension Combination Study of Epoprostenol and Sildenafil (PACES-1) Study Group. Safety and Efficacy of Combination Therapy with Sildenafil and Epoprostenol in Patients with Pulmonary Arterial Hypertension. *Ann Int Med* in press.

Sitbon O., Humbert M., Nunes H. *et al.* (2002) Long-term intravenous epoprostenol infusion in primary pulmonary hypertension: prognostic factors and survival. *JACC* **40**:780–88.

Sitbon O., Humbert M., Nunes H. *et al.* (2002) Clinical efficacy and survival with first-line inhaled iloprost therapy in patients with idiopathic pulmonary arterial hypertension. **40**:780–88.

Van Giersbergen P., Treiber A., Clozel M. *et al.* (2002) In vivo and in vitro studies exploring the pharmacokinetic interaction between bosentan, a dual endothelin receptor antagonist, and glyburide. *Clin Pharmacol Ther* **71**(4):253–62.

8 Interventional and surgical modalities of treatment for pulmonary arterial hypertension

Julio Sandoval and Ramona Doyle

Stanford University Medical Center, California, USA

8.1 Introduction

Medical therapy for pulmonary arterial hypertension (PAH) has undergone a revolution in the last decade and as a result the use of interventional and surgical therapies has changed as well. In the case of PAH related to congenital heart disease many patients are managed surgically early in life and need no further intervention. In some patients medical therapy can now delay or supplant the need for an intervention, but in others, such as those with chronic thromboembolic pulmonary hypertension (CTEPH), the initial choice of therapy may be an intervention or operation. In this chapter we focus on three interventions – atrial septostomy, pulmonary endarterectomy (PEA), lung or heart–lung transplantation – which, despite the growth of

Pulmonary Arterial Hypertension, Edited by Robyn J. Barst
© 2008 John Wiley & Sons, Ltd

effective medical treatment options, may still offer better outcomes in carefully selected subsets of patients.

8.2 Atrial septostomy

Introduction

In patients with advanced idiopathic pulmonary arterial hypertension (IPAH), right ventricular (RV) function is crucial for survival. Parameters that reflect RV dysfunction, such as a low cardiac output (CO), low pulmonary arterial oxygen saturation and, in particular, an elevated mean right atrial pressure (mRAP) are associated with poor prognosis. Likewise, clinical indicators of right ventricular failure (RVF) including NYHA functional class IV, syncope and systemic venous congestion are also markers of poor prognosis (D'Alonzo *et al.*, 1991). Although the pathophysiology of RVF in PAH has not been clearly established (Sandoval *et al.*, 1998), RV dysfunction and failure in PAH is mainly the result of increased, long-standing, right-sided pressure overload. Accordingly, any intervention capable of reducing pulmonary vascular resistance (PVR) and pulmonary arterial pressure (PAP) is a logical and effective way of treatment. Management of the patient with PAH has two main objectives: (1) to alleviate pulmonary microvascular obstruction (decrease PVR) as the primary objective, and (2) to alleviate RVF as a secondary goal. Medical treatments for PAH are reviewed in detail in other chapters in this book. There is no question that therapeutic interventions including the use of oral anticoagulants, calcium channel blockers (CCBs) in appropriate selected patients, long-term intravenous (IV) infusion of prostacyclin and, more recently, other prostacyclin analogues, endothelin receptor antagonists and phosphodiesterase-5 inhibitors have improved the quality of life and survival of patients with PAH (Badesch *et al.*, 2004; Galie *et al.*, 2005). It is also true, however, that despite all of these interventions, RVF may progress or recur in some patients (McLaughlin *et al.*, 2002). Atrial septostomy (AS) represents an additional strategy for the treatment of RVF from severe PAH and several reasons justify its use in this setting:

- the deleterious impact of RVF on survival of patients
- the unpredictable response to medical treatment
- the disparity in the availability of medical therapies throughout the world
- the limited access to lung transplantation.

Here we review the role of AS as an interventional therapy for the management of RVF from severe PAH.

Atrial septostomy: historical background

In 1964, Austen and coworkers were the first to suggest and demonstrate the potential benefit of an AS in PAH treatment (Austen *et al.*, 1964). Working in a canine model of acute and chronic RV hypertension, these authors showed that the creation of an atrial septal defect (ASD) in this setting produced beneficial hemodynamic effects, particularly during exercise, as well as a favorable effect on the survival of the animals. In their conclusions these authors suggested that the surgical creation of an interatrial communication should be considered in the treatment of patients with severe PAH. This operation was never conducted, in part because, two years later, Rashkind and Miller described the catheter-balloon technique for the creation of an atrial septal defect without thoracotomy (Rashkind and Miller, 1966). The technique, indicated to increase pulmonary blood flow in children with transposition of the great vessels or with mitral and pulmonary atresia, had the problem of restenosis of the septostomy and, more importantly, it was difficult to do in older patients with thickened septum. To solve this problem, Park and coworkers, in 1978, developed the Park blade septostomy catheter (Park *et al.*, 1978). Later, the septostomy catheter was optimized and the safety and efficacy of this procedure were demonstrated in a multicenter trial reported in 1982 (Park *et al.*, 1982). Blade balloon atrial septostomy (BBAS) was first reported in 1983 as a palliative therapy for refractory PAH by Rich and Lam (Rich and Lam, 1983).

Rationale for atrial septostomy

The use of AS in PAH is supported by the fact that deterioration in symptoms and death in PAH are associated with obstruction to systemic output and the development of RVF. An AS in this setting would allow right-to-left shunting to increase systemic output, which, in spite of the fall in systemic arterial oxygen saturation ($SaO_2\%$), will produce an increase in systemic oxygen transport (SOT) (Nihill *et al.*, 1991; Kerstein *et al.*, 1995; Rich *et al.*, 1997). In addition, the shunt would allow decompressing the heart resulting in alleviation of RVF. Along with the investigational support stated above (Austen *et al.*, 1964), several clinical observations have also suggested that an interatrial defect may be of benefit in severe PAH. Patients with PAH and with a patent foramen ovale (PFO) had a better survival than those without PFO (Rozkovec *et al.*, 1986). Likewise, patients with Eisenmenger syndrome have a better survival than patients with PAH (Hopkins *et al.*, 1996; Hopkins, 2005).

Atrial septostomy in pulmonary hypertension

The first report of AS for the treatment of refractory PAH was unsuccessful as the patient died 24 hours later as a result of refractory hypoxemia (Rich and Lam, 1983). Subsequent studies (Nihill *et al.*, 1991; Kerstein *et al.*, 1995), however, demonstrated that blade baloon atrial septostomy (BBAS) could be successfully performed in select patients with advanced PAH and result in significant clinical and hemodynamic improvement. Graded balloon dilation atrial septostomy (BDAS), a variant of BBAS introduced by Hausknecht (Hausknecht *et al.*, 1990) and Rothman (Rothman *et al.*, 1993), is the technique most used in recent series (Sandoval *et al.*, 1998;

Table 8.1   Procedure-related mortality in atrial septostomy for pulmonary hypertension

Author	Procedures (Number of patients)	Deaths within 24 hours	Deaths after one month
Sandoval J, *et al.* (1998)	22 (15)	1	1
Rothman A, *et al.* (1999)	13 (12)	0	2
Reichenberger F, *et al.* (2003)	20 (17)	3	5
Kothari SS, *et al.* (2002)	11 (11)	2	3
Vachiery JL, *et al.* (2003)	18 (16)	1	2
Moscussi M, *et al.* (2001)	1 (1)	0	0
Allcock RJ, *et al.* (2003)	12 (9)	0	0
Kurzyna M, *et al.* (2007)	3 (3)	0	1
Chau EM, *et al.* (2004)	1 (1)	0	0
Micheletti A, *et al.* (2006)	22 (20)	0	0
Total	**123 (105)**	**7 (7%)**	**14 (13%)**

Rothman *et al.*, 1999; Moscucci *et al.*, 2001; Kothari *et al.*, 2002; Allcock *et al.*, 2003; Reichenberger *et al.*, 2003; Vachiery JL, 2003; Chau *et al.*, 2004; Micheletti *et al.*, 2006; Kurzyna *et al*, 2007), and has produced similar results to those of BBAS in terms of symptomatic and hemodynamic benefits, but with an apparent reduction in the procedure-related risks. In 123 reported BDAS procedures there were only 7 (6.6%) immediate procedure-related deaths (Table 8.1). However, the likelihood of spontaneous closure is higher with BDAS than with BBAS. Most recently, a cutting balloon catheter with subsequent balloon dilations is being evaluated.

The precise role of AS in the treatment of PAH remains uncertain because most of the knowledge of its use is derived from small series or case reports. The limitations of these studies include:

• the series were all uncontrolled
• the indication for performing the procedures varied between studies
• the etiology of the pulmonary vascular disease was not the same in all patients
• the medical treatment has changed over the past two decades (Barst, 2000).

Despite these limitations, AS appears to have a place as a therapeutic modality for advanced PAH; in fact, the performance of the procedure has steadily increased over the years (Figure 8.1).

The potential beneficial effects and risks of AS in the setting of PAH were addressed in a review derived from a collective analysis of 64 cases from the literature (Sandoval *et al.*, 2001). The knowledge has now expanded with the report of another 100 cases since the late 1990s (Hayden, 1997; Rothman *et al.*, 1999; Moscucci *et al.*, 2001; Kothari *et al.*, 2002; Allcock *et al.*, 2003; Kurzyna *et al.*, 2003; Reichenberger *et al.*, 2003; Vachiery JL, 2003; Chau *et al.*, 2004; Micheletti *et al.*, 2006). Of the total 164 cases reported (age: 27.3 ± 17.2 years), most were performed in women (73%) with severe idiopathic PAH, i.e. in 128 (78%) of the

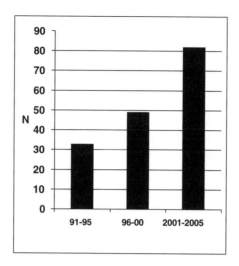

Figure 8.1   Number of atrial septostomy procedures by era: 1991–1995, 1996–2000, 2001–2005.

164 patients. Other etiologies included PAH associated with surgically corrected congenital heart disease (9.1%), PAH associated with connective tissue disease (CTD) (6.7%), peripheral (distal) CTEPH not susceptible to surgical treatment (3%), and other less frequent etiologies (3%). Congestive heart failure (42.5%), syncope (38 %) or both (19.4%) have been the main symptomatic indications for the procedure. The mean NYHA functional class for the group was 3.6. As many as 54 patients who have undergone AS have been regarded as non-responsive to medical treatment, including long-term IV prostacyclin infusion (38) or other prostanoids (5), bosentan (6), prostacyclin plus bosentan (1) or bosentan or prostacyclin combined with sildenafil (4). The simultaneous use of these drugs and AS in these reports as well as the evidence for the safe administration of IV epoprostenol, and subcutaneous treprostinil in the setting of PAH associated to congenital heart disease (Rosenzweig *et al.*, 1999; Simonneau *et al.*, 2002) is supportive of the safety of this potential combination therapy.

Procedure

Two types of atrial septostomy, BBAS and BDAS, have been used in the treatment of PAH. The basic difference between the two procedures is that, in contrast to BBAS, in BDAS, the Park blade septostomy catheter is not used and the interatrial orifice is created by puncture with a Brockenbrough needle and the use of progressively larger balloon catheters in a step-by-step fashion. A 5–10% decrease in $SaO_2\%$ and an increase in left ventricular end-diastolic pressure approaching 18 mm Hg preclude further dilatation (Sandoval *et al.*, 2001). A prospective evaluation of potential differences between the two procedures in regard to hemodynamic results and risk of complications has not been done. The decision to perform BBAS or BDAS should be made in each center based on institutional expertise; however, regardless, the procedure should be performed only in centers experienced in both interventional cardiology and pulmonary hypertension (PH) (Rich *et al.*, 1997; Sandoval *et al.*, 2001). A patient being considered for AS should have a resting arterial O_2 saturation of at least 90% on room air and a hematocrit level greater than 40% to assure maintenance of adequate systemic O_2 transport once the right-to-left shunt is created. Transfusion (with pre-treatment) is not infrequently carried out prior to the procedure. Also, in order to avoid the LV volume overload which would be imposed by the shunt, the patients need to have adequate LV function, as evidenced by the absence of clinically apparent left heart failure and a left ventricular ejection fraction estimated by echocardiography greater than 0.45 (Sandoval and Gaspar, 2004). Optimizing cardiac function before the procedure is also desirable. Some patients with severe RV failure may benefit from a 'preconditioning' regimen with IV dobutamine and diuretics to decrease RV filling pressures, which results in a more favorable hemodynamic condition at the time of the procedure.

There have been some technical modifications to the techniques previously reported. In the most recent one, Micheletti and coworkers introduced a custom-made fenestrated atrial septal device at the end of the procedure in order to keep open the septostomy (Micheletti *et al.*, 2006). By doing this in 7 out of the 20 children, they successfully avoided the spontaneous closure of the defect, a frequent undesirable outcome of BDAS; however, this may increase the risk of a paradoxical embolus if the patient is not adequately anticoagulated.

Outcomes from atrial septostomy

In most of the reported series, AS has been performed in the setting of severe PAH and RVF; accordingly, there is an inherent risk of complications and death during the procedure. In the prior worldwide experience, there was an overall procedure-related mortality of 16.6% and by univariate analysis, a baseline mRAP greater than 20 mm Hg, was the variable most significantly associated with peri-procedural death (Sandoval *et al.*, 2001). Since recommendations to minimize this risk have been established, procedure-related mortality appears to be decreasing (Table 8.1). An mRAP > 20 mm Hg, however, remains a significant risk factor for death (Table 8.2). Causes of immediate death in the 25 out of 164 cases reported so far have been refractory hypoxemia (11), progressive right heart failure (7), procedure-related complications (4), multi-organ failure (1), hemoptysis (1), and unrelated death (dialysis withdrawn, 1).

Symptoms and signs of RVF are improved immediately after AS in the majority of surviving patients (i.e. syncope and systemic venous congestion either disappear or decrease in frequency or intensity) (Sandoval, Rothman *et al.*, 2001). From the total 164 reported cases in the current worldwide experience, 136 (83%) were reported as improved, and from these, 25 (18.4%) were subsequently transplanted.

Table 8.2   Baseline variables associated with procedural death following atrial septostomy

Variable	Alive (*n*)	Dead (*n*)	*p* value
Age (years)	26.4 ± 17.5 (117)	32 ± 15.8 (21)	0.207
Functional class	3.57 ± 0.5 (117)	3.76 ± 0.41	0.089
Mean RAP (mm Hg)	12.7 ± 7 (99)	23.3 ± 9 (16)	0.0001
Mean RAP > 20 mmHg (*n*)	15 / 99 (15%)	12 / 16 (75%)	0.0001
Mean PAP (mm Hg)	63.7 ± 17 (90)	79.8 ± 26 (13)	0.002
CI (l/min/m²)	2.01 ± 0.58 (82)	1.6 ± 0.6 (15)	0.017
PVRI > 55 U m² (*n*)	2 / 89 (2%)	8 / 13 (61.5%)	0.0001

* U Mann-Whitney's Test;   ** Chi-Square's Test (two-tail Fisher's Exact Test).

Exercise endurance, as assessed by the 6-minute walk, was also improved in most of the patients after septostomy in the studies that looked at this (Sandoval *et al.*, 1998; Allcock *et al.*, 2003; Vachiery JL, 2003) (Figure 8.2).

Immediate hemodynamic effects of atrial septostomy

Except for the decrease in SaO_2%, the changes in hemodynamic variables after septostomy are only of moderate magnitude (Sandoval *et al.*, 2001) (Table 8.3). Likewise, the magnitude of hemodynamic changes (increase in CO, and SOT) are not the same for all patients and depend on the level of mRAP. In patients with a

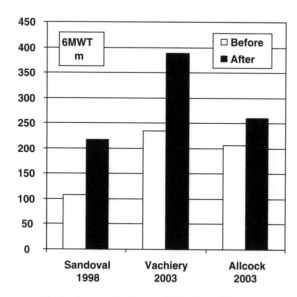

Figure 8.2   Improvement in 6-minute walk distance following atrial septostomy in three studies.

Table 8.3 Hemodynamic changes before and after atrial septostomy ($n = 80$)

Parameter	Before	After	$p <$
Mean RAP (mm Hg)	14 ± 7.4	11 ± 6	0.000
Mean LAP (mm Hg)	6 ± 3	8.5 ± 3	0.000
Cardiac index (l/min/m^2)	2.05 ± 0.54	2.62 ± 0.58	0.000
SaO$_2$ %	93.3 ± 4.4	83.8 ± 7.8	0.000
Mean PAP (mm Hg)	65 ± 16	65.5 ± 17	0.504
Mean SAP (mm Hg)	84 ± 14.5	86.5 ± 14	0.112

From Sandoval, *et al.*, 2001.

RAP < 10 mm Hg, hemodynamic changes are minimal whereas in those with RAP > 20 mm Hg the changes are much more significant. In this last group, however, the risk of procedure-related death is higher. It appears then that the best risk–benefit ratio of AS is for the group with a baseline RAP between 10 and 20 mm Hg (Sandoval *et al.*, 2001; Sandoval and Gaspar, 2004).

Although the immediate hemodynamic changes after septostomy are only moderate (particularly in the group with baseline mRAP less than 10 mm Hg), it has to be stressed that these measurements represent only the resting state. The net hemodynamic effect of septostomy is likely to be different with exercise, as shown in dogs with right ventricular hypertension (Austen *et al.*, 1964). The hemodynamic effects of atrial septostomy during exercise in humans have not been established.

The effect of atrial septostomy on pulmonary blood flow (PBF) and, therefore, on PVR are difficult to assess as, in most of the studies reported so far, a direct measurement of PBF has not been done. Kurzyna and coworkers have reported a significant increase in PVR in some of the patients (Kurzyna *et al.*, 2007). This increase in PVR correlated with the level of mixed venous PO$_2$ after the procedure and it was thought to be responsible in part for the presentation of refractory hypoxemia following AS. In this study, they were able to manage refractory hypoxemia with inhaled iloprost. This most interesting finding deserves future investigation.

Several mechanisms may account for the immediate hemodynamic and observed beneficial clinical effects after AS. These include: decompression of RV chambers at rest, prevention of further RV dilation and dysfunction during exercise and an increase in CO and SOT both at rest and during exercise (via right-to-left shunt). The increase in SOT should also produce beneficial effects on peripheral oxygen utilization and subsequent improvement in exercise capacity (Sandoval *et al.*, 2001; Sandoval and Gaspar, 2004).

It has been shown that PAH patients have an increase in sympathetic nervous activity (SNA) which may, in fact, be one of the pathophysiologic mechanisms leading to RVF (Sandoval and Gaspar, 2004). Ciarka and coworkers have demonstrated a significant decrease in muscle SNA after septostomy in patients with PAH (Ciarka *et al.*, 2006). By decreasing sympathetic overdrive, AS could also improve RV function.

Long-term effects of atrial septostomy

Very little information exists with regard to the long-term hemodynamic effects of AS. In the only study assessing this aspect, Kerstein and coworkers found an improvement in RV function over time in patients who had repeat hemodynamic evaluation 7 to 27 months after septostomy (Kerstein *et al.*, 1995). Their study also raised the possibility of decrease in RV ischemic chest pain owing to a decrease in RV end-diastolic pressure and an increase in right coronary artery driving pressure. Echocardiography studies performed before and six months after AS in patients with PAH by Espínola-Zavaleta and coworkers suggest that AS may also exert beneficial effects on right heart structure and function (Espinola-Zavaleta *et al.*, 1999). One of the findings in this study was a significant decrease in right atrial and RV systolic and diastolic areas after AS, reflecting less right heart dilation after the procedure. This simple decompression effect (decrease in radius) reduces wall stress and may improve RV performance via the La Place relationship (Bristow *et al.*, 1998).

From the clinical point of view, not all patients improve after the procedure. Rothman and coworkers showed that long-term clinical outcome after septostomy seems to depend on the immediate hemodynamic response to the procedure, particularly in terms of the change in cardiac index (CI) and SOT after AS. Compared with patients with no clinical improvement after the procedure, those with significant clinical benefit had a higher and significant increase in CI and SOT immediately after the procedure (Rothman *et al.*, 1999; Sandoval and Gaspar, 2004). Spontaneous closure of the AS appears to occur more often with BDAS than with BBAS. Spontaneous closure also appears to occur more often when the procedure is done for recurrent syncope than for right heart failure as there is a pressure gradient between the RAP and LAP with right heart failure that is more likely to keep the AS open in contrast to patients who have the procedure for recurrent syncope, in whom the RAP is often the same or less than the LAP, increasing the likelihood of spontaneous closure.

Long-term survival following atrial septostomy

The impact of AS on survival of patients with PAH has not been established in prospective and controlled studies. Most reported series, however, have suggested a short-term beneficial effect on the survival of these very sick patients. Long-term survival is limited by late deaths, primarily as a result of progression of the pulmonary vascular disease. By updating the survival estimates of a series of patients reported previously, Sandoval and coworkers found that, after five years of follow-up, the survival of patients diminished considerably (Sandoval *et al.*, 2001). Although limited, the procedure gives the patient a period of time, serving as perhaps a palliative bridge, to other alternatives such as lung transplantation.

Summary of atrial septostomy

Atrial septostomy represents an additional, promising strategy in the treatment of severe PAH. Experience with this procedure is limited, in part because of the relative availability and success of new forms of pharmacological interventions. However, based on analyses of the worldwide experience, several general conclusions can be made:

1 Atrial septostomy can be performed successfully in selected patients with advanced pulmonary vascular disease.
2 In patients with PAH who have undergone successful AS, the procedure has resulted in clinical improvement, beneficial and long-lasting hemodynamic effects at rest, and a trend toward improved survival.
3 The procedure-related mortality is high. Recommendations to minimize this risk are listed below (Sandoval *et al.*, 2001).

  • Atrial septostomy should be performed only at institutions with a track record in the treatment of advanced pulmonary hypertension where atrial septostomy is performed with low morbidity.
  • Atrial septostomy should not be performed in patients with impending death and severe right ventricular failure on maximal cardiorespiratory support. A mRAP > 20 mm Hg, a PVRI > 55 U m^2, and a predicted one-year survival < 40% are all significant predictors of procedure-related death.
  • Before cardiac catheterization, it is important to confirm an acceptable baseline systemic arterial oxygen saturation (> 90% in room air) as well as to optimize cardiac function (adequate right heart filling pressure, additional inotropic support if needed).
  • The following items are mandatory during cardiac catheterization:
    ◦ supplemental oxygen if needed
    ◦ mild and appropriate sedation to prevent anxiety
    ◦ careful monitoring of variables (mLAP, SaO$_2$%, and mRAP)
    ◦ an attempt to use a step-by-step procedure.

After atrial septostomy, it is important to optimize oxygen delivery. Transfusion of packed red blood cells and/or erythropoietin (prior to and following the procedure if needed) may be necessary to increase oxygen content.

  In addition, the consensus is to make the AS perhaps too small (increasing the risk of spontaneous closure with the need to repeat the procedure) rather than risk making the AS too large, resulting in severe hypoxemia with increased mortality and morbidity. Because the disease process in PAH is unaffected by the procedure (late deaths), the long-term effects of an AS must be considered to be palliative. Indications for the procedure include: failure of maximal medical therapy (including oral CCB, prostacyclin analogues, bosentan, and phosphodiesterase-5 inhibitors, alone or combined) with persisting RV failure and/or recurrent syncope, as a bridge to transplantation and, finally, when no other therapeutic options exist (Doyle *et al.*, 2004; Klepetko *et al.*, 2004).

8.3 Pulmonary endarterectomy in chronic thromboembolic pulmonary hypertension

Introduction

Chronic thromboembolic pulmonary hypertension (CTEPH) is a condition characterized by obstruction of the pulmonary vascular bed by single or recurrent organized thromboemboli leading to increased pulmonary vascular resistance,PH and eventually right ventricular failure (Moser *et al.*, 1965). It is generally accepted that pulmonary emboli originating from sites of deep vein thromboses (DVTs) represent the initial event in the pathophysiology of CTEPH, though it is likely that recurrent thromboembolism and/or *in situ* thrombosis contribute in an ongoing fashion to the process (Tapson and Humbert, 2006). Among patients who survive an episode of pulmonary embolism (PE), CTEPH has been estimated to occur in 0.1–0.5% of patients (Dalen and Alpert, 1975; Fedullo and Tapson, 2003), though a more recent study has suggested a much higher incidence of 4% following acute, symptomatic PE (Pengo *et al.*, 2004). Given that venous thromboembolism (VTE) may often be silent, and given the length of time it may take for CTEPH to develop in patients following an inciting event, the true incidence remains difficult to determine. Chronic thromboembolic pulmonary hypertension may in fact represent the most life-threatening end of a spectrum of hemodynamic and anatomic compromise which has the potential to develop in any patient who suffers and survives a PE, but which, in fact, for reasons that are still unclear, occurs in only a minority of patients (Peacock *et al.*, 2006).

Identification of patients with CTEPH is critical because, for many patients with the condition, surgical treatment has been shown to be highly efficacious. Because the clinical presentation of patients with CTEPH, which is characterized by dyspnea and signs of right ventricular failure, may occur long after the acute event, i.e. PE which is often silent and not diagnosed, its clinical course can be indistinguishable from other types of PAH. Radiological imaging plays a central role in making the diagnosis of CTEPH and along with clinical parameters helps determine whether or not a patient is likely to benefit from pulmonary endarterectomy (PEA). This surgical procedure has evolved since the mid 1990s and, while operative mortality was initially quite high, in the current era much lower rates have now been achieved at centers experienced in performing the procedure. Pulmonary endarterectomy has been shown to improve hemodynamics, functional status, quality of life and survival in patients with CTEPH (Mayer and Klepetko, 2006).

Clinical presentation

The clinical presentation of patients with CTEPH may include a history suggesting a prior acute thromboembolic event and/or other known risk factors for VTE, such as a thrombophilia. The presence or absence of co-morbid medical conditions may affect the pace of disease progression in individual patients, affecting their time to presentation and the severity of their symptoms. While CTEPH does not appear to result from any particular thrombophilia, studies have shown higher than normal levels of antiphospholipid antibody and lupus anticoagulant in CTEPH patients (Bonderman *et al.*, 2005; Lang and Kerr, 2006). In addition there is evidence that prothrombotic states such as asplenism or chronic inflammatory disorders may be linked to CTEPH in some patients (Jais *et al.*, 2005). Findings on physical examination, routine diagnostic hematological and blood chemistry tests, pulmonary function tests and echocardiography are similar to those in patients with all forms of PAH (McGoon *et al.*, 2004).

Imaging studies in chronic thromboembolic pulmonary hypertension

Once the diagnosis of PH has been established, the next step is to distinguish large vessel pulmonary vascular disease due to thromboembolism (i.e. CTEPH) from small vessel pulmonary vascular disease. Chest radiographs are likely to have findings consistent with all forms of PH, including enlarged pulmonary arteries and obliteration of the retrosternal airspace owing to enlargement of the right ventricle. Features which may distinguish a patient with CTEPH include irregularly shaped or asymmetrically enlarged pulmonary arteries and evidence of regions of hypoperfusion in the lung parenchyma (Coulden, 2006). A lung ventilation–perfusion scan (V/Q scan) can make the diagnosis of CTEPH and will help determine operability of the patient with CTEPH (Lisbona *et al.*, 1985). In patients with proximal (large vessel) chronic thromboembolic disease, multiple segmental perfusion defects in areas of the lung with normal ventilation are typically seen (Fishman *et al.*, 1983). This is in contrast to findings on V/Q in small vessel pulmonary vascular diseases, such as IPAH, where the pattern of perfusion seen on V/Q scans is less distinct and has been described as mottled. It is important to note, however, that because recanalization can result in the return of some perfusion to some areas of the lung over time, V/Q scans may underestimate the degree of obstruction caused by proximal disease. Mismatched perfusion defects can also be caused by other entities that lead to occlusion or encroachment of the pulmonary arteries, such as mediastinal lymphadenopathy, mediastinal fibrosis or large vessel arteritis (Kerr *et al.*, 1995; Bailey *et al.*, 2000).

While the role of computerized tomography (CT) scanning in diagnosis of CTEPH is not clearly defined, it is of value when alternative explanations for abnormal size or contour of the central pulmonary arteries are being considered, and it can contribute information about the presence or absence of other underlying lung diseases or conditions. A finding of luminal thrombi, occlusions and webs on a CT angiogram may confirm the diagnosis of CTEPH and give some anatomical direction to the surgeon. Contrast-enhanced magnetic resonance (MR) angiography may provide an alternative to a CT angiogram and has shown similar accuracy to V/Q scans in differentiating between patients with IPAH and CTEPH (Bergin *et al.*, 1997) However, one must remain aware that CT angiography has an ~7% false negative rate for diagnosing CTEPH. It is imperative that the radiologist be informed that the procedures are being performed to rule out CTEPH and not just PE. Provision of an adequate surgical 'map' may be obtained by a combination of various noninvasive radiographic techniques, but in most patients pulmonary angiography is still essential to illustrate pulmonary vascular anatomy in enough detail for surgical planning. Pulmonary angioscopy is another useful adjunct to the pre-operative evaluation of patients for PEA and can provide direct visualization of the vascular intima in cases where it is felt that more information on the nature and extent of the organized thromboemboli may influence operability of a borderline candidate for PEA.

Patient selection and assessment of operability

It has been estimated that up to 50% of patients with CTEPH will not be suitable candidates for surgery, due either to the anatomy and pathophysiology of their vascular disease or to the presence of medical co-morbidities. Basic selection criteria for patients being considered for PEA include the following

- NYHA class III or IV symptoms
- a pre-operative PVR > 300 dyn s/cm^5
- a surgically accessible thrombus in the main lobar or segmental pulmonary arteries
- the absence of severe co-morbidities such as severe underlying lung disease (Doyle, McCrory *et al.*, 2004).

In several studies a high pre-operative PVR (> 1000 dyn s/cm^5) has been associated with poor outcomes and increased mortality and such values are considered a relative contraindication to successful PEA (Jamieson *et al.*, 2003; Dartevelle *et al.*, 2004). Assessment for the presence of hemodynamically significant distal disease (either distal thromboembolic obstruction or small vessel pulmonary vascular disease) and ascertainment of its contribution to elevated PVR is a critical element in patient selection (Kim, 2006). For example, if the degree of hemodynamic compromise appears to be out of proportion to the radiographically quantifiable proximal obstruction, then it is likely that distal, inaccessible clot and/or microvascular disease are the predominant contributors to the elevated PVR, making the patient a poor candidate for PEA, as relief of the proximal obstruction may have minimal impact on overall PVR (Thistlethwaite *et al.*, 2002; Kim *et al.*, 2004). There are no precise figures for an acceptable post-operative PVR but given that the greatest risk factor for post-operative mortality in patients undergoing PEA is persistent PH, many experts agree that the operation should only be performed in patients in whom a reduction in PVR of greater than 50% can be expected (Klepetko *et al.*, 2004).

Pulmonary endarterectomy: operative procedure and post-operative management

The pulmonary endarterectomy operation is performed via a median sternotomy and involves total circulatory arrest under conditions of profound hypothermia.

The intraluminal material in CTEPH is inseparable from the intima of the pulmonary artery such that surgical removal requires a true endarterectomy and is thus distinct from a mere thrombectomy or embolectomy (Jamieson *et al.*, 1993; Jamieson *et al.*, 2003) (Plate 7). Two major post-operative complications have been described – reperfusion edema in the endarterectomized parts of the lung and persistent PH, leading to right ventricular failure. Management of post-operative complications following PEA is thus geared towards maneuvers that reduce PVR and optimize right heart function. Ventilator techniques which minimize interactions with the circulatory system, use of inhaled nitric oxide or prostanoids to reduce PVR and inotropes to support RV function, are all treatment strategies which may be helpful (Mares *et al.*, 2000; Kramm *et al.*, 2005). One series has reported successful use of extra corporeal membrane oxidation (ECMO) in post-operative PEA patients with severe reperfusion injury (Thistlethwaite *et al.*, 2006). There is not enough data yet to support a standardized approach to post-operative management of patients undergoing PEA. For select high-risk patients being considered for PEA there is evidence that pre-operative medical therapy may provide an alternative to surgery and, in some patients who do undergo surgery, could help avoid or attenuate some of these post-operative complications (Ghofrani *et al.*, 2003; Bresser *et al.*, 2004; Bonderman *et al.*, 2005).

Outcomes of pulmonary endarterectomy for chronic thromboembolic pulmonary hypertension

PEA leads to significant reductions in PAP and improvements in CO in most patients. For most patients following surgery a near normal CO is achieved with mPAP of 20–30 mm Hg (Jamieson *et al.*, 1993). Marked post-operative improvements in RV size and function with normalization of septal motion and concomitant improvements in LV function have been reported using echocardiography (Menzel *et al.*, 2000). There is also evidence that PEA leads to significant improvements in gas exchange via improvements in V/Q matching post-operatively (Kapitan *et al.*, 1990). In terms of functional outcomes, more than 90% of patients undergoing successful PEA improve from NYHA class III or IV pre-operatively to NYHA class I or II post-operatively. Early attempts at PEA were associated with in-hospital mortality rates as high as 24% and some single-center experiences have continued with similar outcomes (Gilbert *et al.*, 1998). With improvements in patient selection, surgical technique and peri-operative management, experienced centers have reported post-operative mortality in the range of 4% to 8% (Jamieson *et al.*, 2003; Ogino *et al.*, 2006). Major causes of in-hospital mortality include persistent PH and reperfusion edema, which together account for over 50% of deaths (Doyle *et al.*, 2004; Klepetko *et al.*, 2004). Long-term survival data are limited but the UCSD group has reported a 75% six year survival among 308 patients (Archibald *et al.*, 1999) while a recent study from Japan in 88 patients reported an actuarial survival rate of 91% at three years and 86% at five years (Ogino, Ando *et al.*, 2006).

Adjunctive therapy in chronic thromboembolic pulmonary hypertension

While most patients who have successful PEA have stable long-term results, redo operations are not uncommon (Mo *et al.*, 1999). Operative mortality comparable to the initial operation has been reported but hemodynamic improvements were less notable. Risk factors for redo PEA include suboptimal anticoagulation and ineffective caval filtration; thus, while there are no formal studies of their efficacy, inferior vena cava (IVC) filter placement and lifelong anticoagulation are recommended for all patients with CTEPH. In patients in whom surgical therapy is not an option owing to the distal location of their disease, balloon angioplasty has been suggested (Feinstein *et al.*, 2001) but is still considered investigational. New medical therapies may supplant the need for surgery in some CTEPH patients, or may facilitate clinical improvements such that patients deemed too high risk for PEA can become eligible for the operation (Bresser *et al.*, 2004; Bresser *et al.*, 2006). Case series and recent clinical studies also suggest that PAH disease-targeted medical therapies, e.g. prostacyclin analogues, endothelin receptor antagonists, phosphodiesterase type 5 inhibitors, are often effective in patients with inoperable CTEPH and/or significant residual PH following PEA.

8.4 Lung transplantation for pulmonary hypertension

Introduction

Lung transplantation for pulmonary vascular disease began in 1981 when Reitz and colleagues at Stanford performed the first successful heart–lung transplantation (HLT) in a patient with IPAH (Reitz *et al.*, 1982). As this procedure gained acceptance, patients with other pulmonary diseases underwent the operation and, in contrast to patients undergoing single lung transplantation (SLT) in the late 1960s, the survival rates were much better (Doyle and Theodore, 1997). Following the introduction of cyclosporine in 1981 and after a period of research the Toronto group reported success with SLT in patients with pulmonary fibrosis in 1986 (Patterson, 1986). The treatment of patients with septic lung disease and pulmonary vascular diseases helped spur the development of double lung en-bloc transplantation by Patterson and colleagues in 1988 (Patterson *et al.*, 1988). The en-bloc procedure as originally described shortly gave way to the bilateral sequential single lung transplant (BLT), in which two separate bronchial anastomoses were utilized. This improved BLT procedure involved less mediastinal dissection and resulted in superior airway healing owing to the improved vascularization in the donor mainstem bronchi as compared to the trachea (Pasque *et al.*, 1990). Over time it became apparent that, for many patients with pulmonary vascular disease, BLT, or in some cases SLT, could replace HLT. Since the mid-1990s there has been an overall decline in the number of lung or heart-lung transplants performed in patients with PH compared with other indications, likely due to the clinical development of new medical therapies (Plate 8). The decision to pursue transplantation and the choice of the appropriate surgical procedure is based on the patient's diagnosis, their response to therapy and organ availability and is usually at the discretion of the individual transplant center.

Choice of transplant operation in pulmonary hypertension

Idiopathic pulmonary arterial hypertension and PAH in the setting of congenital heart disease (CHD), or Eisenmenger syndrome, are the most common indications for HLT (Trulock et al., 2006). While HLT was the first successful transplant procedure for PAH, given the persistent shortage of organs BLT is the preferred procedure in most patients with IPAH, leaving the donor heart for use for isolated cardiac transplantation (Doyle et al., 2004; Levine, 2004). The severe RV dysfunction seen in PAH is usually reversible after BLT with RV dimensions and function returning to normal or near-normal by three months following transplantation (Kramer et al., 1994; Kasimir et al., 2004). Thus combined HLT is generally only indicated for patients with Eisenmenger's syndrome due to complex CHD, in patients with parenchymal lung disease and in patients with compromised LV function. Patients with simple CHD and PAH can successfully undergo BLT with cardiac repair in most cases. Whether HLT offers a survival benefit over SLT or BLT is unclear, with some studies showing no benefit in survival (Chapelier et al., 1993; Ueno et al., 2000; Mendeloff et al., 2002), while others have shown improved survival with HLT compared to SLT and BLT (Whyte et al., 1999; Franke et al., 2000).

Proponents of SLT for PAH argue that it is an easier operation to perform and allows for more efficient use of organs for transplantation (Gammie et al., 1998). Detractors note the potential for V/Q mismatch and a higher likelihood of reperfusion injury in patients with PAH undergoing SLT (Bando et al., 1994; Bando et al., 1994; Boujoukos et al., 1997). Bilateral lung transplantation for PAH may result in fewer complications in the post-operative period compared to SLT and may also enable the use of more 'marginal' lungs. In addition, by providing better overall lung function at the outset, BLT could be more protective against the physiologic derangements associated with chronic rejection. In a report from Hopkins, survival in IPAH patients who had BLT was better than the survival in those who had SLT. However, the same group found that in patients with PH associated with parenchymal lung disease there was no advantage for BLT over SLT, except in patients in whom mPAP was >40 mm Hg (Conte et al., 2001).

Another larger study from the International Society for Heart and Lung Transplantation (ISHLT) database on the effect of pre-operative pulmonary artery pressure on 90-day mortality following lung transplantation in patients with idiopathic pulmonary fibrosis (IPF) found that patients with a mPAP of ± 35 mm Hg undergoing SLT had a 1.5-fold increase in 90-day mortality (Whelan *et al.*, 2005). In comparing 636 SLT with 194 BLT transplant operations in IPF patients this study also found that BLT, regardless of PAP, was itself a risk factor for 90-day mortality. This is likely due to SLT being a simpler and shorter operation than either BLT or HLT. There are no randomized studies to determine the optimal transplant procedure for PAH, and such studies are unlikely to occur. However, recent guidelines from the ACCP suggest that based on current data and consensus opinion BLT is the transplant procedure of choice in IPAH patients (Doyle *et al.*, 2004). For patients with PH due to parenchymal lung disease the choice of operation is less clear. Older patients in whom mPAP is less than 35 mm Hg might do better with a SLT, i.e. a simpler operation with lower post-operative mortality. The decision, however, about which procedure is indicated in any given patient will largely depend on the availability of organs and the experience of the transplant center.

Timing of transplantation in pulmonary hypertension

The timing of transplantation depends on several factors, including the patient's underlying diagnosis, stage of disease, availability of alternative treatments, response to medical therapy, suitability for an operation, co-morbidities and local waiting time for donors. Data from the US IPAH (previously termed primary PH, PPH) registry estimated the median survival in IPAH patients prior to the availability of disease-specific targeted treatment, i.e. prostacyclin analogues, endothelin receptor antagonists, phosphodiesterase type 5 inhibitors, at 2.8 years from the time of diagnosis, and mean right atrial pressure, CI and mPAP were the variables most closely associated with mortality in that study (D'Alonzo *et al.*, 1991). A mean right atrial pressure of 20 mm Hg or greater was associated with a median one-month survival. The emergence of IV epoprostenol in the 1990s dramatically changed the paradigm for the evaluation and listing of most patients with PAH, and improvement in survival in PAH with the use of long-term IV epoprostenol has clearly impacted center practices (Conte *et al.*, 1998; Robbins *et al.*, 1998). Prior to the epoprostenol era it was generally recommended that all PH patients who were in NYHA Classes III or IV should be referred for transplantation. It is now recommended that referral should be initiated in those patients who fail to show a benefit after three months of therapy with long-term IV epoprostenol. However, referring physicians should factor in the time needed to complete a proper evaluation of transplant candidates as well as the potential waiting time for a donor (Doyle *et al.*, 2004).

There are hemodynamic parameters generally accepted as indications for transplant in patients with PAH and these include a mPAP > 55 mm Hg, a mean right atrial pressure (RAP) > 15 mm Hg, and a CI < 2 l/min/m^2 (Glanville *et al.*, 1987). Similar levels of PAP are associated with lower RAP, a better CI and a better prognosis in patients with PAH related to CHD, and many of these patients may live into their adult years despite severe hemodynamic derangements. In contrast to PAH, natural history studies for patients with Eisenmenger syndrome have demonstrated 80% five-year survival and 40% 25-year survival. Since hemodynamic parameters are less helpful in these patients as guidelines, the presence of progressive signs and symptoms such as hemoptysis, chest pain, dizziness, arrhythmias, worsening shortness of breath and functional deterioration to NYHA Class III or IV may signal a significant decline. Special consideration should be given to listing any PH patient who presents with exertional syncope, life-threatening hemoptysis or malignant arrhythmias.

Frequently the identification of a critical turning point in a patient's disease which signals an accelerated decline is key to the timing of transplantation. Prior to the advent of IV epoprostenol these critical turning points for patients with PAH were perhaps unfortunately easier to identify and more predictable. It is likely that, even in the era of improved medical therapies, parameters of RV function (CI, RAP) are still highly predictive of death in PH patients, but the timing of transplant may now be more problematic. For example in the case of a patient who has been on long-term IV epoprostenol therapy (five years or longer) and appears to be declining it is unclear if it is realistic or appropriate to potentially delay transplantation while adding new therapies. Delays due to the use of combined medical therapies could prove detrimental if they fail and/or if sicker patients undergo transplant, potentially leading to worse outcomes. As more data on the impact of new therapies on survival in PAH accumulate, hopefully these questions can be answered.

Timing of transplantation in pulmonary hypertension and organ allocation

Another variable that must be considered in the timing of transplantation is the organ allocation system in the country in which the patient is seeking transplantation and the local waiting times involved. In the US, a new UNOS Lung Allocation System was implemented in 2005 for patients 12 years and older in the hope that allocation of organs could be based primarily on medical urgency, while avoiding futile transplants. The Lung Allocation Score (LAS) for each listed patient is calculated using the following measures: (1) waitlist urgency measure, (2) post-transplant survival measure. The waitlist urgency measure and the post-transplant survival measure are generated using Cox proportional hazards models (Table 8.4). Factors used to predict the risk of death on the transplant list (waitlist urgency measure) include forced vital capacity (FVC), insulin-dependent diabetes, age, body mass index (BMI), NYHA class, 6-minute walk test, ventilator use and diagnosis. Factors used to predict one-year survival (post-transplant survival measure) after transplant include FVC, ventilator use, age, creatinine, NYHA class and diagnosis. The final LAS, which is meant to reflect the overall transplant benefit, incorporates these two elements of the equation. Clinical variables on which the LAS is based must be updated every six months at a minimum but can be updated more frequently. The LAS

Table 8.4 Clinical variables used for UNOS Lung Allocation Score (LAS) calculation

Characteristics for waitlist urgency measure	Characteristics for post-transplant survival measure
Age (years)	Age at transplant (years)
Body mass index (kg/m^2)	Creatinine at transplant (mg/dl)
Diabetes	New York Heart Association functional class
New York Heart Association functional class	Forced vital capacity for groups B and D (% predicted)
Forced vital capacity (% predicted)	Pulmonary capillary wedge pressure mean 20 mm Hg for group D
Pulmonary arterial systolic pressure for diagnosis groups A, C, and D	Mechanical ventilation
Oxygen requirements at rest (l/min)	Diagnosis groups*
6-minute walk distance	Detailed diagnosis**
Continuous mechanical ventilation	
Diagnosis groups*	
Detailed diagnosis *	

*Diagnosis groups: **A** = Obstructive lung disease; **B** = Pulmonary vascular disease; **C** = Cystic fibrosis or immunodeficiency disorder; **D** = Restrictive lung disease.
** Detailed diagnosis: Bronchiectasis; Eisenmenger syndrome; Lymphangioleiomyomatosis; Obliterative bronchiolitis; Pulmonary fibrosis; Sarcoidosis with mPAP > 30 mm Hg; Sarcoidosis with mPAP < 30 mm Hg.

does not contain variables for clinical events important to PAH patients such as syncope, hemoptysis or arrhythmias and thus patients with these symptoms may receive an LAS score which is not reflective of the severity of their illness. In cases where a center feels this is the case an appeal can be made to the UNOS Lung Review Board. Unfortunately this may frequently be the case for patients with PAH in whom cardiac function, which is not currently assessed in the LAS, is the main determinant of survival. Given concerns about the LAS as it pertains to PH patients, in the fall of 2006 an amendment was passed by UNOS which stated that PH patients with a CI < 1.8 l/min/m^2 and/or a RAP > 15 mm Hg and evidence of clinical right heart failure, upon appeal to the Lung Review Board, could be granted a higher LAS.

Selection of candidates for transplantation

Selection of patients for transplantation is based on objective clinical data derived from an evaluation of each individual patient and a critical assessment of diagnostic studies, e.g. complete pulmonary function testing, 6-minute walk test, chest radiographs and CT scans, echocardiograms and hemodynamic parameters obtained from cardiac catheterization. In terms of laboratory studies, a pre-operative serum creatinine level should be less than 1.5 mg/dl and a 24-h creatinine clearance greater than 50 ml/min. Patients in whom impaired renal function can be attributed to poor cardiac output may be an exception to this rule. Hyperbilirubinemia of greater than 2.5 mg/dl has been shown to be a marker of poor outcome in patients with PAH undergoing transplantation (Jamieson *et al.*, 1984; Kramer *et al.*, 1991a; Kramer, Marshall *et al.*, 1991b) and may be encountered frequently in PAH patients, owing to passive hepatic congestion.

Donor matching

Donor matching in lung and heart–lung transplantation is based on size and ABO compatibility alone, and human leukocyte antigens (HLA) matching is not possible, though mismatches at particular loci have been shown to be detrimental and are known to impact outcome (Trulock *et al.*, 2006). Extensive laboratory evaluations, including a panel reactive antibody (PRA) screen, are performed in all potential transplant recipients to exclude the presence of preformed antibodies. A PRA > 10% has been associated with worse outcomes after transplantation (Gammie *et al.*, 1997; Hadjiliadis *et al.*, 2005). A variety of maneuvers aimed at reducing preformed antibodies prior to transplant are available to highly sensitized patients but depending on the type of antibodies may prove more or less efficacious in individual patients. Patients in whom this screening test is positive undergo direct cross-match from the donor prospectively prior to transplantation. Screening for infectious diseases including hepatitis, human immunodeficiency virus (HIV), cytomegalovirus (CMV), Epstein-Barr virus (EBV), varicella-zoster virus (VZV) and herpes simplex virus (HSV) is also performed prior to transplantation. The seroprevalence of CMV in the general population varies from 40% to 90% (Ljungman *et al.*, 2002) but when possible donor and recipient are matched for CMV status. The incidence of CMV disease is 50%–80% in lung and heart–lung transplant recipients, and the major risk factor for CMV disease in solid organ transplantation is a seronegative recipient and a seropositive donor (van der Bij and Speich, 2001). In CMV-exposed patients, aggressive prophylaxis for CMV following transplantation is used to attenuate the impact of serious CMV infection on the transplant recipient.

General criteria

Contraindications to transplantation include the presence of uncontrolled systemic disease such as sepsis or thrombophilia, malignancy or diseases resulting in multiple end organ damage or failure (Maurer *et al.*, 1998; Orens *et al.*, 2006) These are listed below.

- significant systemic or multisystem disease
- active extrapulmonary infection
- significant hepatic disease
- significant renal disease
- cachexia or obesity
- current cigarette smoking
- inability or unwillingness to comply with therapeutic plan

- drug or alcohol abuse
- age > 65 years
- symptomatic osteoporosis
- severe chest wall deformity
- hepatitis B or C infection
- malignancy precluding long-term survival

A psychosocial assessment is done to help ascertain the adequacy of the patient's social support system and their ability to cope with the stress of the operative and post-operative period. An inability or an unwillingness to comply with recommended treatments and any ongoing substance abuse or smoking are considered contraindications to transplantation. There is a requirement for routine health maintenance exams (e.g. PAP smear, mammography, colon cancer screening, prostate cancer screening) which should be performed using guidelines established for the general population. Osteoporosis leading to fractures with pain and impaired mobility is a significant cause of morbidity in patients following transplantation and should be screened for and treated aggressively (Aris *et al.*, 1996). Clinical symptoms suggestive of gastroesophageal reflux disease (GERD) should be evaluated as indicated, as significant GERD following transplantation may adversely impact graft survival and function (Berkowitz *et al.*, 1995)

Age

Age is an important determinant of outcomes following lung or heart–lung transplantation; thus age limits for transplantation are a reasonable criteria for patient selection. In the ISHLT analysis from 1995–2005 there was no significant difference in survival among age groups at three months, but by one year survival was significantly better in the younger age cohorts (18 to 34 year olds and 35 to 49 year olds) compared to the older age cohorts (50 to 59, 60 to 64 and > 65 years). After five years, survival rates for recipients less than 49 years old were 10–14% higher than those for patients greater than 60 years of age at the time of transplant (Trulock *et al.*, 2006). Age limits by procedure which have been used are: HLT – 50 years, BLT – 55 years, SLT – 60 years (based on data demonstrating no survival benefit with transplant over survival without transplant in patient > 65 years). Some centers may use more strict, and others more liberal, age criteria but co-morbidities associated with increasing age impact long-term survival and would favor the former approach over the latter.

Post-operative management of lung and heart–lung recipients

Following lung and heart–lung transplantation, patients are kept euvolemic to hypovolemic to protect the pulmonary allograft, which is susceptible to pulmonary edema. This is due to the absence of lymphatic drainage and the presence of at least some degree of reperfusion injury, which increases pulmonary capillary permeability. Barring the development of severe reperfusion injury (also known as primary graft dysfunction (PGD)) most patients are extubated within 24 to 48 hours following surgery. Aggressive respiratory therapy and sufficient pain control are employed to allow for early mobilization of patients. Prophylactic antibiotics are frequently given in the first 5–7 days after transplant. Initial immunosuppression includes steroids, azathioprine or mycophenolate mofetil (MMF), and cyclosporine or tacrolimus. Cytolytic induction therapy with rabbit antithymocyte globulin (RATG, when it is used) is given intravenously on post-operative days one, two and three. In the ISHLT Registry, induction therapy with a polyclonal ATG reduced the incidence of rejection in the first year when compared to either no induction or to induction with monoclonal IL-2 receptor antagonists (Trulock *et al.*, 2006). Patients receive a pulse of IV methylpred-nisolone within 24 hours of the transplant, then oral prednisolone is begun and slowly tapered to a maintenance dose of 1.0 mg/kg; patients remain on steroids, azathioprine or MMF, and cyclosporine or tacrolimus, indefinitely. Rejection episodes are treated with pulsed IV methylprednisolone 1 g/day for three days, followed by an increase in oral prednisolone for approximately four weeks.

Complications and outcomes following lung transplantation

Primary graft dysfunction

Primary graft dysfunction is characterized by hypoxia, impaired ventilation, hypercapnia and diffuse chest radiograph infiltrates, and occurs in about 10–20% of patients following lung transplantation, usually within the first 72 hours (Christie *et al.*, 2003). A pre-operative diagnosis of PAH has been cited as a risk factor for PGD (Barr *et al.*, 2005) and recent data suggest that this could be due to the impaired thrombolytic system common in pulmonary vas-cular disease, leading to increased microthromboses and graft dysfunction (Christie *et al.*, 2007). The management of PGD is supportive including appro-priate ventilatory and hemodynamic maneuvers. Inhaled nitric oxide (NO) may be useful for treating established PGD when mild to moderate PH and hypoxia are both present but it does not appear effective as prophylaxis against PGD (Shargall *et al.*, 2005).

Acute rejection

Acute rejection is diagnosed using transbronchial lung biopsy specimens obtained during fiberoptic bronchoscopy. Acute rejection can be subtle and indistinguishable from other complications, including infection. Acute rejection is often character-ized by low-grade fevers, impaired oxygenation and new findings on chest radi-ograph, including new parenchymal infiltrates and/or subtle bilateral effusions.

Acute rejection can also occur in the absence of clinical or functional deterioration; thus routine surveillance lung biopsies with bronchoalveolar lavage are performed at two and four weeks and then at two, three, six and twelve months after transplantation (Glanville, 2006).

Infection

Bacterial infection is the most common cause of early post-operative death following lung transplantation and remains an important source of mortality beyond the first year. Following lung or heart–lung transplantation, patients are particularly susceptible to pneumonia owing to the combined effects of immune suppression and alterations in natural defense mechanisms such as cough and mucociliary clearance. Cytomegalovirus infection is a very common problem in the first year following transplantation but with the use of prophylactic treatment outcomes have improved. Cytomegalovirus infection is extremely common in lung allografts but can also cause disease in other organs such as the gastrointestinal tract. Fungi are significant pathogens in lung transplant, and in the case of aspergillus can represent a life-threatening infection. Aspergillus infection in the lung transplant recipient can present as a bronchitis, an invasive pneumonia or as disseminated disease and in the latter case carries a high mortality (Westney *et al.*, 1996). The introduction of regular oral prophylaxis with trimethoprim/sulfamethoxazole has reduced the incidence of infection with *Pneumocystis jirovecii* (formerly known as *Pneumocystis carinii* or PCP), once a significant cause of pneumonia following lung transplantation.

Malignancy

Immune suppression following lung transplantation can lead to malignant complications, with lymphoid neoplasms and skin cancers the most common. Post-transplant lymphoproliferative disease (PTLD), a B-cell Non-Hodgkin's lymphoma associated with the EBV, generally appears in the allograft and usually responds to a reduction in the level of immune suppression and treatment of the EBV with acyclovir (Ramalingam *et al.*, 2002; Gao *et al.*, 2003; Reams *et al.*, 2003). Depending, however, on the aggressiveness of the PTLD and whether or not it is disseminated at the time of diagnosis, conventional chemotherapy and chemotherapy using anti-CD 20 agents may be required (Knoop *et al.*, 2006).

Renal dysfunction

Renal dysfunction is common following lung transplantation and is due in large part to the effects of chronic use of the calcineurin antagonists, tacrolimus and cyclosporine. These drugs are a cornerstone of therapy following lung transplantation

Table 8.5 The cumulative prevalence of systemic hypertension, renal dysfunction, hyperlipidemia and diabetes in survivors after lung transplantation within one and five years post transplant

Outcome	Within one year (%)	Within five years (%)
Systemic hypertension	51.3	85.5
Renal dysfunction	25.7	39.4
Abnormal creatinine < 2.5 mg/dl	16.2	22.7
Creatinine > 2.5 mg/dl	7.6	12.8
Chronic dialysis	1.9	3.2
Renal transplant	0.0	0.7
Hyperlipidemia	18.8	49.3
Diabetes	22.6	31.5

Data from ISHLT Registry: April 1994 to June 2005.

such that attempts to employ immune suppressive regimens without them have by and large proven unsuccessful. In patients who develop renal insufficiency, the decline in renal function typically begins within the first three to six months and stabilizes within the first year after transplantation. Reducing the dose of the calcineurin inhibitor usually results in improvement in renal function, although in some patients the renal damage is irreversible and progressive. Strategies to minimize renal damage include close monitoring of drug levels and maintenance of low therapeutic trough levels of the calcineurin inhibitors. Among patients who survive at least five years following lung transplantation, renal dysfunction is very common (Table 8.5).

Diabetes, hyperlipidemia and hypertension

Diabetes mellitus is common following lung transplantation and is due to the adverse effects of immunosuppressive drugs, including prednisone. Cyclosporine and tacrolimus are associated with impaired glucose tolerance, independent of corticosteroid therapy. Immunosuppressive agents, particularly cyclosporine and prednisone are also implicated in the development of hyperlipidemia following transplantation. Systemic hypertension is very common following solid organ transplantation and generally requires treatment.

Chronic rejection

Chronic rejection of the lung allograft, known as bronchiolitis obliterans syndrome (BOS), is characterized by progressive irreversible airflow obstruction which, over a period of months, can lead to respiratory failure and death (Estenne *et al.*, 2002). It is the major limiting factor in the long-term survival of patients following lung transplantation, affecting approximately 50% of lung transplant recipients who survive to five years (Levine and Bryan, 1995; Trulock *et al.*, 2006). It is generally unresponsive to treatment, though some patients may respond to augmented immune suppression (Glanville *et al.*, 1987) with improvements or stabilization of lung function for some period of time.

Outcomes and survival following lung transplantation

Major causes of early death after transplantation include technical complications, graft failure and infection. Major causes of late death include infection and BOS, i.e. chronic rejection. Although any injury to the lung may contribute to the development of BOS, including infection, reperfusion injury or acute rejection, the relationship of BOS to the recipient's diagnosis and type of transplant procedure is unclear. Survival for all lung transplant recipients in the ISHLT database from 1994 through 2004 was 78% at one year, 61% at three years 49% at five years and 25% at ten years. Survival in SLT and BLT recipients is comparable at one year but BLT appeared to have better survival further out in this analysis. However BLT and SLT recipients likely have differences with regard to age and indications for transplant, and these differences are not accounted for in this analysis. Pre-transplant diagnosis can affect early peri-operative mortality but late mortality is caused mainly by complications from the transplant itself, not from issues related to pre-transplantation disease. This is important in PAH, which has been traditionally associated with poor one-year survival, but where conditional survival analyses reveals that recipients with PAH have comparable survival to other recipients at five years and significantly better survival out to ten years compared to those with IPF and COPD (Trulock *et al.*, 2006). In terms of heart–lung transplantation, early survival rates have improved compared with previous eras and one-year and five-year survival of 73% and 44% have been reported. In the ISHLT registry, among pulmonary vascular diseases pretransplant diagnosis appears to be a major determinant of survival, with survival rates out to ten years the highest among patients with Eisenmenger's syndrome, intermediate for IPAH and lowest for PAH associated with other conditions such as CTDs.

The UNOS Registry provides survival data from all transplants in the US. In the UNOS Registry for heart–lung transplant recipients with a diagnosis of IPAH, the one-, three- and five-year survival is reported as 83%, 61% and 49%, respectively (www.unos.org, February 2007). For heart–lung recipients with a diagnosis of PAH related to CHD, survival at one, three and five years is 61%, 52% and 38%, respectively. For patients with IPAH undergoing lung transplantation alone, one-, three- and five-year survival is reported at 75%, 60% and 48%, respectively. It has also been shown that lung transplantation can improve health-related quality of life in patients (TenVergert *et al.*, 1998). In one report at least 80% of lung or heart–lung transplant survivors reported no limitation in activity at one year, three years and five years following transplantation, and 50% were working either full-time or part-time (Hertz *et al.*, 2003) (Plate 9).

8.5   Conclusions

While medical therapy for PAH has advanced significantly since the mid-1990s, many patients may, in the course of their treatment, require further intervention. Atrial septostomy is one intervention used in the treatment of severe PAH when maximal medical therapy has failed and when no other therapeutic options exist. Since procedure-related mortality is high, selection of patients is critical. Atrial septostomy should be performed at centers experienced in the procedure and in the management of patients with advanced pulmonary vascular disease. Successful AS can result in a significant clinical improvement but its long-term effects must be considered palliative. The clinical presentation of patients with CTEPH can be indistinguishable from other types of PAH. Radiological imaging plays a pivotal role in the identification and characterization of patients with CTEPH and is key to identifying patients who will benefit from PEA. Pulmonary endarterectomy has been shown to improve hemodynamics, functional status, quality of life and survival in patients with CTEPH. Lung or heart–lung transplantation is indicated in patients with PAH who are declining despite aggressive medical therapy and/or other interventions. While BLT is the transplant procedure of choice in most IPAH patients, the decision about the appropriate operative procedure depends on the availability of organs and the experience of the transplant center. Chronic rejection of the lung allograft is characterized by progressive irreversible airflow obstruction, which can lead to respiratory failure and death. It affects up to 50% of patients at five years following transplantation and is the major limiting factor in the long-term survival of patients following lung or heart–lung transplantation.

References

Allcock, R.J., J.J. O'Sullivan *et al.* (2003). Atrial septostomy for pulmonary arterial hypertension. *Heart* **89**(11): 1344–7.

Archibald, C.J., W.R. Auger *et al.* (1999). Long-term outcome after pulmonary thromboendarterectomy. *Am J Respir Crit Care Med* **160**(2): 523–8.

Aris, R.M., I.P. Neuringer *et al.* (1996). Severe osteoporosis before and after lung transplantation. *Chest* **109**(5): 1176–83.

Austen, W.G., A.G. Morrow *et al.* (1964). Experimental Studies of the Surgical Treatment of Primary Pulmonary Hypertension. *J Thorac Cardiovasc Surg* **48**: 448–55.

Badesch, D.B., S.H. Abman *et al.* (2004). Medical therapy for pulmonary arterial hypertension: ACCP evidence-based clinical practice guidelines. *Chest* **126**(1 Suppl): 35S-62S.

Bailey, C.L., R.N. Channick *et al.* (2000). 'High probability' perfusion lung scans in pulmonary venoocclusive disease. *Am J Respir Crit Care Med* **162**(5): 1974–8.

Bando, K., J.M. Armitage *et al.* (1994). Indications for and results of single, bilateral, and heart-lung transplantation for pulmonary hypertension. *J Thorac Cardiovasc Surg* **108**(6): 1056–65.

Bando, K., R.J. Keenan *et al.* (1994). Impact of pulmonary hypertension on outcome after single-lung transplantation. *Ann Thorac Surg* **58**(5): 1336–42.

Barr, M.L., S.M. Kawut *et al.* (2005). Report of the ISHLT Working Group on Primary Lung Graft Dysfunction part IV: recipient-related risk factors and markers. *J Heart Lung Transplant* **24**(10): 1468–82.

Barst, R.J. (2000). Role of atrial septostomy in the treatment of pulmonary vascular disease. *Thorax* **55**(2): 95–6.

Bergin, C.J., J. Hauschildt *et al.* (1997). Accuracy of MR angiography compared with radionuclide scanning in identifying the cause of pulmonary arterial hypertension. *AJR Am J Roentgenol* **168**(6): 1549–55.

Bergin, C.J., C.B. Sirlin *et al.* (1997). Chronic thromboembolism: diagnosis with helical CT and MR imaging with angiographic and surgical correlation. *Radiology* **204**(3): 695–702.

Berkowitz, N., L.L. Schulman *et al.* (1995). Gastroparesis after lung transplantation. Potential role in postoperative respiratory complications. *Chest* **108**(6): 1602–7.

Bonderman, D., J. Jakowitsch *et al.* (2005). Medical conditions increasing the risk of chronic thromboembolic pulmonary hypertension. *Thromb Haemost* **93**(3): 512–6.

Bonderman, D., R. Nowotny *et al.* (2005). Bosentan therapy for inoperable chronic thromboembolic pulmonary hypertension. *Chest* **128**(4): 2599–603.

Boujoukos, A.J., G.D. Martich *et al.* (1997). Reperfusion injury in single-lung transplant recipients with pulmonary hypertension and emphysema. *J Heart Lung Transplant* **16**(4): 439–48.

Bresser, P., P.F. Fedullo *et al.* (2004). Continuous intravenous epoprostenol for chronic thromboembolic pulmonary hypertension. *Eur Respir J* **23**(4): 595–600.

Bresser, P., J. Pepke-Zaba *et al.* (2006). Medical therapies for chronic thromboembolic pulmonary hypertension: an evolving treatment paradigm. *Proc Am Thorac Soc* **3**(7): 594–600.

Bristow, M.R., L.S. Zisman *et al.* (1998). The pressure-overloaded right ventricle in pulmonary hypertension. *Chest* **114**(1 Suppl): 101S-106S.

Chapelier, A., P. Vouhe *et al.* (1993). Comparative outcome of heart-lung and lung transplantation for pulmonary hypertension. *J Thorac Cardiovasc Surg* **106**(2): 299–307.

Chau, E.M., K.Y. Fan *et al.* (2004). Combined atrial septostomy and oral sildenafil for severe right ventricular failure due to primary pulmonary hypertension. *Hong Kong Med J* **10**(4): 281–4.

Christie, J.D., R.M. Kotloff *et al.* (2003). Clinical risk factors for primary graft failure following lung transplantation. *Chest* **124**(4): 1232–41.

Christie, J.D., N. Robinson *et al.* (2007). Association of protein C and type 1 plasminogen activator inhibitor with primary graft dysfunction. *Am J Respir Crit Care Med* **175**(1): 69–74.

Ciarka A, V.J., Stoupel E *et al* (2006). Atrial septostomy and muscle sympthetic nerve activity in pulmonary arterial hypertension. *Kardiol Pol* **64**(5 (Suppl 1)): B29.

Conte, J.V., M.J. Borja *et al.* (2001). Lung transplantation for primary and secondary pulmonary hypertension. *Ann Thorac Surg* **72**(5): 1673–9; discussion 1679–80.

Conte, J.V., S.P. Gaine *et al.* (1998). The influence of continuous intravenous prostacyclin therapy for primary pulmonary hypertension on the timing and outcome of transplantation. *J Heart Lung Transplant* **17**(7): 679–85.

Coulden, R. (2006). State-of-the-Art Imaging Techniques in Chronic Thromboembolic Pulmonary Hypertension. *Proc Am Thorac Soc* **3**(7): 577–583.

D'Alonzo G.E., R.J. Barst, S.M. Ayres *et al* (1991). Survival in patients with primary pulmonary hypertension. Results of a national prospective study. *Ann Int Med* **115**: 343–349.

Dalen, J.E. and J.S. Alpert (1975). Natural history of pulmonary embolism. *Prog Cardiovasc Dis* **17**(4): 259–70.

Dartevelle, P., E. Fadel *et al.* (2004). Chronic thromboembolic pulmonary hypertension. *Eur Respir J* **23**(4): 637–48.

Doyle, R.L., D. McCrory *et al.* (2004). Surgical treatments/interventions for pulmonary arterial hypertension: ACCP evidence-based clinical practice guidelines. *Chest* **126**(1 Suppl): 63S-71S.

Doyle, R.L. and J. Theodore (1997). Current status of lung transplantation. *West J Med* **166**(1): 67–8.

Espinola-Zavaleta, N., J. Vargas-Barron *et al.* (1999). Echocardiographic Evaluation of Patients with Primary Pulmonary Hypertension Before and After Atrial Septostomy. *Echocardiography* **16**(7, Pt 1): 625–634.

Estenne, M., J.R. Maurer *et al.* (2002). Bronchiolitis obliterans syndrome 2001: an update of the diagnostic criteria. *J Heart Lung Transplant* **21**(3): 297–310.

Fedullo, P.F. and V.F. Tapson (2003). Clinical practice. The evaluation of suspected pulmonary embolism. *N Engl J Med* **349**(13): 1247–56.

Feinstein, J.A., S.Z. Goldhaber *et al.* (2001). Balloon Pulmonary Angioplasty for Treatment of Chronic Thromboembolic Pulmonary Hypertension. *Circulation* **103**(1): 10–13.

Fishman, A.J., K.M. Moser *et al.* (1983). Perfusion lung scans vs pulmonary angiography in evaluation of suspected primary pulmonary hypertension. *Chest* **84**(6): 679–83.

Franke, U., K. Wiebe *et al.* (2000). Ten years experience with lung and heart-lung transplantation in primary and secondary pulmonary hypertension. *Eur J Cardiothorac Surg* **18**(4): 447–52.

Galie, N., H.A. Ghofrani *et al.* (2005). Sildenafil citrate therapy for pulmonary arterial hypertension. *N Engl J Med* **353**(20): 2148–57.

Gammie, J.S., R.J. Keenan *et al.* (1998). Single- versus double-lung transplantation for pulmonary hypertension. *J Thorac Cardiovasc Surg* **115**(2): 397–402; discussion 402–3.

Gammie, J.S., S.M. Pham *et al.* (1997). Influence of panel-reactive antibody on survival and rejection after lung transplantation. *J Heart Lung Transplant* **16**(4): 408–15.

Gao, S.Z., S.V. Chaparro *et al.* (2003). Post-transplantation lymphoproliferative disease in heart and heart-lung transplant recipients: 30-year experience at Stanford University. *J Heart Lung Transplant* **22**(5): 505–14.

Ghofrani, H.A., R.T. Schermuly *et al.* (2003). Sildenafil for long-term treatment of nonoperable chronic thromboembolic pulmonary hypertension. *Am J Respir Crit Care Med* **167**(8): 1139–41.

Gilbert, T.B., S.P. Gaine *et al.* (1998). Short-term outcome and predictors of adverse events following pulmonary thromboendarterectomy. *World J Surg* **22**(10): 1029–32; discussion 1033.

Glanville, A.R. (2006). The role of bronchoscopic surveillance monitoring in the care of lung transplant recipients. *Semin Respir Crit Care Med* **27**(5): 480–91.

Glanville, A.R., J.C. Baldwin *et al.* (1987). Obliterative bronchiolitis after heart-lung transplantation: apparent arrest by augmented immunosuppression. *Ann Intern Med* **107**(3): 300–4.

Glanville, A.R., C.M. Burke *et al.* (1987). Primary pulmonary hypertension. Length of survival in patients referred for heart-lung transplantation. *Chest* **91**(5): 675–81.

Hadjiliadis, D., C. Chaparro *et al.* (2005). Pre-transplant panel reactive antibody in lung transplant recipients is associated with significantly worse post-transplant survival in a multicenter study. *J Heart Lung Transplant* **24**(7 Suppl): S249–54.

Hausknecht, M.J., R.E. Sims *et al.* (1990). Successful palliation of primary pulmonary hypertension by atrial septostomy. *Am J Cardiol* **65**(15): 1045–6.

Hayden, A. (1997). Balloon atrial septostomy incfreases cardiac index and may reduce mortality among pulmonary hypertension patients awaiting lung transplantation. *J Transp Coord* **7**: 131–133.

Hertz, M.I., P.J. Mohacsi *et al.* (2003). The registry of the International Society for Heart and Lung Transplantation: introduction to the Twentieth Annual Reports–2003. *J Heart Lung Transplant* **22**(6): 610–5.

Hopkins, W.E. (2005). The remarkable right ventricle of patients with Eisenmenger syndrome. *Coron Artery Dis* **16**(1): 19–25.

Hopkins, W.E., L.L. Ochoa *et al.* (1996). Comparison of the hemodynamics and survival of adults with severe primary pulmonary hypertension or Eisenmenger syndrome. *J Heart Lung Transplant* **15**(1 Pt 1): 100–5.

Jais, X., V. Ioos *et al.* (2005). Splenectomy and chronic thromboembolic pulmonary hypertension. *Thorax* **60**(12): 1031–4.

Jamieson, S.W., W.R. Auger *et al.* (1993). Experience and results with 150 pulmonary thromboendarterectomy operations over a 29-month period. *J Thorac Cardiovasc Surg* **106**(1): 116–26; discussion 126–7.

Jamieson, S.W., D.P. Kapelanski *et al.* (2003). Pulmonary endarterectomy: experience and lessons learned in 1,500 cases. *Ann Thorac Surg* **76**(5): 1457–62; discussion 1462–4.

Jamieson, S.W., E.B. Stinson *et al.* (1984). Heart-lung transplantation for irreversible pulmonary hypertension. *Ann Thorac Surg* **38**(6): 554–62.

Kapitan, K.S., J.L. Clausen *et al.* (1990). Gas exchange in chronic thromboembolism after pulmonary thromboendarterectomy. *Chest* **98**(1): 14–9.

Kasimir, M.T., G. Seebacher *et al.* (2004). Reverse cardiac remodelling in patients with primary pulmonary hypertension after isolated lung transplantation. *Eur J Cardiothorac Surg* **26**(4): 776–81.

Kerr, K.M., W.R. Auger *et al.* (1995). Large vessel pulmonary arteritis mimicking chronic thromboembolic disease. *Am J Respir Crit Care Med* **152**(1): 367–73.

Kerstein, D., P.S. Levy *et al.* (1995). Blade balloon atrial septostomy in patients with severe primary pulmonary hypertension. *Circulation* **91**(7): 2028–35.

Kim, N.H., P. Fesler *et al.* (2004). Preoperative partitioning of pulmonary vascular resistance correlates with early outcome after thromboendarterectomy for chronic thromboembolic pulmonary hypertension. *Circulation* **109**(1): 18–22.

Kim, N.H. S. (2006). Assessment of Operability in Chronic Thromboembolic Pulmonary Hypertension. *Proc Am Thorac Soc* **3**(7): 584–588.

Klepetko, W., E. Mayer *et al.* (2004). Interventional and surgical modalities of treatment for pulmonary arterial hypertension. *J Am Coll Cardiol* **43**(12 Suppl S): 73S-80S.

Knoop, C., A. Kentos *et al.* (2006). Post-transplant lymphoproliferative disorders after lung transplantation: first-line treatment with rituximab may induce complete remission. *Clin Transplant* **20**(2): 179–87.

Kothari, S.S., A. Yusuf *et al.* (2002). Graded balloon atrial septostomy in severe pulmonary hypertension. *Indian Heart J* **54**(2): 164–9.

Kramer, M.R., S.E. Marshall *et al.* (1991a). The distribution of ventilation and perfusion after single-lung transplantation in patients with pulmonary fibrosis and pulmonary hypertension. *Transplant Proc* **23**(1 Pt 2): 1215–6.

Kramer, M.R., S.E. Marshall *et al.* (1991b). Clinical significance of hyperbilirubinemia in patients with pulmonary hypertension undergoing heart-lung transplantation. *J Heart Lung Transplant* **10**(2): 317–21.

Kramer, M.R., H.A. Valantine *et al.* (1994). Recovery of the right ventricle after single-lung transplantation in pulmonary hypertension. *Am J Cardiol* **73**(7): 494–500.

Kramm, T., B. Eberle *et al.* (2005). Inhaled iloprost to control residual pulmonary hypertension following pulmonary endarterectomy. *Eur J Cardiothorac Surg* **28**(6): 882–8.

Kurzyna, M., M. Dabrowski *et al.* (2003). Atrial septostomy for severe primary pulmonary hypertension - report on two cases. *Kardiol Pol* **58**(1): 27–33.

Kurzyna M, D.M., Bielecki D *et al* (2007). Atrial septostomy in the treatment of end-stage right heart failure in patients with pulmonary hypertension. *Chest* **131**:877–83.

Lang, I. and K. Kerr (2006). Risk Factors for Chronic Thromboembolic Pulmonary Hypertension. *Proc Am Thorac Soc* **3**(7): 568–570.

Levine, S.M. (2004). A survey of clinical practice of lung transplantation in North America. *Chest* **125**(4): 1224–38.

Levine, S.M. and C.L. Bryan (1995). Bronchiolitis obliterans in lung transplant recipients. The thorn in the side of lung transplantation. *Chest* **107**(4): 894–7.

Lisbona, R., H. Kreisman *et al.* (1985). Perfusion lung scanning: differentiation of primary from thromboembolic pulmonary hypertension. *AJR Am J Roentgenol* **144**(1): 27–30.

Ljungman, P., P. Griffiths *et al.* (2002). Definitions of cytomegalovirus infection and disease in transplant recipients. *Clin Infect Dis* **34**(8): 1094–7.

Mares, P., T.B. Gilbert *et al.* (2000). Pulmonary artery thromboendarterectomy: a comparison of two different postoperative treatment strategies. *Anesth Analg* **90**(2): 267–73.

Maurer, J.R., A.E. Frost *et al.* (1998). International guidelines for the selection of lung transplant candidates. The International Society for Heart and Lung Transplantation, the American Thoracic Society, the American Society of Transplant Physicians, the European Respiratory Society. *Transplantation* **66**(7): 951–6.

Mayer, E. and W. Klepetko (2006). Techniques and outcomes of pulmonary endarterectomy for chronic thromboembolic pulmonary hypertension. *Proc Am Thorac Soc* **3**(7): 589–93.

McGoon, M., D. Gutterman *et al.* (2004). Screening, early detection, and diagnosis of pulmonary arterial hypertension: ACCP evidence-based clinical practice guidelines. *Chest* **126**(1 Suppl): 14S-34S.

McLaughlin, V.V., A. Shillington *et al.* (2002). Survival in primary pulmonary hypertension: the impact of epoprostenol therapy. *Circulation* **106**(12): 1477–82.

Mendeloff, E.N., B.F. Meyers *et al.* (2002). Lung transplantation for pulmonary vascular disease. *Ann Thorac Surg* **73**(1): 209–219.

Menzel, T., S. Wagner *et al.* (2000). Pathophysiology of impaired right and left ventricular function in chronic embolic pulmonary hypertension: changes after pulmonary thromboendarterectomy. *Chest* **118**(4): 897–903.

Micheletti, A., A.A. Hislop *et al.* (2006). Role of atrial septostomy in the treatment of children with pulmonary arterial hypertension. *Heart* **92**(7): 969–72.

Mo, M., D.P. Kapelanski *et al.* (1999). Reoperative pulmonary thromboendarterectomy. *Ann Thorac Surg* **68**(5): 1770–6; discussion 1776–7.

Moscucci, M., I.T. Dairywala *et al.* (2001). Balloon atrial septostomy in end-stage pulmonary hypertension guided by a novel intracardiac echocardiographic transducer. *Catheter Cardiovasc Interv* **52**(4): 530–4.

Moser, K.M., V.N. Houk *et al.* (1965). Chronic, massive thrombotic obstruction of the pulmonary arteries. Analysis of four operated cases. *Circulation* **32**(3): 377–85.

Nihill, M.R., M.P. O'Laughlin *et al.* (1991). Effects of atrial septostomy in patients with terminal cor pulmonale due to pulmonary vascular disease. *Cathet Cardiovasc Diagn* **24**(3): 166–72.

Ogino, H., M. Ando *et al.* (2006). Japanese single-center experience of surgery for chronic thromboembolic pulmonary hypertension. *Ann Thorac Surg* **82**(2): 630–6.

Orens, J.B., M. Estenne *et al.* (2006). International guidelines for the selection of lung transplant candidates: 2006 update–a consensus report from the Pulmonary Scientific Council of the International Society for Heart and Lung Transplantation. *J Heart Lung Transplant* **25**(7): 745–55.

Park, S.C., W.H. Neches *et al.* (1982). Blade atrial septostomy: collaborative study. *Circulation* **66**(2): 258–66.

Park, S.C., W.H. Neches *et al.* (1978). Clinical use of blade atrial septostomy. *Circulation* **58**(4): 600–6.

Pasque, M.K., J.D. Cooper *et al.* (1990). Improved technique for bilateral lung transplantation: rationale and initial clinical experience. *Ann Thorac Surg* **49**(5): 785–91.

Patterson, A. (1986). Unilateral lung transplantation for pulmonary fibrosis. Toronto Lung Transplant Group. *N Engl J Med* **314**(18): 1140–5.

Patterson, G.A., J.D. Cooper *et al.* (1988). Technique of successful clinical double-lung transplantation. *Ann Thorac Surg* **45**(6): 626–33.

Peacock, A., G. Simonneau *et al.* (2006). Controversies, Uncertainties and Future Research on the Treatment of Chronic Thromboembolic Pulmonary Hypertension. *Proc Am Thorac Soc* **3**(7): 608–614.

Pengo, V., A.W. Lensing *et al.* (2004). Incidence of chronic thromboembolic pulmonary hypertension after pulmonary embolism. *N Engl J Med* **350**(22): 2257–64.

Ramalingam, P., L. Rybicki *et al.* (2002). Posttransplant lymphoproliferative disorders in lung transplant patients: the Cleveland Clinic experience. *Mod Pathol* **15**(6): 647–56.

Rashkind, W.J. and W.W. Miller (1966). Creation of an atrial septal defect without thoracotomy. A palliative approach to complete transposition of the great arteries. *Jama* **196**(11): 991–2.

Reams, B.D., H.P. McAdams *et al.* (2003). Posttransplant lymphoproliferative disorder: incidence, presentation, and response to treatment in lung transplant recipients. *Chest* **124**(4): 1242–9.

Reichenberger, F., J. Pepke-Zaba *et al.* (2003). Atrial septostomy in the treatment of severe pulmonary arterial hypertension. *Thorax* **58**(9): 797–800.

Reitz, B.A., J.L. Wallwork *et al.* (1982). Heart-lung transplantation: successful therapy for patients with pulmonary vascular disease. *N Engl J Med* **306**(10): 557–64.

Rich, S., E. Dodin *et al.* (1997). Usefulness of atrial septostomy as a treatment for primary pulmonary hypertension and guidelines for its application. *Am J Cardiol* **80**(3): 369–71.

Rich, S. and W. Lam (1983). Atrial septostomy as palliative therapy for refractory primary pulmonary hypertension. *Am J Cardiol* **51**(9): 1560–1.

Robbins, I.M., B.W. Christman *et al.* (1998). A survey of diagnostic practices and the use of epoprostenol in patients with primary pulmonary hypertension. *Chest* **114**(5): 1269–75.

Rosenzweig, E.B., D. Kerstein *et al.* (1999). Long-term prostacyclin for pulmonary hypertension with associated congenital heart defects. *Circulation* **99**(14): 1858–65.

Rothman, A., D. Beltran *et al.* (1993). Graded balloon dilation atrial septostomy as a bridge to lung transplantation in pulmonary hypertension. *Am Heart J* **125**(6): 1763–6.

Rothman, A., M.S. Sklansky *et al.* (1999). Atrial septostomy as a bridge to lung transplantation in patients with severe pulmonary hypertension. *Am J Cardiol* **84**(6): 682–6.

Rozkovec, A., P. Montanes *et al.* (1986). Factors that influence the outcome of primary pulmonary hypertension. *Br Heart J* **55**(5): 449–58.

Sandoval, J., J. Gaspar *et al.* (1998). Graded balloon dilation atrial septostomy in severe primary pulmonary hypertension. A therapeutic alternative for patients nonresponsive to vasodilator treatment. *J Am Coll Cardiol* **32**(2): 297–304.

Sandoval, J. and J. Gaspar (2004). Atrial septostomy. *Pulmonary Circulation*, 2nd edn (eds A.J. Peacock and L.J. Rubin), Edward Arnold Publishers, pp. 319–333.

Sandoval, J., A. Rothman *et al.* (2001). Atrial septostomy for pulmonary hypertension. *Clin Chest Med* **22**(3): 547–60.

Shargall, Y., G. Guenther *et al.* (2005). Report of the ISHLT Working Group on Primary Lung Graft Dysfunction part VI: treatment. *J Heart Lung Transplant* **24**(10): 1489–500.

Simonneau, G., R.J. Barst *et al.* (2002). Continuous subcutaneous infusion of treprostinil, a prostacyclin analogue, in patients with pulmonary arterial hypertension: a double-blind, randomized, placebo-controlled trial. *Am J Respir Crit Care Med* **165**(6): 800–4.

Tapson, V.F. and M. Humbert (2006). Incidence and Prevalence of Chronic Thromboembolic Pulmonary Hypertension: From Acute to Chronic Pulmonary Embolism. *Proc Am Thorac Soc* **3**(7): 564–567.

TenVergert, E.M., M.L. Essink-Bot *et al.* (1998). The effect of lung transplantation on health-related quality of life: a longitudinal study. *Chest* **113**(2): 358–64.

Thistlethwaite, P.A., M.M. Madani *et al.* (2006). Venovenous extracorporeal life support after pulmonary endarterectomy: indications, techniques, and outcomes. *Ann Thorac Surg* **82**(6): 2139–45.

Thistlethwaite, P.A., M. Mo *et al.* (2002). Operative classification of thromboembolic disease determines outcome after pulmonary endarterectomy. *J Thorac Cardiovasc Surg* **124**(6): 1203–11.

Trulock, E.P., L.B. Edwards *et al.* (2006). Registry of the International Society for Heart and Lung Transplantation: twenty-third official adult lung and heart-lung transplantation report–2006. *J Heart Lung Transplant* **25**(8): 880–92.

Ueno, T., J.A. Smith *et al.* (2000). Bilateral sequential single lung transplantation for pulmonary hypertension and Eisenmenger's syndrome. *Ann Thorac Surg* **69**(2): 381–7.

Vachiery JL, S.E. Boonstra A, Naeije R (2003). Balloon atrial septostomy for pulmonary hypertension in the prostacylcin era. *Am J Respir Crit Care Med* **167**: A692.

van der Bij, W. and R. Speich (2001). Management of cytomegalovirus infection and disease after solid-organ transplantation. *Clin Infect Dis* **33 Suppl 1**: S32–7.

Westney, G.E., S. Kesten *et al.* (1996). Aspergillus infection in single and double lung transplant recipients. *Transplantation* **61**(6): 915–9.

Whelan, T.P., J.M. Dunitz *et al.* (2005). Effect of preoperative pulmonary artery pressure on early survival after lung transplantation for idiopathic pulmonary fibrosis. *J Heart Lung Transplant* **24**(9): 1269–74.

Whyte, R.I., R.C. Robbins *et al.* (1999). Heart-lung transplantation for primary pulmonary hypertension. *Ann Thorac Surg* **67**(4): 937–41; discussion 941–2.

9 End points and clinical trial design in pulmonary arterial hypertension: Clinical and regulatory perspectives

Andrew J. Peacock

Scottish Pulmonary Vascular Unit, Western Infirmary, Glasgow, UK

9.1 Introduction

Pulmonary arterial hypertension (PAH) is a disease of the peripheral pulmonary arteries. The pathoetiology of the condition can vary from infection (such as HIV) to genetic (BMPR2 mutation) to mechanical loading (congenital heart disease) to an association with autoimmune connective tissue diseases or an association with portal hypertension. Despite these varying etiologies, the histological features of the peripheral pulmonary arteries are similar. The end effect, i.e. death from right heart failure, is also the same and responses to treatment (with the exception of

Pulmonary Arterial Hypertension, Edited by Robyn J. Barst
© 2008 John Wiley & Sons, Ltd

connective tissue disease associated with PAH which has a worse prognosis) are also similar. These similarities have meant that, in the past, trials in pulmonary hypertension have included cases of PAH from various etiologies, and drugs used for treating the condition, though not perfect, have similar effects no matter what the etiology.

Up until the 1990s, most reports of treatment of PAH, which is a rare disease, were anecdotal case series, and most treatments were found to be ineffective. The first report of successful treatment of PAH was a single case report that described the use of continuous intravenous prostacyclin (Higgenbottam *et al.*, 1984). Subsequently in the 1990s three randomized clinical trials of continuous intravenous epoprostenol (in IPAH and PAH associated with the scleroderma spectrum of disease), showed improvements in exercise capacity and survival (in IPAH (IPAH)) (Barst *et al.*, 1994; Barst *et al.*, 1996; Rubin *et al.*, 1990; Badesch *et al.*, 2000). In 1992 Rich showed that there was a marked variability in the survival of patients with IPAH (previously termed primary pulmonary hypertension) (Rich, Kaufmann and Levy, 1992). For example, those unresponsive to an acute vasodilator, and untreated, had a 28% two-year survival, whereas those who were responsive to an acute vasodilator and were treated with both anticoagulation and high-dose calcium antagonists had a two-year survival approaching 100%. These case reports and case series resulted in a renewed interest in PAH. With that interest came new science and new therapies based on that science – in particular the endothelin receptor antagonists, the prostacyclin analogues and the phosphodiesterase-5 inhibitors. Remarkably, for a rare disease, almost 1500 patients were randomized between 2000 and 2003 in placebo-controlled trials. At the time of writing, eleven of these trials have been published and seven therapies are now licensed for PAH (see Table 9.1). This is remarkable success by any medical standard and has led in turn to many more trials of different therapies and combinations of therapies (see Table 9.2). Given the enormous interest in the treatment of PAH, it is appropriate to consider the **design of trials** of new therapies or combinations of therapy for PAH and also to consider the **end points** that will be measured when trying to decide whether a drug or combination of drugs is effective or not. In this chapter we shall deal with some aspects of clinical trial design, consider end points used in previous and current studies and consider what end points might be used in the future. Treatments for PAH are always expensive, sometimes invasive and liable to have significant side-effects. To convince patients, treating physicians, funding agencies and regulatory bodies of the value of the treatment, it is extremely important to conduct trials of appropriate design using end points of appropriate quality.

9.2 Trial design

Intravenous epoprostenol was approved at least in the United States for the treatment of PAH a number of years ago, but the first oral therapy for the treatment of the condition was bosentan, an oral endothelin A and B receptor antagonist.

Table 9.1 Reported placebo-controlled trials in pulmonary arterial hypertension

Trial name	Intervention	Number of patients	Duration	Primary end points	Secondary end points	References
PPH-SG	Epoprostenol Intravenous	192	12 weeks	6MWD	QOL, Survival, HD, Safety (NYHA, Dyspnoea score)	Badesch et al., 2000; Barst et al., 1996, Rubin et al., 1990[4]
AIR	Iloprost inhaled	203	12 weeks	NYHA, 6MWD	Δ6MWD, Dyspnoea score, HD, TTW, QOL	Olschewski et al., 2002
TSG	Treprostinil subcutaneous	470	12 weeks	6MWD	PH signs / symptoms, TTW, Borg, HD, QOL	Simonneau et al., 2002
Bosentan pilot 351	Bosentan oral	32	16 weeks	6MWD	HD, Borg, WHO, TTW	Channick et al., 2001
BREATHE-1	Bosentan oral	213	16 weeks	6MWD	Borg, WHO, TTW, Safety	Rubin et al., 2002
ALPHABET	Beraprost oral	130	12 weeks	6MWD	Borg, NYHA, HD, TTW, Safety	Galie et al., 2002
BSG	Beraprost oral	116	1 year	Survival, TTW, VO2	6MWD, Borg, NYHA, HD, QOL	Barst et al., 2003
STRIDE-1	Sitaxsentan oral	178	12 weeks	VO2	6MWD, NYHA, QOL, HD, TTW, CPET	Barst et al., 2004
STRIDE-2	Sitaxsentan oral	247	18 weeks	6MWD	WHO, TTW, Borg	Barst et al., 2006
SUPER-1	Sildenafil oral	278	12 weeks	6MWD	HD, Borg, WHO, TTW	Galie et al., 2005
Terbogrel	Terbogrel oral	135(71)	12 weeks	6MWD	HD, Safety, Circulating prostanoids	Langleben et al., 2002
ARIES 1 & 2	Ambrisentan	202/192	12 weeks	6MWD	Borg, WHO, CW	Rubin et al., 2006
STEP	Bosentan / inhaled iloprost	67	12 weeks	Safety	6MWD, HD, CW	McLaughlin et al., Annals 2006
PACES-1	IV epoprostenol / sildenafil	267	12 weeks	6MWD	HD, CW, QOL, Borg	Simonneau et al., 2008

6MWD: 6-minute walk distance. HD: Resting haemodynamics. CW: time to clinical worsening. WHO: WHO functional class. Borg: Borg dyspnoea index score. QOL: quality of life CPET: Cardiopulmonary exercise test data.

Table 9.2 Current/proposed clinical trial protocols for pulmonary arterial hypertension

Sponsor	Trial name	Intervention	Duration	Primary end points	Secondary end points
Lung Rx	TRIUMPH 1	Inhaled treprostinil	12 weeks	6MWD	Borg, WHO, QOL, CW
United Therapeutics	FREEDOM-M	Oral treprostinil	12 weeks	6MWD	Borg, WHO, Safety, ECG
	FREEDOM-C	Bosentan / sildenafil / oral treprostinil	16 weeks	6MWD	Borg, WHO, Safety, ECG
Actelion	BENEFIT	Bosentan (Inoperable CTEPH)	16 weeks	6MWD, HD	WHO, CW
Actelion	EARLY	Bosentan	6 months	6MWD	HD, WHO, QOL
Actelion	COMPASS 1, 2 &3	Bosentan / Sildenafil	16 weeks	6MWD, TTW	WHO, Borg, QOL, CW, Survival
Pfizer	A1481243	Sildenafil / Bosentan	12 weeks	6MWD	Borg, WHO, HD, QOL, TTW
Lilly ICOS	PHIRST-1	Tadalafil	16 weeks	6MWD	WHO, Borg, HD, QOL, CW
University of Cincinnati	ISAPH	Iloprost (Sarcoid PAH)	16 weeks	6MWD	QOL, HD, PFTs, Safety
Imperial College London and University Hospital, Giessen	—	Simvastatin	6 months	HD, cMRI	6MWD, NT-BNP, other biomarkers, Echo, Safety
NHLBI (John Hopkins and Columbia University)	—	Simvastatin / Aspirin	6 months	6MWD	WHO, CW, Safety, Platelet and endothelial function
Assitance Publique – Hopitaux de Paris	—	Escitalopram	16 weeks	6MWD	HD, WHO, Borg, QOL, CW
Northern Therapeutics Inc	PHACeT	NO synthase transfected endothelial prog cells	3 months	Safety	HD, 6MWD, QOL
Biogen idec	VIRTUE-1	Aviptadil	12 months	6MWD	—
Novartis	CST1571E2203	Imatinib	6 months	6MWD, Safety	WHO, Borg, HD, CW, Biomarkers

6MWD: 6-minute walk distance; HD: Resting haemodynamics; CW: time to clinical worsening; WHO: WHO functional class. Borg: Borg dyspnoea index score; QOL: quality of life

Following its approval a range of questions needed to be asked about trial design:

(1) Can we continue to do placebo-controlled studies?
(2) Is it possible to do non-inferiority studies in PAH?
(3) Can we do withdrawal studies in PAH?

All these issues and also the issues of the appropriateness or otherwise of specific end points were considered at a workshop in Gleneagles, Scotland, May 1–4, 2003 and subsequently at the 3rd World Symposium on Pulmonary Arterial Hypertension Meeting (Venice 2003). These workshops and other meetings have led to a number of publications dealing specifically with trial design and end points in PAH (Peacock *et al.*, 2004; Kawut and Palevsky, 2004; Rich, 2006; Barst, 2007).

Placebo-controlled studies (superiority)

All the currently approved therapies for PAH have been subjected to placebo-controlled studies, to demonstrate superiority against placebo. These were major and remarkable undertakings given the rarity of disease, and required a degree of multinational cooperation rarely seen in modern medicine. At the time of writing the following are licensed for treatment of PAH (Barst *et al.*, 1996; Simmoneau *et al.*, 2002; Oudiz *et al.*, 2004; Badesch *et al.*, 2000; Olschewski *et al.*, 2002; Rubin *et al.*, 2002; Channick *et al.*, 2001; Barst *et al.*, 2006; Barst, 2007):

- intravenous (IV) epoprostenol WHO Class III and IV IPAH (FDA and EMEA) and PAH related to connective tissue disease (FDA)
- subcutaneous treprostinil WHO Class II, III and IV PAH (FDA) and Class II and III PAH (EMEA)
- intravenous treprostinil WHO Class II, III and IV PAH (FDA) and Class II and III PAH (EMEA)
- intravenous iloprost WHO Class III and IV PAH (New Zealand)
- inhaled iloprost WHO Class III PAH (EMEA) and Class III and IV PAH (FDA)
- bosentan WHO Class III PAH (EMEA) and Class III and IV PAH (FDA).
- sildenafil WHO Class II and III PAH (FDA and EMEA)
- sitaxsentan WHO Class III PAH (EMEA)
- beraprost WHO Class II and III PAH (Japan and Korea)
- ambrisentan WHO class II and III PAH (FDA and EMEA)

All these studies looked at morbidity in the form of exercise capacity with various other secondary end points (Table 9.1). Only IV epoprostenol has been shown to improve survival compared with placebo (Barst *et al.*, 1996). Most experts believe that placebo-controlled mortality studies are no longer ethical and if we are to see survival studies in the future then these will need to be done using IV epoprostenol as comparator. Clearly, survival is an extremely important end point for these studies and in order to try and get around the ethical problem, some authors (McLaughlin, Shillington and Rich, 2002; McLaughlin *et al.*, 2005) have recently compared survival of patients on therapy with survival based on data from the NIH registry, which was of course formulated in the pre-treatment era (McLaughlin, Shillington and Rich, 2002; McLaughlin *et al.*, 2005; D'Alonzo *et al.*, 1991). These are not true comparative survival studies because they were not designed as such; however, given the ethical considerations, they are likely to be the best that we can achieve.

Since we now consider that placebo-controlled survival studies are not possible, we must also consider whether in the future placebo-controlled morbidity studies are ethical. All the early trials were placebo-controlled, and indeed one or two of the studies being performed currently are also placebo-controlled, but most studies which lasted between three and four months have shown a significant deterioration in the placebo group. The current view is that, if we are to do placebo-controlled studies in the future, these will need to be combinations studies where the patients are always receiving an active ingredient even if the additional ingredient is a placebo. A possible exception to this rule is the patients with WHO Class II function, where it might be reasonable to plan a placebo-controlled study. This would need to be done with very tight control such that, if there is any deterioration, patients can be put on treatment. Another possibility – this has been exploited by the imatinib study – is to do a placebo-controlled study of both morbidity and mortality with the new drug where patients are already on maximal available combination therapy. Whether or not patients wish to be recruited to such a study is not known.

Non-comparative (non-inferiority) studies

Clearly it will not be possible to do comparative **superiority** studies between drugs because of the very large numbers of patients needed. An alternative approach is the comparative **non-inferiority** study where Drug A is compared with Drug B and the sponsors need to show that it is not worse than the original therapy. Although the numbers needed are not as great as are needed for superiority studies, they are still considerable and it is very unlikely that any company will wish to sponsor such a study, which will involve considerable expense with an indeterminate outcome. Furthermore, non-inferiority studies can only be performed using identical investigational conditions (inclusion criteria, exclusion criteria, patient population, study protocol, end points, etc.) as the original comparator (Galie, 2001; Galie, Manes and Branzi, 2002). Given all these constraints and the relatively large numbers of patients involved it is unlikely that we will see non-inferiority studies in the field of PAH.

Withdrawal studies

The world's experts in PAH were rather surprised when the regulatory agencies (FDA and EMEA) asked whether we would consider doing **withdrawal** studies in patients on established therapy. The reasons for asking for withdrawal studies are sensible, specifically when a study has shown only marginal benefit or benefits of low clinical importance. Although this may be an interesting academic question, most experts feel that withdrawal studies are unethical for the following reasons:

- We already know that patients treated with placebo deteriorate over time and hence we would be subjecting patients to the possibility of deterioration.
- Experts are concerned that if a patient should deteriorate when a drug is withdrawn, re-introduction of the drug may not restore the patient to their baseline state.

Possible alternatives to withdrawal studies are **transition** or **switch** studies, in which one drug is withdrawn and another drug is substituted. This approach, though valid, has not found favor with most experts and currently there are no published trials of such an approach. In most cases, if a patient deteriorates, drugs are simply added so that the patient is on a combination of two or more therapies. There are good reasons, however, for considering switch studies in the future:

- If the patient improved on drug A but subsequently deteriorates again it is unknown if drug A is actually having an effect.
- Drugs for PAH are extraordinarily expensive and the funding agencies need to be convinced that the combination approach is more effective than the switch approach. At the time of writing only one switch study has been done and, to our knowledge, none are currently planned.

9.3 End points in trials of therapy for pulmonary arterial hypertension

From the tables of past (Table 9.1) and current (Table 9.2) trials it can be seen that the most frequently used primary end point is the 6-minute walk distance (6MWD). However, in the current trials additional end points such as hemodynamics and quality of life are also being used. This change reflects the fact many people feel the traditional end points (e.g. 6MWD) are inadequate to describe the effect of therapy. When considering these issues we must develop some definitions. At the Gleneagles Meeting (Peacock *et al.*, 2004) we defined an end point as 'a measurement used by investigators conducting a drug trial to determine whether patients with PAH would benefit by drug administration.' Although this definition can be generally accepted, there are a number of categories of end points and different levels of importance are given to each of these categories.

A primary end point is one that is clinically meaningful. In the context of PAH, the most clinically meaningful end point is survival but, for the reasons stated above, it is unlikely we will see survival trials in the future. Another clinically meaningful end point is exercise capacity. Most trials have measured exercise endurance using the 6MWD. There are advantages and disadvantages to the 6-minute walk (see below).

A secondary end point is also called a surrogate end point (Kawut and Palevsky, 2004). These may be hemodynamic variables, blood biomarkers, imaging, quality of life or others. Both the FDA and the EMEA permit the use of surrogate end points for the licensing of drugs for PAH but they must be convinced that this end point will predict clinical benefit based on epidemiological, therapeutic or pathophysiological evidence. The strengths of secondary (surrogate) end points are:

- They are continuous variables, therefore smaller numbers are required for adequately powered studies when compared with categoric end points (e.g. survival).
- They can be repeated over time and rate of change incorporated.
- They may shed light on the mechanism of disease and be more biologically relevant than a clinical end point.

The disadvantages of secondary (surrogate) end points are:

- The treatment may improve the secondary end point but not improve the patient. For example, cardiac output is an important physiological end point in PAH. This could be improved either by improving pulmonary vascular resistance with secondary improvement in cardiac output (clinical beneficial) or directly stimulate the failing muscle (by using inotropes, which is possibly harmful).
- Secondary (surrogate) end points may miss an important change, e.g. because they are performed at the wrong time.

Many people, including the authors of this chapter, feel that the current end points used in clinical trials of PAH are not as valid as they might be. This frustration has been articulated by Rich (2006). While the regulatory authorities may come to the view that the only thing that really matters is quality of life and that all other end points are simply surrogates, this does not appeal to clinicians with physiological training, who feel that in PAH the problem is primarily in the small peripheral arteries of pulmonary circulation and secondarily in the right heart. For most treating physicians, a therapy that influences neither of these two variables, even if it does improves quality of life, is not the way forward.

Problems with the current end points for PAH trials are as follows:

- They are inaccurate (not proportional to the status of disease).
- They are incomplete (ignore important components of disease).
- They are insensitive (have a low signal-to-noise ratio).
- They are difficult to determine (expensive, invasive, time-consuming, require a high level of expertise or need long-term periods to show change).

An ideal end point might have the following characteristics:

- It should be heart or lung specific.
- It should be abnormal in PAH.
- Sample collection should be simple.
- The markers should be easy to measure (ideally bedside).

- Values should be reproducible.
- Values should follow the course of the disease (increasing if patients deteriorate and falling if patients improve).
- Abnormal values should be indicative of poor survival.

What is clear, however, is that since the trials of currently licensed therapies most-ly used combination of 6-minute walk, functional class and hemodynamics, all new studies will more likely than not require at least these variables before they will be approved. Any new end point would need to be tested alongside traditional end points and shown to be demonstrably better if it is to be considered a primary or first-level secondary end point in the future.

It is worth now considering the various end points that have been or could be used in the assessment of patients with PAH.

Exercise testing

The most common symptoms for patients with PAH are shortness of breath and fatigue. These symptoms appear initially only on exercise and it is only later that they are present at rest as the patient transitions from WHO Class II through III to Class IV. The progressive nature of symptoms and hemodynamic derangement is shown in Figure 9.1. From this diagram it is clear that, in the initial stages, as the peripheral pulmonary arterial disease develops, pulmonary artery pressure rises but cardiac out-put is maintained. At this point there are no symptoms. Later, as pulmonary vascular resistance increases, symptoms develop with exercise because the cardiac output can-not increase adequately with exercise. Finally, in the later stages, although the pul-monary artery pressure may not rise further, there is a decline in cardiac output

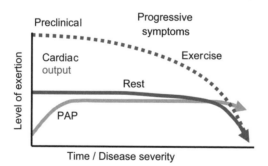

Figure 9.1 Disease progression in pulmonary arterial hypertension. In the early phase of dis-ease patients have an asymptomatic rise in pulmonary artery pressure, with preservation of car-diac output at rest and on exertion. As disease progresses, resting cardiac ouput remains stable but the ability to raise stroke volume & cardiac output on exercise is progressively impaired – resulting in progressive exertional symptoms. In the later stages of disease advanced right ven-tricular failure results in a fall in resting cardiac output with fatigue and breathlessness at rest and right heart failure.

because of the high outflow impedance and there are symptoms even at rest. At this point the pulmonary artery pressure may actually fall. This fall in pulmonary artery pressure with advanced disease has confused the non-expert who may feel that treatments has been effective because of the fall of pressure when in reality the fall in pressure is a consequence of the diminishing cardiac output and cardiac reserve. Given that the cardiac output is so critical to the maintenance of wellbeing, and cardiac failure is the normal mode of death, end points need to reflect cardiac output.

A measure of exercise capacity (6-minute walk test) has been used in nearly all clinical trials in PAH. A 6-minute walk test is really just a measure of steady state exercise capacity. To measure the variables that are likely to be affected by PAH, namely physiological dead space, oxygen delivery to the tissues, arterial hypoxemia and early anaerobic threshold necessitates a full cardiopulmonary exercise test.

Cardiopulmonary exercise testing

Cardiopulmonary exercise tests are feasible in patients – even quite ill patients – with PAH and are routinely done in most pulmonary circulation centers. As expected, patients with PAH have decreased maximum oxygen consumption, increased ventilatory equivalents for oxygen and CO_2 (reflecting increased physiological dead space) and decreased oxygen pulse reflecting diminishing stroke volume on exercise (Deboeck et al., 2004). Pulmonary hypertension can be predicted when screening patients by an increased ventilatory equivalent for CO_2. Furthermore, variables measured during cardiopulmonary exercise tests predict survival. In particular, Wensel and coworkers showed in 86 patients with IPAH that a decreased peak VO_2 (which, interestingly, was associated with a decreased systemic blood pressure at peak exercise) related to survival (Wensel et al., 2002). Cardiopulmonary exercising is the best current method of exercise testing, but it is expensive, time-consuming and prone to technical error. This was shown in a beraprost trial and in a sitaxsentan trial when patients were examined by cardiopulmonary exercise test (CPET) and 6MWD and it was found that the drugs improved 6MWD but not VO_2 max (Barst et al., 2004, Barst et al., 2003).

Six-minute walk test

Six-minute walk distance was shown to be proportional to peak oxygen consumption (Figure 9.2), ventilatory equivalents for CO_2, cardiac output but not to mean pulmonary artery pressure (Miyamoto et al., 2000). In addition, this study also showed that distance walked in six minutes was proportional to survival: those that managed a 6MWD greater than the median of 332 m had considerably improved survival over those that walked less than 332 m. The 6-minute walk test is ubiquitous but once again must be performed correctly using the appropriate guidelines (ATS, 2002). There are concerns that the 6MWD is affected by a number of factors other than pulmonary hypertension, including age, gender, height, weight and

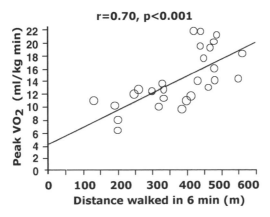

Figure 9.2 Peak VO$_2$ (as measured on an incremental cardiopulmonary exercise test using cycle ergometry) correlates well with the distance walked in six minutes. (Reproduced with permission from Miyamoto *et al.* (2000). Clinical correlates and prognostic significance of six-minute walk test in patients with primary pulmonary hypertension. *Am J Resp Crit Care Med*, **161**:487–92. ©American Thoracic Society.)

musculo-skeletal conditioning (Rich, 2006). Furthermore, it has been shown that the 6-minute walk can improve considerably with simple rehabilitory measures without the addition of treatment (Mereles *et al.*, 2006) and, since the trials have relied on quite small improvements (treatment effect) of 6MWD, it is pertinent to ask whether these improvements were really due to therapy or were simply a consequence of improved technique and volition. The average improvement in these trials was approximately 50 m from baseline of approximately 350 m, so one must question the clinical relevance of relatively small improvements. Certainly the 6-minute walk test has its supporters. Naeije's group in particular consider it a good test of submaximal exercise performance and interestingly have shown that within 3–4 min a steady state VO$_2$ is achieved that may actually be higher than the VO$_2$ max achieved during CPET (Figure 9.3) (Deboeck *et al.*, 2004).

Given the concerns about the 6-minute walk test it is reasonable to ask whether it could actually be improved. Rather surprisingly, there are no studies looking at the effect of age, gender, height, weight, etc. on 6MWD in patients with PAH but one group has looked to see whether other variables measured during the 6-minute walk test, in particular maximum oxygen saturation and heart rate, offer additional information. They evaluated eighty-three patients with IPAH and associated PAH before and after approximately five months of treatment and found that, following treatment, the changes in 6MWD were significantly related to changes in chronotropic response in both IPAH and associated PAH (Provencher *et al.*, 2006). It is clear that patients with PAH are unable to adequately increase their stroke volume with exercise (see section on magnetic resonance imaging) so that the chronotropic response remains the primary mechanism by which they can increase

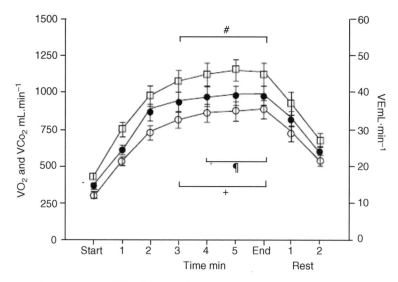

Figure 9.3 Oxygen uptake (VO_2; filled circle) carbon dioxide output (VCO_2; open square) and minute ventilation (VE; open circle) during the 6-min walk test in 20 patients with pulmonary arterial hypertension. A steady state for these ventilatory variables was achieved after 3–4 min. (Reproduced with permission from Deboeck *et al.* (2004), *Eur Respir J* **23**(5):747–51. ©European Respiratory Society Journals Ltd.)

cardiac output. It therefore seems logical that the chronotropic response would be important for these patients; thus monitoring chronotropic response may be a useful addition to our standard techniques. It is clear that from an exercise point of view cardiac output is the most important variable and we need a good non-invasive method of measuring it. In the meantime, the Naeije group maintain that the 6MWD is a useful surrogate for cardiac output using the following logic:

- VO_2 max = flow (cardiac output) × arterial–venous oxygen difference.
- VO_2 max is proportional to 6MWD.
- Arterial–venous oxygen difference is constant during the 6-minute walk test.
- Therefore cardiac output is reflected by 6MWD.

Certainly survival does seem to relate to the 6-minute walk (Miyamoto *et al.*, 2000; Sitbon *et al.*, 2002) and it seems likely therefore that we will continue to use this measurement, hopefully under more strictly controlled conditions, at least for monitoring patients in our clinics. It will also remain an important, if not primary, end point in drug trials.

Biological markers

The ideal biological marker would be one that reflected directly the ongoing activity of the disease process at the level of the pulmonary vasculature. Ideally we would have a blood test that reflected increased or decreased vasoconstrictive and remodeling activity, and this marker would be exquisitely sensitive to improvements rendered by new therapies. The currently available markers of vascular function are largely markers of endothelial cell and/or platelet dysfunction. Proteomic studies are underway, with the aim of identifying new PAH biomarkers (Abdul-Salam *et al.*, 2006). None of these, on current evidence, can be used as end points.

Thus far the most useful markers have been those which assess right ventricular function and dysfunction, in particular the natriuretic peptides. It is known that stretching of the atria or the ventricles releases natriuretic peptides, particularly brain natriuretic peptides (BNPs). NT-pro BNP can be measured in the peripheral blood, levels are relatively unaffected by acute activity (unlike BNP) and thus no special conditions of posture or rest are necessary. Serial measurement of plasma NT-pro BNP has great attractions as an end point. Its presence in the blood is related to the problem (i.e. right ventricular dysfunction) and it is simple to measure and relatively cheap. Some remarkable relationships between plasma BNP/NT-pro BNP and various elements of right ventricular dysfunction have been shown. For example, BNP/NT-pro BNP is proportional to WHO Class (Nagaya *et al.*, 2000), is proportional to pulmonary hemodynamics including pressures and cardiac output (Nagaya *et al.*, 1998) and is also proportional to VO_2 max and 6MWD (Leuchte *et al.*, 2004). Improvements in hemodynamic function lead to improvements in BNP (Nagaya *et al.*, 1998; Andreassen *et al.*, 2006). Deterioration in right ventricular function is associated with an increase in levels (Leuchte *et al.*, 2006). It would appear that BNP/NT-pro BNP measurement is a dynamic measurement reflecting the current state of the right ventricle. Furthermore there appears to be a threshold for severe cardiac dysfunction. For NT-pro BNP this has been shown to be approximately 1400 pg/ml whether measured by echocardiography (Fijalkowska *et al.*, 2006) or by magnetic resonance imaging (MRI) (Blyth *et al.*, 2006). Blyth found that there was a linear relationship between levels of BNP and right ventricular function as assessed by cardiac MRI. This relationship manifested only above the threshold, and thus it would appear that BNP may be a sensitive measure of the onset of right heart dysfunction before there are significant symptoms or signs. Thus it could be used as a screening test in patients with PAH in whom clinicians might be considering more aggressive therapy.

BNP/NT-pro BNP levels are proportional to survival whether measured at baseline or at follow-up on treatment (Nagaya *et al.*, 2000). Interestingly, serum troponin, usually a measure of myocardial damage following myocardial infarction, is also proportional to survival in PAH (Torbicki *et al.*, 2003). From the above it would appear that we have easily performed blood tests which can indicate the onset of right ventricular dysfunction and which may have potential to track right ventricular dysfunction in both deteriorating and improving patients. Furthermore, this measurement is proportional to all the relevant variables as well as survival, our ultimate end point. Not surprisingly, this good press has meant that BNP or NT-pro

BNP levels are now used routinely in nearly all expert centers around the world. We wait for further large-scale studies to see whether these promises are fulfilled.

Quality of life

It has been suggested, not least by the regulatory agencies, that quality of life is the most important end point in measurements of the efficacy of drug therapy. Unfortunately, it has always been very difficult to objectify quality of life measurements and, until recently, there were no specific health-related quality of life measures in PAH. Previously, quality of life in PAH has been evaluated by generic health status measures such as the 36-item short-form health survey (Ware and Sherbourne, 1992), Nottingham Health Profile (Hunt, McEwen and McKenna, 1986), European Quality of Life Scale (EuroQol Group, 1990) and living with heart failure Minnesota questionnaire (Rector and Cohn, 1992). Shafazand and coworkers used a number of these questionnaires in 53 patients with PAH and found that compared with population norms the participants reported moderate to severe impairment in multiple domains of heath-related quality of life, including physical mobility, emotional reaction, pain, energy, sleep and social isolation (Shafazand *et al.*, 2004). Clearly these findings are important but it is unproven whether generic questionnaires are useful for describing specific symptoms in PAH. In an attempt to overcome this deficiency the Cambridge Group developed a specific quality of life (symptoms and function) scale for PAH (McKenna *et al.*, 2006). They did this by interviewing 35 patients and analyzing their responses. They found good internal consistency and reproducibility but as yet this questionnaire has not been compared with the previous generic questionnaires nor has it been used in clinical trials. There is some preliminary evidence that the findings relate to 6MWD but we await definitive proof. Quality of life is undoubtedly important and if we can find ways to make it an objective measure it is likely it will be more useful as an end point in clinical trials in the future.

Hemodynamics

Invasive catheterization of the right heart has been available for over 100 years (Fishman, 2004) and is still considered essential for diagnosis and staging of patients with PAH (Anon, 2001; McGoon *et al.*, 2004; Galie *et al.*, 2004). Routinely, measurements of pulmonary artery pressure and blood flow are made allowing calculation of pulmonary vascular resistance. However, the relationships between these measurements and clinical state, functional class, exercise capacity and prognosis are not tight. For example, Miyamoto found that there was little relationship between pulmonary artery pressure and 6-minute walk (Miyamoto *et al.*, 2000) and Kawut found that hemodynamics were similar when comparing patients with IPAH and those with connective tissue disease associated with PAH even though survival was considerably worse in the latter (Kawut *et al.*, 2003). The main problems with routine right heart catheterization as currently practiced are:

* The measurements are made with the patient supine and at rest.
* The measurements are made in unfamiliar and possibly frightening circumstances (the cardiac catheterization laboratory).

A number of attempts have been made to try and improve the information available from invasive haemodynamics:

* Pressure flow relationships – Single-point measures of pressure and flow to calculate vascular resistance can either underestimate or overestimate because of assumptions that are made about the zero crossing of the pressure flow relationship. Multipoint measurements are better (McGregor and Sniderman, 1985) and it has been shown that patients who have no change in pulmonary vascular resistance as measured by single-point estimation may actually have a change in the slope of the line describing pressure vs flow, indicating that there has been improvement (Castelain *et al.*, 2002).
* Measurement of vascular properties – In PAH there is change in the actual function of the vessel wall. Reeves and coworkers measured a distensibility quotient called alpha and showed that, whereas in acute hypoxic pulmonary hypertension there was no change in distensibility, in chronic hypoxia or in an ageing subject, this decreased (Reeves, Linehan and Stenmark, 2005). It appears also that the function of the major vessels can dictate prognosis. Mahapatra and coworkers showed in patients with IPAH that the pulmonary artery capacitance as measured by stroke volume divided by pulmonary artery pulse pressure was predictive of survival (Mahapatra *et al.*, 2006).
* Ambulatory pulmonary artery pressure – Given the concerns about single measurements of pulmonary artery pressure, it is tempting to try and measure pulmonary artery pressure over a prolonged period, preferably during normal physical activity. Raeside showed that pulmonary artery pressure can more than double during exercise in patients with PAH or during sleep in patients with chronic hypoxic lung disease (Raeside *et al.*, 1998; Raeside *et al.*, 2000; Raeside *et al.*, 2002). These measurements are, however, specialized, requiring a micromanometer-tipped pulmonary artery catheter which is attached to an online processing system. Clearly these measurements will be used to validate other techniques rather than be used widely in the pulmonary hypertension community. However, ongoing investigation of an implantable monitor which provides continuous right ventricular and pulmonary artery hemodynamics may provide a more reliable means of assessing the course of disease in selected patients.

Ultimately we will need noninvasive techniques, particularly for the measurement of cardiac output as this is so fundamental in the assessment of status in patients with PAH.

Echocardiography

Echocardiography was, and is likely to remain for some time, the most important screening tool for patients with suspected pulmonary hypertension (Mukerjee *et al.*, 2004; Bossone *et al.*, 2005). In most developed countries a patient referred with unexplained breathlessness will have an echocardiogram. Abnormal echo findings are often the first indication of pulmonary hypertension and these should prompt referral to a pulmonary hypertension center. Using echocardiography it is routinely possible to estimate right ventricular systolic pressure from the pressure difference across the tricuspid valve, the flow of blood in the pulmonary outflow tract and the size of the cardiac chambers and to document the presence of a pericardial effusion. Echocardiography has the appeal that it is widely available and relatively easy to perform and repeat, though considerable technical expertise is required for good and reproducible results. Some studies have also shown that echocardiographic variables are proportional to outcome. For example, Raymond showed that survival in patients with PAH was reduced when there was right atrial enlargement, septal shift or pericardial effusion (Raymond *et al.*, 2002). Since the usual measure of pulmonary artery pressure quoted in the literature is mean pulmonary artery pressure, attempts have been made to calculate this using echocardiography (Abbas *et al.*, 2003a). In fact, however, there is a tight mathematical relationship between mean pulmonary artery pressure and systolic pulmonary artery pressure under all conditions, and thus it should be possible to estimate mean PA pressure from right ventricular systolic pressure measurements made in the echocardiography laboratory (Syyed and Peacock, 2004; Chemla *et al.*, 2004). There have also been attempts to measure pulmonary vascular resistance by echocardiography. For example, Abbas and coworkers found that the ratio of peak tricuspid regurgitation velocity to right ventricular outflow tract × velocity integral compared well with pulmonary vascular resistance measured by cardiac catheterization (Abbas *et al.*, 2003b).

The main problem with echocardiography has been the semi-subjective nature of the findings, making objective analysis difficult. Additionally several mathematical assumptions must be made to describe chamber size and shape and flow. Positive effects on echo-variables including right ventricular size, left ventricular size, right ventricular systolic function and left ventricular early diastolic filling were, however, confirmed in a study of the effects of bosentan (Galie *et al.*, 2003).

New techniques in the future such as amplification of echocardiographic signals by hypoxia, dobutamine and/or exercise, or the new technologies of three-dimensional echocardiography and tissue Doppler echocardiography may alter our perception but, currently, the place of echocardiography is largely for screening.

Magnetic resonance imaging

Magnetic resonance imaging (MRI) with a cardiac package allowing measurements throughout the cardiac cycle both at rest and with exercise is now held to be the 'gold standard' in right heart imaging in patients with pulmonary hypertension. Magnetic resonance imaging is, of course, expensive. Some patients suffer claustrophobia and the presence of a high powered magnet means that patients cannot be studied with any sort of metal in place. It does however offer great possibilities.

- It can be used to measure right ventricular mass, which is likely to be a function of both right ventricular outflow impedence and other variables that promote muscular hypertrophy. Right ventricular mass relates well to mean pulmonary artery pressure measured by catheterization, particularly when mass is expressed as the 'ventricular mass index' i.e. right ventricular mass/left ventricular mass (Saba *et al.*, 2002). Currently it appears that right ventricular mass changes little with therapy for pulmonary hypertension (Roeleveld *et al.*, 2004) but we do not yet know enough to know whether this is a good or bad thing. The studies conducted thus far which have assessed the effects of disease-targeted treatment on right ventricular mass have variously found improvement (Wilkins *et al.*, 2005; van Wolferen *et al.*, 2006) or stability (Roeleveld *et al.*, 2004) of right ventricular mass with (apparently beneficial) therapy.
- It can be used to measure chamber size of all four chambers during a cardiac cycle, at rest and with exercise. These measurements have been particularly fruitful and have shown that when patients with PAH exercise, the normal increase in right ventricular stroke volume does not occur (Figure 9.4) (Holverda *et al.*, 2006). Using dynamic images from MRI videos the relationship between right ventricular size, intraventricular septal shift and left ventricular size can be studied during the cardiac cycle (Figure 9.5). We know that septal shift into the left ventricle is proportional to systolic pulmonary artery pressure (Roeleveld *et al.*, 2005) . Improvements in these indices with disease-targeted treatments have been confirmed in small studies (Roeleveld *et al.*, 2004; van Wolferen *et al.*, 2006).

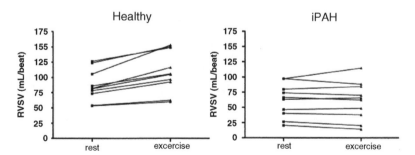

Figure 9.4 Right ventricular stroke volume (RVSV) at rest and during exercise in healthy controls and patients with idiopathic pulmonary arterial hypertension (iPAH). Right ventricular stroke volume in the patient group was lower at rest ($p = 0.06$), and did not change during exercise. In contrast to the patient group, RVSV was significantly increased during exercise ($p < 0.05$) in healthy controls. (Reproduced from *J Am Coll Cardiol.*, **47**(8), Holverda *et al.*, 1732–1733, Copyright (2006) with permission from the American College of Cardiology.)

Specifically, significant changes in left ventricular filling and stroke volume are sometimes seen, and these are likely the cause of exertional syncope in patients with PAH. It is possible to detect improvement in these parameters after three to six months of therapy (Figure 9.5; McLure *et al*, 2007)

- Magnetic resonance imaging can also show evidence of right ventricular myocardial damage. For example, Blyth and coworkers showed a pattern of delayed gadolinium contrast enhancement in patients with severe pulmonary hypertension. This contrast enhancement was concentrated at the right ventricular insertion points and in the interventricular septum, and the extent of this correlated with right ventricular function and pulmonary hemodynamics, suggesting that this may be a useful prognostic marker (Blyth *et al*., 2005). Interestingly, this pattern of delayed contrast enhancement matches the pattern of atrial natriuretic peptide staining in ventricles of chronic hypoxic rats (McKenzie *et al*., 1994).

We need longitudinal studies of right ventricular mass and chamber size after long-term therapy; a large scale European project is currently underway (the Euro MR project) to examine these changes. We also need to validate MRI-derived measures of cardiac output and pulmonary arterial flow. In the future it is likely that MRI will be more widely available and will be used for follow up of patients with PAH. In

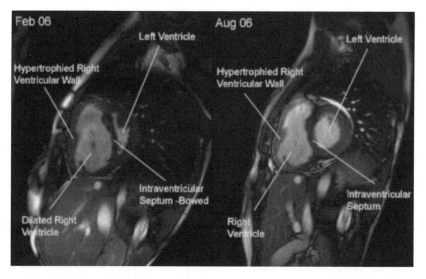

Figure 9.5 End-diastolic short axis cardiac MRI images from a patient with idiopathic pulmonary arterial hypertension at time of baseline assessment (Febuary 2006) and following 6 months of bosentan therapy (August 2006). Notable features at baseline are the severe dilatation of the right ventricle, bowing of the intraventricular at rest and near-obliteration of the left ventricular cavity. Follow up scan following a good clinical response to therapy shows significant improvement in right ventricular dilatation and septal bowing with normalization of left ventricular morphology (From McLure *et al*, in preparation)

the meantime, there is evidence that MRI variables in PAH patients do relate to NT-pro BNP measurement (Blyth *et al.*, 2006) and thus BNP may be a surrogate for the abnormalities in right ventricular function detected on MR.

9.4 Conclusions

Further clinical trials in PAH are probably going to be of combination therapies which may include patients at an earlier stage of disease (WHO Class II). Clinical trial design will therefore be more difficult if we wish to come to firm conclusions about the advisability or otherwise of combination therapy or early therapy with extremely expensive drugs. To convince patients, their doctors, the financiers and the regulators of the benefits of these therapies our end points will need to be increasingly sophisticated. Currently available are a number of techniques which help us evaluate directly and non-invasively the right ventricular and pulmonary circulatory function. These techniques must prove themselves alongside more traditional end points.

References

Abbas AE, Fortuin FD, Schiller NB, *et al.* (2003a) Echocardiographic determination of mean pulmonary artery pressure. *Am J Cardiol*; **92**(11):1373–1376.

Abbas AE, Fortuin FD, Schiller NB, *et al.* (2003b) A simple method for noninvasive estimation of pulmonary vascular resistance. *J Am Coll Cardiol*; **41**(6):1021–1027.

Abdul-Salam VB, Paul GA, Ali JO, *et al.* (2006) Identification of plasma protein biomarkers associated with idiopathic pulmonary arterial hypertension. *Proteomics*; **6**(7):2286–2294.

Andreassen AK, Wergeland R, Simonsen S, *et al.* (2006) N-terminal pro-B-type natriuretic peptide as an indicator of disease severity in a heterogeneous group of patients with chronic precapillary pulmonary hypertension. *Am J Cardiol*; **98**(4):525–529.

Anon, (2001) Recommendations on the management of pulmonary hypertension in clinical practice. *Heart*; 86 Suppl 1:I1–13.

ATS statement: guidelines for the six-minute walk test. (2002) *Am J Respir Crit Care Med*; **166**(1):111–117.

Badesch DB, Tapson VF, McGoon MD, *et al.* (2000) Continuous intravenous epoprostenol for pulmonary hypertension due to the scleroderma spectrum of disease. A randomized, controlled trial. *Ann Intern Med*; **132**(6):425–434.

Barst RJ, Rubin LJ, McGoon MD, *et al.* (1994) Survival in primary pulmonary hypertension with long-term continuous intravenous prostacyclin. *Ann Intern Med*; **121**(6):409–415.

Barst RJ, Rubin LJ, Long WA, *et al.* (1996) A comparison of continuous intravenous epoprostenol (prostacyclin) with conventional therapy for primary pulmonary hypertension. The Primary Pulmonary Hypertension Study Group. *N Engl J Med*; **334**(5):296–302.

Barst RJ, McGoon M, McLaughlin V, *et al.* (2003) Beraprost therapy for pulmonary arterial hypertension. *J Am Coll Cardiol*; **41**(12):2119–2125.

Barst RJ, Langleben D, Frost A, *et al.* (2004) Sitaxsentan therapy for pulmonary arterial hypertension. *Am J Respir Crit Care Med*; **169**(4):441–447.

Barst RJ, Langleben D, Badesch D, *et al.* (2006) Treatment of pulmonary arterial hypertension with the selective endothelin-A receptor antagonist sitaxsentan. *J Am Coll Cardiol*; **47**(10):2049–2056.

Barst RJ (2007) A review of pulmonary arterial hypertension: role of ambrisentan. *Vasc Health Risk Manag*; **3**(1):11–22.

Blyth KG, Groenning BA, Martin TN, *et al.* (2005) Contrast enhanced-cardiovascular magnetic resonance imaging in patients with pulmonary hypertension. *Eur Heart J.*; **28**:1993–1999.

Blyth KG, Groenning BA, Mark PB, *et al.* (2007) NT-proBNP can be used to detect RV systolic dysfunction in pulmonary hypertension. *Eur Respir J*; **29**:737–744.

Bossone E, Bodini BD, Mazza A, *et al.* (2005) Pulmonary arterial hypertension: the key role of echocardiography. *Chest*; **127**(5):1836–1843.

Castelain V, Chemla D, Humbert M, *et al.* (2002) Pulmonary artery pressure-flow relations after prostacyclin in primary pulmonary hypertension. *Am J Respir Crit Care Med*; **165**(3): 338–340.

Channick RN, Simonneau G, Sitbon O, *et al.* (2001) Effects of the dual endothelin-receptor antagonist bosentan in patients with pulmonary hypertension: a randomised placebo-controlled study. *Lancet*; **358**(9288):1119–1123.

Chemla D, Castelain V, Humbert M, *et al.* (2004) New formula for predicting mean pulmonary artery pressure using systolic pulmonary artery pressure. *Chest*; **126**(4):1313–1317.

D'Alonzo GE, Barst RJ, Ayres SM, *et al.* (1991) Survival in patients with primary pulmonary hypertension. Results from a national prospective registry. *Ann Intern Med*; **115**(5): 343–349.

Deboeck G, Niset G, Lamotte M, *et al.* (2004) Exercise testing in pulmonary arterial hypertension and in chronic heart failure. *Eur Respir J*; **23**(5):747–751.

EuroQol Group, (1990) EuroQol – a new facility for the measurement of health-related quality of life. *Health Policy*; **16**(3):199–208.

Fijalkowska A, Kurzyna M, Torbicki A, *et al.* (2006) Serum N-terminal brain natriuretic peptide as a prognostic parameter in patients with pulmonary hypertension. *Chest*; **129**(5):1313–1321.

Fishman AP, (2004) A century of pulmonary hemodynamics. *Am J Respir Crit Care Med*; **170**(2):109–113.

Galie N, (2001) Do we need controlled clinical trials in pulmonary arterial hypertension? *Eur Respir J*; **17**(1):1–3.

Galie N, Manes A, Branzi A, (2002) The new clinical trials on pharmacological treatment in pulmonary arterial hypertension. *Eur Respir J*; **20**(4):1037–1049.

Galie N, Humbert M, Vachiery JL, *et al.* (2002) Effects of beraprost sodium, an oral prostacyclin analogue, in patients with pulmonary arterial hypertension: a randomized, double-blind, placebo-controlled trial. *J Am Coll Cardiol.* May 1 2002; **39**(9):1496–1502.

Galie N, Hinderliter AL, Torbicki A, *et al.* (2003) Effects of the oral endothelin-receptor antagonist bosentan on echocardiographic and doppler measures in patients with pulmonary arterial hypertension. *J Am Coll Cardiol*; **41**(8):1380–1386.

Galie N, Torbicki A, Barst R, *et al.* (2004) Guidelines on diagnosis and treatment of pulmonary arterial hypertension. The Task Force on Diagnosis and Treatment of Pulmonary Arterial Hypertension of the European Society of Cardiology. *Eur Heart J*; **25**(24):2243–2278.

Higenbottam T, Wheeldon D, Wells F, *et al.* (1984) Long-term treatment of primary pulmonary hypertension with continuous intravenous epoprostenol (prostacyclin). *Lancet*; **1**(8385): 1046–1047.

Holverda S, Gan CT, Marcus JT, *et al.* (2006) Impaired stroke volume response to exercise in pulmonary arterial hypertension. *J Am Coll Cardiol*; **47**(8):1732–1733.

Hunt S, McEwen J, McKenna S. (1986) *Measuring health status*. London: Croom Helm.

Kawut SM, Palevsky HI, (2004) Surrogate end points for pulmonary arterial hypertension. *Am Heart J*; **148**(4):559–565.

Kawut SM, Taichman DB, Archer-Chicko CL, *et al*. (2003) Hemodynamics and survival in patients with pulmonary arterial hypertension related to systemic sclerosis. *Chest*; **123**(2):344–350.

Langleben D, Christman BW, Barst RJ, *et al*. (2002) Effects of the thromboxane synthetase inhibitor and receptor antagonist terbogrel in patients with primary pulmonary hypertension. *Am Heart J*; **143**(5):E4.

Leuchte HH, Neurohr C, Baumgartner R, *et al*. (2004) Brain natriuretic peptide and exercise capacity in lung fibrosis and pulmonary hypertension. *Am J Respir Crit Care Med*; **170**(4):360–365.

Leuchte HH, Baumgartner RA, Nounou ME, *et al*. (2006) Brain natriuretic peptide is a prognostic parameter in chronic lung disease. *Am J Respir Crit Care Med*; **173**(7):744–750.

Mahapatra S, Nishimura RA, Sorajja P, *et al*. (2006) Relationship of pulmonary arterial capacitance and mortality in idiopathic pulmonary arterial hypertension. *J Am Coll Cardiol*; **47**(4):799–803.

McGoon M, Gutterman D, Steen V, *et al*. (2004) Screening, early detection, and diagnosis of pulmonary arterial hypertension: ACCP evidence-based clinical practice guidelines. *Chest*; **126**(1 Suppl):14S–34S.

McGregor M, Sniderman A, (1985) On pulmonary vascular resistance: the need for more precise definition. *Am J Cardiol*; **55**(1):217–221.

McKenna SP, Doughty N, Meads DM, *et al*. (2006) The Cambridge Pulmonary Hypertension Outcome Review (CAMPHOR): a measure of health-related quality of life and quality of life for patients with pulmonary hypertension. *Qual Life Res*; **15**(1):103–115.

McKenzie JC, Kelley KB, Merisko-Liversidge EM, *et al*. (1994) Developmental pattern of ventricular atrial natriuretic peptide (ANP) expression in chronically hypoxic rats as an indicator of the hypertrophic process. *J Mol Cell Cardiol*; **26**(6):753–767.

McLaughlin VV, Shillington A, Rich S, (2002) Survival in primary pulmonary hypertension: the impact of epoprostenol therapy. *Circulation*; **106**(12):1477–1482.

McLaughlin VV, Sitbon O, Badesch DB, *et al*. (2005) Survival with first-line bosentan in patients with primary pulmonary hypertension. *Eur Respir J*; **25**(2):244–249.

McLure *et al*. (2007) Personal Communication.

Mereles D, Ehlken N, Kreuscher S, *et al*. (2006) Exercise and respiratory training improve exercise capacity and quality of life in patients with severe chronic pulmonary hypertension. *Circulation*; **114**(14):1482–1489.

Miyamoto S, Nagaya N, Satoh T, *et al*. (2000) Clinical correlates and prognostic significance of six-minute walk test in patients with primary pulmonary hypertension. Comparison with cardiopulmonary exercise testing. *Am J Respir Crit Care Med*; **161**(2 Pt 1):487–492.

Mukerjee D, St George D, Knight C, *et al*. (2004) Echocardiography and pulmonary function as screening tests for pulmonary arterial hypertension in systemic sclerosis. *Rheumatology (Oxford)*; **43**(4):461–466.

Nagaya N, Nishikimi T, Okano Y, *et al*. (1998) Plasma brain natriuretic peptide levels increase in proportion to the extent of right ventricular dysfunction in pulmonary hypertension. *J Am Coll Cardiol*; **31**(1):202–208.

Nagaya N, Nishikimi T, Uematsu M, *et al*. (2000) Plasma brain natriuretic peptide as a prognostic indicator in patients with primary pulmonary hypertension. *Circulation*; **102**(8):865–870.

Olschewski H, Simonneau G, Galie N, *et al*. (2002) Inhaled iloprost for severe pulmonary hypertension. *N Engl J Med*; **347**(5):322–329.

Oudiz RJ, Schilz RJ, Barst RJ, *et al*. (2004) Treprostinil, a prostacyclin analogue, in pulmonary arterial hypertension associated with connective tissue disease. *Chest*; **126**(2):420–427.

Peacock A, Naeije R, Galie N, *et al*. (2004) End points in pulmonary arterial hypertension: the way forward. *Eur Respir J*; **23**(6):947–953.

Provencher S, Chemla D, Herve P, *et al*. (2006) Heart rate responses during the 6-minute walk test in pulmonary arterial hypertension. *Eur Respir J*; **27**(1):114–120.

Raeside DA, Chalmers G, Clelland J, *et al*. (1998) Pulmonary artery pressure variation in patients with connective tissue disease: 24 hour ambulatory pulmonary artery pressure monitoring. *Thorax*; **53**(10):857–862.

Raeside DA, Smith A, Brown A, *et al*. (2000) Pulmonary artery pressure measurement during exercise testing in patients with suspected pulmonary hypertension. *Eur Respir J*; **16**(2): 282–287.

Raeside DA, Brown A, Patel KR, *et al*. (2002) Ambulatory pulmonary artery pressure monitoring during sleep and exercise in normal individuals and patients with COPD. *Thorax*; **57**(12): 1050–1053.

Raymond RJ, Hinderliter AL, Willis PW, *et al*. (2002) Echocardiographic predictors of adverse outcomes in primary pulmonary hypertension. *J Am Coll Cardiol*; **39**(7):1214–1219.

Rector TS, Cohn JN, (1992) Assessment of patient outcome with the Minnesota Living with Heart Failure questionnaire: reliability and validity during a randomized, double-blind, placebo-controlled trial of pimobendan. Pimobendan Multicenter Research Group. *Am Heart J*; **124**(4):1017–1025.

Reeves JT, Linehan JH, Stenmark KR, (2005) Distensibility of the normal human lung circulation during exercise. *Am J Physiol Lung Cell Mol Physiol*; **288**(3):L419–425.

Rich S, (2006) The current treatment of pulmonary arterial hypertension: time to redefine success. *Chest*; **130**(4):1198–1202.

Rich S, Kaufmann E, Levy PS, (1992) The effect of high doses of calcium-channel blockers on survival in primary pulmonary hypertension. *N Engl J Med*; **327**(2):76–81.

Roeleveld RJ, Vonk-Noordegraaf A, Marcus JT, *et al*. (2004) Effects of epoprostenol on right ventricular hypertrophy and dilatation in pulmonary hypertension. *Chest*; **125**(2):572–579.

Roeleveld RJ, Marcus JT, Faes TJ, *et al*. (2005) Interventricular Septal Configuration at MR Imaging and Pulmonary Arterial Pressure in Pulmonary Hypertension. *Radiology*; **234**(3):710–717.

Rubin LJ, Mendoza J, Hood M, *et al*. (1990) Treatment of primary pulmonary hypertension with continuous intravenous prostacyclin (epoprostenol). Results of a randomized trial. *Ann Intern Med*; **112**(7):485–491.

Rubin LJ, Badesch DB, Barst RJ, *et al*. (2002) Bosentan therapy for pulmonary arterial hypertension. *N Engl J Med*; **346**(12):896–903.

Saba TS, Foster J, Cockburn M, *et al*. (2002) Ventricular mass index using magnetic resonance imaging accurately estimates pulmonary artery pressure. *Eur Respir J*; **20**(6):1519–1524.

Shafazand S, Goldstein MK, Doyle RL, *et al*. (2004) Health-related quality of life in patients with pulmonary arterial hypertension. *Chest*; **126**(5):1452–1459.

Simonneau G, Barst RJ, Galie N, *et al*. (2002) Continuous subcutaneous infusion of treprostinil, a prostacyclin analogue, in patients with pulmonary arterial hypertension: a double-blind, randomized, placebo-controlled trial. *Am J Respir Crit Care Med*; **165**(6):800–804.

Simonneau G., Rubin LJ., Galie N. *et al*. (2008) For the Pulmonary Arterial Hypertension Combination Study of Epoprostenol and Sildenafil (PACES-1) Study Group. Safety and Efficacy of Combination Therapy with Sildenafil and Epoprostenol in Patients with Pulmonary Arterial Hypertension. *Ann Int Med* in Press.

Sitbon O, Humbert M, Nunes H, *et al*. (2002) Long-term intravenous epoprostenol infusion in primary pulmonary hypertension: prognostic factors and survival. *J Am Coll Cardiol*; **40**(4):780–788.

Syyed R, Peacock A, (2004) The relationship between systolic and diastolic and mean pulmonary artery pressures are conserved in man under differeing physiological and pathophysiological conditions [abstract]. *Am J Respir Crit Care Med*; 161:A56.

Torbicki A, Kurzyna M, Kuca P, *et al.* (2003) Detectable serum cardiac troponin T as a marker of poor prognosis among patients with chronic precapillary pulmonary hypertension. *Circulation*; **108**(7):844–848.

van Wolferen SA, Boonstra A, Marcus JT, *et al.* (2006) Right ventricular reverse remodelling after sildenafil in pulmonary arterial hypertension. *Heart*; **92**(12):1860–1861.

Ware JE, Jr., Sherbourne CD, (1992) The MOS 36-item short-form health survey (SF-36). I. Conceptual framework and item selection. *Med Care*; **30**(6):473–483.

Wensel R, Opitz CF, Anker SD, *et al.* (2002) Assessment of survival in patients with primary pulmonary hypertension: importance of cardiopulmonary exercise testing. *Circulation*; **106**(3):319–324.

Wilkins MR, Paul GA, Strange JW, *et al.* (2005) Sildenafil versus Endothelin Receptor Antagonist for Pulmonary Hypertension (SERAPH) study. *Am J Respir Crit Care Med*; **171**(11):1292–1297.

10 Comparative analysis of clinical trials and evidence-based treatment algorithm for pulmonary arterial hypertension

Nazzareno Galiè,[1] Alessandra Manes,[1] Naushad Hirani[2] and Robert Naeije[3]

[1]*Institute of Cardiology, University of Bologna, Italy*
[2]*Department of Cardiology, University of Calgary, Calgary, Canada*
[3]*Erasme University Hospital, Brussels, Belgium*

10.1 Introduction

Pulmonary arterial hypertension (PAH) encompasses a group of disorders characterized by a progressive increase in pulmonary vascular resistance leading to right ventricular failure and premature death (Farber and Loscalzo, 2004). PAH includes

Pulmonary Arterial Hypertension, Edited by Robyn J. Barst
© 2008 John Wiley & Sons, Ltd

idiopathic pulmonary arterial hypertension (IPAH, formerly known as primary pulmonary hypertension or PPH) and pulmonary hypertension associated with conditions such as connective tissue diseases, congenital systemic-to-pulmonary shunts, portal hypertension and human immunodeficiency virus (HIV) infection (Simonneau *et al.*, 2004). Since the early 1990s, significant advances in our understanding of the pathobiology of PAH have led to the development of several possible treatment options for this devastating condition (Humbert, Sitbon and Simonneau, 2004; Galiè *et al.*, 2004a). Despite these rapid and encouraging therapeutic advances, there remains no cure for IPAH.

In 1980, the National Institutes of Health (NIH) established an IPAH Registry that described the characteristics of IPAH and its natural history over a five-year period. The median survival was 2.8 years, with survival rates of 68%, 48% and 34% at one, three and five years, respectively (D'Alonzo *et al.*, 1991). These mortality rates rival those of patients with advanced metastatic carcinomas, particularly in the case of those most severely afflicted, or World Health Organization (WHO) functional class IV patients. Analysis of the survival of patients with PAH associated with differing etiologies suggests that the prognosis is worse for PAH associated with HIV and connective tissue diseases, but may be slightly better for PAH associated with portal hypertension (McLaughlin *et al.*, 2004). Patients with PAH related to congenital left-to-right cardiac shunts seem to have the best long-term prognosis overall, and may represent a somewhat distinct pathophysiologic subset.

A historical review reveals that therapeutic developments in this field have been accelerating. Between 1990 and 2000, there were three randomized clinical trials (RCTs) published in the literature (Rubin *et al.*, 1990; Barst *et al.*, 1996; Badesch *et al.*, 2000) compared with 15 RCTs published from 2001 to 2007 (Channick *et al.*, 2001; Langleben *et al.*, 2002; Simonneau *et al.*, 2002; Rubin *et al.*, 2002; Galiè *et al.*, 2002; Olschewski *et al.*, 2002; Barst *et al.*, 2003; Humbert *et al.*, 2004; Barst *et al.*, 2004; Sastry *et al.*, 2004; Galiè *et al.*, 2005; Galiè *et al.*, 2006; Barst *et al.*, 2006a; McLaughlin *et al.*, 2006; Singh *et al.*, 2006) (Tables 10.1 and 10.2). The wealth of recent literature has enabled the adoption of evidence-based guidelines to assist with the therapeutic approach to WHO class III and IV patients with PAH (Galiè *et al.*, 2004a; Badesch *et al.*, 2004; Badesch *et al.*, 2007). Additional long-term studies have provided insights into the maintenance of beneficial effects seen in short-term studies and into the survival of treated cohorts (Table 10.3)

This chapter will comparatively analyze both Randomized Controlled Studies and Long-term Continuation Studies (> six months to years) with the new treatments reported in the literature and will propose a current, evidence-based treatment algorithm.

Table 10.1 Randomized controlled trials with PAH monotherapies

Class	Reference	Agent	n	6MWD (m) Treatment effect
Prostanoids	Rubin *et al.*, 1990	epoprostenol	23	45
	Barst *et al.*, 1996	epoprostenol	81	47
	Badesch *et al.*, 2000	epoprostenol	111[a]	94
	Simonneau *et al.*, 2002	treprostinil	469	16[†]
	Olschewski *et al.*, 2002	iloprost	203	36
	Galiè *et al.*, 2002	beraprost	130	25
	Barst *et al.*, 2003	beraprost	116	31[b]
TXA$_2$I	Langleben *et al.*, 2002	terbogrel	71	0
ERA	Channick *et al.*, 2001	bosentan	32	76
	Rubin *et al.*, 2002	bosentan	213	44
	Barst *et al.*, 2004	sitaxsentan	178	33
	Barst *et al.*, 2006a	sitaxentan	247	31
	Galiè *et al.*, 2006	bosentan	54[c]	53
PDE5I	Sastry *et al.*, 2004	sildenafil	22	44%[d]
	Galiè *et al.*, 2005a	sildenafil	278	50
	Singh *et al.*, 2006	sildenafil	20	66
	Oudiz *et al.*, 2007a	ambrisentan	202	31, 51[e]
	Olschewski *et al.*, 2006	ambrisentan	192	32, 59[f]

ERA: endothelin receptor antagonists; PAH: pulmonary arterial hypertension; PDE5I: phosphodiesterase-5 inhibitors; 6MWD: 6-minute walk distance; TXA$_2$I: thromboxane synthetase inhibitor/receptor antagonist.

[a] patients with sclerodermia spectrum of diseases; [b] median values; [c] patients with Eisenmenger Syndrome; [d] exercise time improvement; [e] 2 doses; [f] 2 doses.

Table 10.2 Randomized controlled trials with PAH combination therapies

Classes	Reference	Agents	n	6MWD (m) Treatment effect
Prostanoid + ERA	Humbert *et al.*, 2003	epoprostenol + bosentan	33	ns
Prostanoid + PDE5I	Simonneau *et al.*, 2007	epoprostenol + sildenafil	267	26
ERA + Prostanoid	Hoeper *et al.*, 2007	bosentan + iloprost	40[a]	ns
	McLaughlin *et al.*, 2006	bosentan + iloprost	67	26

ERA: endothelin receptor antagonists; PDE5I: phosphodiesterase-5 inhibitors; 6MWD: 6-minute walk distance; ns: no statistically significant difference detected; [a] study terminated early.

Table 10.3 Long-term studies with PAH therapies in IPAH

Drug class	Reference	Agent	n	Long-term (≥ 1 year) increase in 6MWD (m)	Reported survival (%)			
					1 yr	3 yr	4 yr	5 yr
Supportive therapy	D'Alonzo et al., 1991	—	194	—	68	48		34
CCB (vasoreactivity responders)	Rich, Kaufmann and Levy, 1992	CCB	17	—	94	94		94
Prostanoids	Sitbon et al., 2005a	CCB	38	87	100	97		97
	Nagaya et al., 1999	beraprost	24	—	96	76		
	Hoeper et al., 2000	iloprost	24	85	100			
	McLaughlin, Shillington and Rich, 2002	epoprostenol	162	—	88	63		
	Sitbon et al., 2002	epoprostenol	178	142	85	63		55
	Kuhn et al., 2003a	epoprostenol	41	55	85	65		
	Barst et al., 2003a	beraprost	60	23b	98b			
	Opitz et al., 2005	iloprost	76	—	79	59	59	49
	Lang et al., 2006a,c	treprostinil	122	65	89		66	
	Barst et al., 2006a	treprostinil	332	—	91	76	72	
ERA	Benza et al., 2006a	sitaxsentan	92	—	94			
	McLaughlin et al., 2005c	bosentan	169	—	96	86		
	Sitbon et al., 2005bc	bosentan	139	—	97			
	Provencher et al., 2006d	bosentan	103	41	92	79		
	Oudiz et al., 2007ba	ambrisentan	383	36	92			
PDE5I	Galiè et al., 2005a	sildenafil	149	51	94			

IPAH: idiopathic pulmonary arterial hypertension; n: number of patients receiving active treatment; 6MWD: 6-minute walk distance; CCB: calcium channel blockers; ERA: endothelin receptor antagonists; PDE5I: phosphodiesterase-5 inhibitors.

[a] These studies include also patients with associated types of PAH in addition to IPAH.

[b] Not significantly different from placebo-control group.

[c] This study includes also patients with non-operable chronic thromboembolic pulmonary hypertension.

[d] The survival rates include significant numbers of patients that received combination therapy.

10.2 Randomized controlled studies (Table 10.1)

Exercise capacity

The first agent to be studied using an RCT design was epoprostenol. Although the trials were placebo-controlled, for logistical and ethical reasons the trials were not double blind, avoiding the application of a tunnelized catheter and portable pumps in the placebo patients; protocols were third party blind (for efficacy end points) (Rubin *et al.*, 1990; Barst *et al.*, 1996; Badesch *et al.*, 2000). The Barst study (Barst *et al.*, 1996) used a 12-week timeframe and demonstrated that continuous intravenous (IV) epoprostenol increased 6-minute walk distance by 47 m over conventionally treated patients. Although it was not designed to address mortality, it did suggest a significant survival benefit in NYHA functional class III and IV patients. In this study, the baseline 6-minute walk distance was correlated with survival, a correlation that has been verified by other authors (Miyamoto *et al.*, 2000; Paciocco *et al.*, 2001; Sitbon *et al.*, 2002). In addition, regulatory authorities have accepted the short-term 6-minute walk distance change as the primary end point for designing studies intended to demonstrate efficacy and to achieve official approval for the treatment of PAH patients. All recent studies using prostanoids (Simonneau *et al.*, 2002; Galiè *et al.*, 2002; Olschewski *et al.*, 2002; Barst *et al.*, 2004), endothelin receptor antagonists (Channick *et al.*, 2001; Rubin *et al.*, 2002; Barst *et al.*, 2004; Galiè *et al.*, 2006; Barst *et al.*, 2006a; Olschewski *et al.*, 2006; Oudiz *et al.*, 2007) and phosphodiesterase-5 inhibitors (Galiè *et al.*, 2005; Singh *et al.*, 2006) have shown a statistically significant improvement of the 6-minute walk distance, ranging from 16 to 76 m. The importance of this benefit in 6-minute walk distance cannot be downplayed given its relationship with mortality, but the average final 6-minute walk distance of most trials is approximately 360–400 m after three to four months of therapy. This still represents a severe impairment in exercise capacity, as the normal predicted 6-minute walk distance for the typical subject would range from 606 m (female, age 50, weight 55 kg, height 1.68 m) to 655 m (male, age 55, weight 75 kg, height 1.78 m) (Enright and Sherril, 1998).

Functional capacity

Functional capacity is an inherently more subjective outcome measure than exercise capacity, although changes with therapy may provide ancillary corroborative data for improvement or deterioration (Peacock *et al.*, 2004). The Bosentan Randomized Trial of Endothelin Antagonist THErapy (BREATHE-1) study showed that 42% of patients improved at least one functional class with 16 weeks of bosentan while 30% of those who received placebo did the same (Rubin *et al.*, 2002). The Sitaxsentan To Relieve ImpaireD Exercise (STRIDE-1) trial suggested that 30% of patients receiving sitaxsentan improved functional class compared to 15% in the placebo group at 12 weeks (Barst *et al.*, 2003), but STRIDE-2 suggested these values to be closer to 13% and 10%, respectively, at 18 weeks (Barst *et al.*, 2006a). A similar analysis with increasing doses of sildenafil in the Sildenafil Use in Pulmonary Arterial HypERtension (SUPER-1) trial indicated the proportion of patients who improved functional class ranged between 28 and 42% at 12 weeks, compared with only 7% with placebo (Galiè et al., 2005). With inhaled iloprost, 24% of patients improved one WHO functional class, whereas 13% improved on placebo (Olschewski et al., 2002). Although these results are not very compelling overall given that between 7 and 30% of placebo-treated patients also improve across trials, it appears that 15 to 40% of patients can improve by one functional class at three to four months with PAH-specific monotherapy. Conversely, this suggests that the majority of patients in fact do not improve functional capacity to an extent that is clearly detectable.

Clinical worsening

The combined end point of time-to-clinical-worsening is commonly defined as the time between enrollment and the need for PAH-related hospitalization, the need for escalation of therapy (e.g. IV epoprostenol or lung transplantation), or death (Peacock et al., 2004). The BREATHE-1 study showed that 6% of bosentan-treated patients vs 20% of placebo-treated patients had deteriorated by week 28; the effect was statistically significant after 16 weeks but not at 12 weeks (Rubin et al., 2002). In the Aerosolized Iloprost Randomized (AIR) study, investigators reported that 5% vs 12% of patients deteriorated or died in the inhaled iloprost vs placebo groups, respectively, although this was not a statistically significant difference (Olschewski et al., 2002). If total withdrawals from the protocol for all reasons were included, Kaplan–Meier curves did suggest a difference between the two groups at 12 weeks. The most recent study with sitaxsentan did not corroborate these early data, with no significant difference demonstrated between either of the endothelin receptor antagonists (the study included an open-label bosentan arm) and placebo at 18 weeks (Barst et al., 2006a). The time-to-clinical-worsening results were significant for ARIES-2 but not for ARIES-1. The time-to-clinical-worsening results were not statistically significant at 12 weeks with sildenafil, although there may have been a difference in the hospitalization rate between the placebo and active treatment groups (Galiè et al., 2005). The different results observed in these trials could be explained by a diverse efficacy of the compounds. However, other reasons could explain the data: including differences in inclusion criteria, enrichment (or lack thereof) of the patient population, baseline characteristics, definition of clinical worsening and study duration. In addition, time-to-clinical-worsening was a secondary end point in these studies and therefore the results should only be considered supportive or unsupportive of the primary end points.

Hemodynamics

The hemodynamic consequences of PAH have been well documented, and data from the NIH registry has suggested that survival is correlated particularly with initial mean right atrial pressure (RAP), mean pulmonary arterial pressure (mPAP), and cardiac index (D'Alonzo *et al.*, 1991). The changes in these parameters with PAH-specific therapies in the short term have been small, loosely correlated with clinical outcomes and sometimes difficult to demonstrate (Peacock *et al.*, 2004; Galiè *et al.*, 2004b). For example, with IV epoprostenol, mPAP decreased from 61.0 to 58.6 mm Hg for a fall of 2.4 mm Hg, but a fall of 1.4 mm Hg was also seen in the conventional therapy group, resulting in a statistically insignificant difference (Badesch *et al.*, 2000). Similarly small changes in mPAP, RAP and cardiac index have been noted in the short-term components of studies with bosentan (Channick *et al.*, 2001), sitaxsentan (Barst *et al.*, 2004), ambrisentan (Galiè *et al.*, 2005b), iloprost (Olschewski *et al.*, 2002) and sildenafil (Galiè *et al.*, 2005a), although statistical significance has been demonstrated. In general, the increase in cardiac index appears to be of a greater magnitude (approximately 10–20%) than the 2–6% reduction seen in mPAP, suggesting that this may in fact be the physiologic mechanism most responsible for clinical improvement. Interestingly, no study has demonstrated a significant improvement in the important parameter RAP. Therefore, despite definite exercise, functional and clinical improvements, the short-term effects of the new compounds on hemodynamics have been disappointing.

Quality of life

Quality of life has not been addressed in many PAH trials, but more recent studies have included it as an outcome measure using the Short Form-36 (SF-36) survey instrument. This tool uses questions designed to assess the impact of illness (including the burdens of treatment) on eight domains of the quality of life of patients, and has been used as a measure of impairment and disability in several disease settings, including PAH (Stahl *et al.*, 2005; Pepke-Zaba *et al.*, 2005). Data from the SUPER-1 trial suggested that at 12 weeks sildenafil was associated with improvements in SF-36 scores over placebo in three of the eight domains, particularly in the physical functioning and general health domains (Pepke-Zaba *et al.*, 2005). Absolute scores, however, remained low at the end of the study, again supporting the concept that although monotherapy with PAH-specific agents is associated with improvements, they are of an inadequate degree in the short term. Instruments designed to assess health-related quality of life more specifically for PAH patients are under development, and will hopefully provide more insight into therapeutic outcomes in the future (Doughty *et al.*, 2005; McKenna *et al.*, 2006).

10.3 Long-term continuation studies (Table 10.2)

Long-term data from cohorts of PAH patients treated with emerging agents are accumulating daily, and recent studies have described the outcomes of treatment for up to several years or more. However, these studies have numerous limitations, including their open-label nature, patient drop-outs, treatment changes and the absence of contemporary placebo comparison groups.

Exercise capacity

A long-term cohort analysis of patients treated with IV epoprostenol in France suggested that the 142-m improvement in walk distance achieved in severe patients by three months was maintained at one year (Sitbon *et al.*, 2002). A one-year study with inhaled iloprost had suggested an impressive benefit in 6-minute walk distance in IPAH patients (Hoeper *et al.*, 2000), although a more thorough recent analysis of up to five years of experience after the AIR trial has shown less favorable results (Opitz *et al.*, 2005). A recent study of the long-term experience with subcutaneous (SC) treprostinil in Europe suggested that the improvement in exercise capacity after 12 months of therapy was 73 m, a substantial increase over the short-term results that may have been related to underdosing during the short-term RCT (Lang *et al.*, 2006). The long-term experience with oral beraprost also underscores the importance of continually re-analyzing outcomes, since the apparent benefits to exercise capacity at three (Galiè *et al.*, 2002) and six (Barst *et al.*, 2003) months were not maintained at the end of a subsequent one-year RCT (Barst *et al.*, 2003). It should be noted that this is the only study with a double-blind and randomized phase of 12 months' duration.

In an extension of the original bosentan pilot study, Sitbon and coworkers demonstrated that 19 patients treated with blinded and then open-label bosentan for more than one year maintained the 60 m gains that they had achieved in 6-minute walk distance (Sitbon *et al.*, 2003). This was the first evidence that exercise endurance gains can be maintained for longer than three to four months with an oral agent, and it has been replicated, although with a one-year improvement of 41 m in a larger cohort (Provencher *et al.*, 2006). A one-year follow-up study of 10 Canadian patients who received sitaxsentan also suggested persistence of a 50-m treatment effect (Benza *et al.*, 2006). The experience with the selective endothelin-A receptor antagonist ambrisentan is more recent, but data from 64 patients indicated that 6-minute walk distance improvements of over 50 m were maintained up to 48 weeks (Galiè *et al.*, 2005c).

With sildenafil, the 149 patients who completed the one-year open-label extension (SUPER-2) of the SUPER-1 study maintained an average benefit of 51 m in 6-minute walk distance (Rubin *et al.*, 2005). Taken together, it appears as if the short-term improvements in exercise capacity seem to be maintained from 6–12 months, although this still only represents approximately 60% of the predicted normal exercise capacity for most patients.

Functional capacity

The experience from McLaughlin and coworkers with IV epoprostenol demonstrated that 72–90% of patients improved functional class after approximately 17 months of treatment (McLaughlin, Shillington and Rich, 2002). From the data of

Sitbon and coworkers with epoprostenol (Sitbon *et al.*, 2002), at least 63% of patients improved functional capacity at one year. In the cohort observed by Kuhn and others, it was seen that a majority of the survivors also improved functional class with epoprostenol (Kuhn *et al.*, 2003). Also, a recent intention-to-treat analysis of long-term SC treprostinil-treated patients suggested that functional class improved from a mean of 2.5 to 3.2 at one year (Lang *et al.*, 2006).

With bosentan, 41% of the 29 patients who participated in the open-label extension of the pilot study were in a better WHO functional class at the end of one year (Sitbon *et al.*, 2006), and 48% of a 91-patient cohort improved (Provencher *et al.*, 2006). In the 10-patient cohort that was exposed to sitaxsentan for over one year, 9 patients improved functional class (Benza *et al.*, 2006). The ambrisentan data have shown 35% of patients having a better functional class at 48 weeks (Galiè *et al.*, 2005c), which is similar to what has been seen with sildenafil (Rubin *et al.*, 2005).

Of course, the interpretation of such cohort analyses is limited by the lack of an adequate control group and possible selection or survival bias. Taking into account these limitations, there appears to be a suggestion for sustained benefit in functional capacity for at least a proportion of patients treated with newer agents, although it seems that one-half or more are not likely to benefit and therefore remain in functional classes III or IV.

Hemodynamics

The benefits of continuous IV epoprostenol on cardiac index, mean RAP, and mPAP were demonstrated by McLaughlin and coworkers at 17 months in 115 patients, with maintenance of the benefits to 47 months in 61 of these patients (McLaughlin, Shillington and Rich, 2002). Other analyses of the long-term experience with epoprostenol have shown similar sustained benefits at up to the three-year mark (Sitbon *et al.*, 2002; Kuhn *et al.*, 2003). The initial positive results on hemodynamics from the initial cohort of iloprost-treated patients (Olschewski *et al.*, 2002) have not been reproduced in longer-term analyses (Opitz *et al.*, 2005). Similarly, there was no difference between the placebo and treatment group hemodynamic variables at the end of the one-year beraprost trial (Barst *et al.*, 2003).

There were positive hemodynamic changes noted in most of the 11 patients treated with a mean of 15 months of bosentan in the cohort described by Sitbon and coworkers (Sitbon *et al.*, 2003), as well as in 48 patients in a more recent cohort (Provencher *et al.*, 2006), helping to corroborate the positive clinical findings.

Despite a suggestion for maintenance of the short-term hemodynamic benefit exerted by PAH-specific treatments, the extent of the favorable long-term effect remains limited.

Survival

Given the constraints on trial design mentioned above, recent studies have attempted to address the issue of survival by comparing cohorts of treated patients either with matched historical controls or with the expected survival extrapolated from baseline hemodynamic parameters using the NIH registry equation (D'Alonzo *et al.*, 1991). The advantage of using this approach is that the expected survival can be calculated for each patient, thereby more accurately accounting for baseline severity. However, there are numerous limitations: the data used to derive the NIH equations were collected in the early 1980s, when clinical practice may have differed substantially; only a minority of patients (20%) were on anticoagulant therapy, which is not the case in more recent cohorts; the data were limited to IPAH patients; entry into the registry did not require stringent inclusion criteria, as modern clinical trials do. These limitations make such comparative studies suboptimal, and the insights gained from them cannot be considered definitive. However, they remain valuable to reassure clinicians that emerging agents are not detrimental to their patients and that improvement in survival is occurring over time with newer treatment strategies.

In 1992, the dramatic improvement in survival demonstrated by Rich and coworkers in their non-randomized cohort study using high-dose calcium channel blockers (CCBs) suggested for the first time that in a subset of PAH patients mortality rates could be altered (Rich, Kaufmann and Levy, 1992). A five-year survival of 94% was shown in treated patients who were previously identified as acute vasodilator responders, an impressive achievement in comparison to historical controls and conventionally managed non-responders. Observations in cohorts of responders have verified this over several years (Sitbon *et al.*, 2005a). However, the use of CCBs has been occasionally associated with catastrophic outcomes (Partanen *et al.*, 1993) if initiated without an acute vasoreactivity test (Galiè *et al.*, 1995), and this procedure is mandatory to identify the subgroup of subjects who will likely respond to CCBs (Galiè *et al.*, 2004a). Review of years of experience seems to suggest that this subset of patients is smaller than initially thought (Sitbon *et al.*, 2005a, Galiè *et al.*, 1995), and long-term treatment with CCBs has been of great benefit to a relatively small number of patients. This has lead to a tightening of the definition of 'acute vasodilator response,' and has altered the current recommended indications for the use of CCBs (Galiè *et al.*, 2004a). The evolution of the role of CCBs highlights the importance of continued vigilance and documentation of the experience with promising therapies in this area.

Apart from the landmark RCT with IV epoprostenol in which there were no deaths in the treatment group vs eight in the conventionally managed group (Barst *et al.*, 1996), three other studies have reported survival in patients treated with epoprostenol (Sitbon *et al.*, 2002; McLaughlin, Shillington and Rich, 2002; Kuhn *et al.*, 2003). Two of these (McLaughlin, Shillington and Rich, 2002; Kuhn *et al.*, 2003) compared the prospectively followed cohort survival rates with the predicted NIH registry prediction equation (D'Alonzo *et al.*, 1991), and one (Sitbon *et al.*, 2002) used a matched historical cohort. All three studies suggest an improvement in survival at the three-year point from the predicted 33–39% to approximately 63–65%. Similarly, two more recent publications (Lang *et al.*, 2006; Barst *et al.*, 2006b) suggest that the four-year survival with SC treprostinil is 66–72%, with one of these studies (Barst *et al.*, 2006b) reporting a corresponding NIH predicted survival to be 38% at four years. The long-term survival initially seemed quite favorable in a retrospective analysis of 24 patients receiving oral beraprost therapy compared to 34 consecutive conventionally managed patients in 1999 (Nagaya *et al.*, 2006), but the year-long RCT with beraprost and placebo did not verify this first impression (Barst *et al.*, 2003). The survival data with inhaled iloprost up to five years were published recently, and although there was an improvement over the predicted survival – 49% vs. 32% using the NIH registry prediction equation – the overall analysis suggests that the role of inhaled iloprost as a monotherapy is questionable (Opitz *et al.*, 2005).

The most recent long-term observational study of 103 IPAH patients treated with bosentan estimated the three-year survival rate to be 79% vs an NIH registry predicted survival of 51% (Provencher *et al.*, 2006). However, this study included 45 patients who were also eventually treated with prostanoids, and thus was more akin to an evaluation of the strategy of initial monotherapy with bosentan than a true survival cohort. The results were in keeping with the experience of McLaughlin and coworkers, who estimated the three-year IPAH survival with first-line bosentan to be 86% (McLaughlin *et al.*, 2005). With sitaxsentan, preliminary survival rates from the STRIDE-2 study show an observed one-year survival of 94% in IPAH patients vs an NIH Registry predicted 73% (Benza *et al.*, 2006). Similarly, with ambrisentan, preliminary survival rates from the pooled experience show an observed one-year survival of 92% in IPAH patients vs an NIH Registry predicted 74% (Galiè *et al.*, 2005c). The one-year survival results with 141 IPAH sildenafil-treated patients were 96% vs predicted 71% (Galiè *et al.*, 2005d).

Table 10.3 illustrates the striking difference between the dismal survival of IPAH patients enrolled in the NIH registry and the subsequent series. It confirms the very good long-term survival of the vasoreactive patients who respond favorably to chronic CCB treatment, a clearly distinct subset of patients who are likely to have a unique underlying pathobiology. The more recent series with new targeted therapies show similar survival patterns that appear to be better as compared to the NIH registry cohort. However, given the suboptimal study designs, the observed improvements in survival could conceivably be attributed to many factors, including diverse inclusion/diagnostic criteria and different contemporary supportive treatment strategies in addition to the possible favorable effect of the novel therapies. Even if the methodological limitations thus far have hindered the determination of the absolute benefits of individual agents, there is a suggestion that the evaluated strategies with first-line targeted compounds appear to be providing PAH patients with options that are extending survival much longer than would have been possible in the 1980s.

10.4 Combination studies

Combination therapy with different classes of targeted PAH therapies is the subject of ongoing studies, although four randomized trials (McLaughlin *et al.*, 2006;

Humbert *et al.*, 2003; Hoeper *et al.*, 2006; Simonneau *et al.*, 2007) (Table 10.2) and several uncontrolled, open label studies have been reported (Hoeper *et al.*, 2006; Hoeper *et al.*, 2003; Ghofrani *et al.*, 2003; Hoeper *et al.*, 2004; Mathai *et al.*, 2007). Most of these studies have used an incremental approach when monotherapy has been considered inadequate. The determination of efficacy on various end points with combination therapy has proven difficult, with somewhat inconclusive results from two small, likely underpowered RCTs, despite trends toward improvements in exercise capacity and hemodynamics (Humbert *et al.*, 2003; Hoeper *et al.*, 2006). More recently, two larger, international, multicenter combination trials have demonstrated more significant improvements in hemodynamics and 6-minute walk distance, but of a notably smaller magnitude than with the monotherapy trials (McLaughlin *et al.*, 2006; Simonneau *et al.*, 2007). The reasons for this may relate to limitations of the outcome measure of 6-minute walk distance (i.e. a 'ceiling-effect'), the numerous difficulties in trial design with combination therapy in a rare disease setting, or to true problems with incremental efficacy of the combinations and strategies tested. Given the extensive positive – albeit uncontrolled – collective experience with combination therapies targeting multiple pathobiologic pathways in PAH (Hoeper, 2007), the latter seems unlikely, but further RCTs with refinements of trial design and outcome measures may help clarify the issue. However, the positive outcomes of the two more recent larger studies on combination therapy suggest upgrading the recommendation for the use of combination therapy as outlined in the following treatment algorithm (McLaughlin *et al.*, 2006; Simonneau *et al.*, 2007).

10.5   Evidence-based treatment algorithm

The treatment algorithm is shown in Figure 10.1 and color plate 10 (Galiè *et al.*, 2004a; Badesch *et al.*, 2004; Badesch *et al.*, 2007; Galiè *et al.*, 2004b). The algorithm is appropriate for patients with IPAH or PAH associated to connective tissue diseases. Extrapolation of these recommendations to the other PAH subgroups should be done with caution. The suggested initial approach is the adoption of the general measures and initiation of the supportive therapy. Oral anticoagulant treatment is initiated in patients with IPAH. The proposed target international normalized ratio (INR) varies somewhat between 1.5 and 3.0. The anticoagulation of other forms of PAH is also suggested if no bleeding-risk factors are present. Appropriate diuretic treatment in case of right heart failure allows clear symptomatic and clinical benefits. Although no consistent data are currently available on long-term supplemental oxygen treatment in PAH, the consensus is to maintain oxygen saturations at $> 90\%$. The usefulness of digitalis is controversial and IV inotropes such as dobutamine may be used in end-stage right heart failure. Owing to the complexity of the acute vasoreactivity tests, and of the treatment options available, it is recommended that consideration be given to referral of patients with PAH to a specialized center. A positive acute response to vasoreactivity test is defined as a fall in mPAP

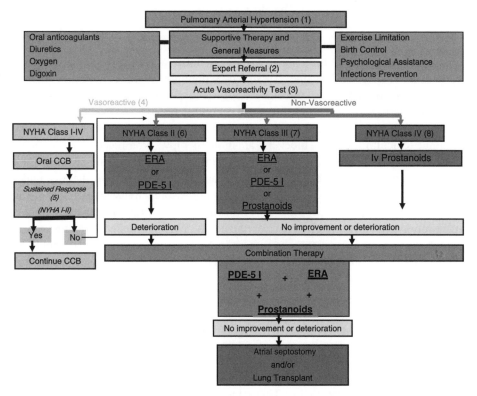

Figure 10.1 Pulmonary arterial hypertension treatment algorithm. A full color version of the figure is reproduced in the color plate section of this book.

(1) Different treatments have been evaluated mainly in sporadic idiopathic pulmonary arterial hypertension patients (IPAH), and in PAH associated with scleroderma or to anorexigen use. Extrapolation of these recommendations to the other PAH subgroups should be done with caution.

(2) Owing to the complexity of the acute vasoreactivity tests, and of the treatment options available, it is strongly recommended that consideration be given to referral of patients with PAH to a specialized center.

(3) Acute vasoreactivity test should be performed in all patients with PAH even if the greater incidence of positive response is achieved in patients with IPAH and PAH associated to anorexigen use.

(4) A positive acute response to vasodilators is defined as a fall in mean pulmonary artery pressure of at least 10 mm Hg to less than or equal to 40 mm Hg, with an increase or no change in cardiac output during acute challenge with inhaled NO or IV epoprostenol.

(5) Sustained response to calcium channel blockers (CCB) is defined as patients being in NYHA functional class I or II with near-normal hemodynamics after several months of treatment.

(6) In patients in NYHA functional class II, first line therapy may include phosphodiesterase-5 inhibitors or oral endothelin receptor antagonists

(7) In patients in NYHA functional class III, first line therapy may include phosphodiesterase-5 inhibitors, oral endothelin receptor antagonists, chronic IV epoprostenol or prostanoid analogues.

(8) Most experts consider that NYHA functional class IV patients (regardless of response with acute vasoreactivity testing) should be treated with IV prostanoids (survival improvement, worldwide experience and rapidity of action).

CCB: calcium channel blockers; ERA: endothelin receptor antagonists; IV: continuous intravenous; PDE5 I: phosphodiesterase-5 inhibitors; BAS: balloon atrial septostomy.

of at least 10 mm Hg to less than or equal to 40 mm Hg, with an increase or unchanged cardiac output during acute challenge with inhaled NO, IV epoprostenol, or IV adenosine. Treatment with high doses of calcium channel blockers is recommended in NYHA class I–III responders to acute vasoreactivity tests; long-term response (after three to six months) needs to be evaluated and subjects in NYHA classes I and II and with marked hemodynamic improvement can continue calcium channel blockers as monotherapy. Non-responders to acute vasoreactivity testing who are in NYHA functional class I with no signs of poor prognosis should continue with general measures and supportive therapy under close clinical follow-up. Non-responders to acute vasoreactivity testing who are in NYHA functional class II may be initiated with an oral phosphodiesterase-5 inhibitor or an oral endothelin receptor antagonist. Non-responders to acute vasore-activity testing, or responders who remain in NYHA functional class III should be considered candidates for treatment with either an endothelin receptor antagonist, an oral phosphodiesterase type 5 inhibitor or a prostanoid.

As no head-to-head comparisons between the three classes of drugs are available it is not possible to define the 'first line compound' to be used. Therefore the choice of the drug is dependent on a variety of factors, including the approval status, route of administration, side-effect profile, patient's preferences, physician's experience and costs.

Combination therapy may be considered for patients who fail to improve or deteriorate with first-line treatment. This strategy should be implemented in experienced referral centers.

Continuous IV prostanoids are most often considered as first line therapy for patients in NYHA functional class IV because of the demonstrated survival benefit in this subset. However, these patients should be considered for concurrent listing for lung transplantation and subsequently delisted if significant improvement is demonstrated on long-term PAH therapy; close serial follow-up evaluation is needed as sudden onset of rapid deterioration is not uncommon in patients with PAH. Although both oral bosentan and SC/IV treprostinil are approved in NYHA class IV patients, most experts consider these treatments as a second line for severely ill patients. Also in this case, combination therapy should be implemented in case of no response or deterioration. Atrial septostomy is performed in severely ill patients as a palliative bridge to lung transplantation. Double lung or heart–lung transplantation are indicated in patients with advanced NYHA class III and class IV symptoms that are refractory to available medical treatments.

10.6   Conclusions

In the early 1990s PAH was uniformly fatal, with a median life expectancy of only a few years. However, since then, a total of 18 multicenter, randomized, controlled, trials of prostacyclin derivatives, endothelin receptor antagonists and a phosphodiesterase-5 inhibitor have been reported in a total of 2248 patients, with favorable results. This is a remarkable achievement given the rarity and severity of the disease. All these trials, with the exception of one interrupted because of side effects, have reported a moderate but significant increase in exercise capacity, together with improvements in functional class, clinical stability, hemodynamics and quality of life, though less consistently and often to a minor degree. None of the treatments tested so far has offered a cure. Long-term continuation studies have shown a persistent improvement in exercise capacity and a better survival, but in approximately half of the patients after one to two years, the functional handicap remains excessive and quality of life limited. Accordingly, randomized, controlled trials of combination therapies have been undertaken, up to a total of four reported until now, though with inconclusive results. No head-to-head comparison between classes of drugs shown efficacious in PAH has been reported. Therefore the choice of the 'first-line' compound remains a patient-tailored clinical decision. In general, the best results have been obtained in patients with IPAH. A reasonable expert consensus evidence-based step-by-step treatment algorithm can be proposed on the basis of initial functional impairment and iterative evaluations, starting with an oral drug, either an endothelin receptor antagonist or a phosphodiesterase-5 inhibitor, then combining them, and eventually adding a parenteral prostacyclin derivative until consideration of atrial septostomy and lung transplantation.

References

Badesch DB, Tapson VF, McGoon MD *et al.* (2000) Continuous intravenous epoprostenol for pulmonary hypertension due to the scleroderma spectrum of disease. A randomized, controlled trial. *Ann Intern Med*; **132**(6):425–434.

Badesch BD, Abman SH, Ahearn GS *et al.* (2004) Medical Therapy for Pulmonary Arterial Hypertension. ACCP Evidence-Based Guidelines for Clinical Practice. *Chest*; **126**: 35S–62S.

Badesch DB, Abman SH, Simonneau G *et al.* (2007) Medical Therapy for Pulmonary Arterial Hypertension: Updated ACCP Evidence-Based Clinical Practice Guidelines. *Chest*; **131**(6):1917–1928.

Barst RJ, Rubin LJ, Long WA *et al.* (1996) A comparison of continuous intravenous epoprostenol (prostacyclin) with conventional therapy for primary pulmonary hypertension. The Primary Pulmonary Hypertension Study Group. *New Engl J Med*; **334**(5):296–302.

Barst RJ, McGoon M, Mc Laughlin VV *et al.* (2003) Beraprost Therapy for Pulmonary Arterial Hypertension. *J Am Coll Cardiol*; **41**:2119–2125.

Barst RJ, Langleben D, Frost A *et al.* (2004) Sitaxsentan therapy for pulmonary arterial hypertension. *Am J Respir Crit Care Med*; **169**(4):441–447.

Barst RJ, Langleben D, Badesch D *et al.* (2006a) Treatment of Pulmonary Arterial Hypertension With the Selective Endothelin-A Receptor Antagonist Sitaxsentan. *J Am Coll Cardiol*; **47**(10):2049–2056.

Barst RJ, Galie N, Naeije R *et al.* (2006b) Long-term outcome in pulmonary arterial hypertension patients treated with subcutaneous treprostinil. *Eur Respir J*; 28(6):1195–1203.

Benza R, Frost A, Girgis R *et al.* on behalf of the STRIDE-2X Study Group. (2006) Chronic Treatment of Pulmonary Arterial Hypertension (PAH) with Sitaxsentan and Bosentan. *Proc Am Thor Soc*; **3**:A729.

Channick RN, Simonneau G, Sitbon O *et al.* (2001) Effects of the dual endothelin-receptor antagonist bosentan in patients with pulmonary hypertension: a randomised placebo-controlled study. *Lancet*; **358**(9288):1119–1123.

D'Alonzo GE, Barst RJ, Ayres SM *et al.* (1991) Survival in patients with primary pulmonary hypertension. Results from a national prospective registry. *Ann Intern Med*; **115**(5):343–349.

Doughty N, McKenna P, Meads D *et al.* (2005) The CAMPHOR: Correlations with Objective Measures of Severity of Pulmonary Hypertension. *Proc Am Thor Soc*; **2**:A801.

Enright PL, Sherril DL. (1998) Reference equations for the six-minute walk in healthy adults. *Am J Resp Crit Care Med*; **158**:1384–1387.

Farber HW, Loscalzo J. (2004) Pulmonary Arterial Hypertension. *New Engl J Med*; **351**(16):1655–1665.

Galie N, Ussia G, Passarelli P *et al.* (1995) Role of pharmacologic tests in the treatment of primary pulmonary hypertension. *Am J Cardiol*; 19;**75**(3):55A–62A.

Galie N, Humbert M, Vachiery JL *et al.* (2002) Effects of beraprost sodium, an oral prostacyclin analogue, in patients with pulmonary arterial hypertension: a randomised, double-blind placebo-controlled trial. *J Am Coll Cardiol*; **39**:1496–1502.

Galie N, Torbicki A, Barst R *et al.* (2004a) Guidelines on diagnosis and treatment of pulmonary arterial hypertension: The Task Force on Diagnosis and Treatment of Pulmonary Arterial Hypertension of the European Society of Cardiology. *Eur Heart J*; **25**(24):2243–2278.

Galie N, Seeger W, Naeije R *et al.* (2004b) Comparative Analysis of Clinical Trials and Evidence-Based Treatment Algorithm in Pulmonary Arterial Hypertension. *J Am Coll Cardiol*; **43**:S81–S88.

Galie N, Ghofrani HA, Torbicki A *et al.* (2005a) Sildenafil Citrate Therapy for Pulmonary Arterial Hypertension. *New Engl J Med*; **353**(20):2148–2157.

Galie N, Badesch BD, Oudiz R *et al.* (2005b) Ambrisentan therapy for pulmonary arterial hypertension. *J Am Coll Cardiol*; **46**:529–535.

Galie N, Keogh A, Frost A *et al.* (2005c) Ambrisentan Long-Term Safety and Efficacy in Pulmonary Arterial Hypertension – One Year Follow-Up. *Proc Am Thor Soc*; **2**:A299.

Galie N, Burgess G, Parpia T, Rubin L. (2005d) Effects of sildenafil on 1-year survival of patients with idiopathic pulmonary arterial hypertension (PAH). *Eur Heart J*; **26**: 612.

Galie N, Beghetti M, Gatzoulis MA *et al.* (2006) Bosentan Therapy in Patients With Eisenmenger Syndrome: A Multicenter, Double-Blind, Randomized, Placebo-Controlled Study. *Circulation*; **114**(1):48–54.

Ghofrani HA, Rose F, Schermuly RT *et al.* (2003) Oral sildenafil as long-term adjunct therapy to inhaled iloprost in severe pulmonary arterial hypertension. *J Am Coll Cardiol*; **42**(1):158–164.

Hoeper MM. (2007) Observational trials in pulmonary arterial hypertension: low scientific evidence but high clinical value. *Eur Respir J*; **29**(3):432–434.

Hoeper MM, Schwarze M, Ehlerding S *et al.* (2000) Long-term treatment of primary pulmonary hypertension with aerosolized iloprost, a prostacyclin analogue. *New Engl J Med*; **342**(25):1866–1870.

Hoeper M, Taha N, Bekjarova A, Spiekerkoetter E. (2003) Bosentan treatment in patients with primary pulmonary hypertension receiving non-parenteral prostanoids. *Eur Respir J*; **22**:330–334.

Hoeper MM, Faulenbach C, Golpon H *et al.* (2004) Combination therapy with bosentan and sildenafil in idiopathic pulmonary arterial hypertension. *Eur Respir J*; **24**(6):1007–1010.

Hoeper M, Leuchte H, Halank M, *et al.* (2007) Combining inhaled iloprost with bosentan in patients with idiopathic pulmonary arterial hypertension. *Eur Resp J*; **4**(28):691–694.

Humbert M, Barst R, Robbins I *et al.* (2003) Safety and Efficacy of Bosentan Combined with Epoprostenol in Patients with Severe Pulmonary Arterial Hypertension. *Am J Resp Crit Care Med*; **167**:A441.

Humbert M, Sitbon O, Simonneau G. (2004) Treatment of Pulmonary Arterial Hypertension. *New Engl J Med*; **351**(14):1425–1436.

Humbert M, Barst RJ, Robbins IM *et al.* (2004) Combination of bosentan with epoprostenol in pulmonary arterial hypertension: BREATHE-2. *Eur Respir J*; **24**(3):353–359.

Kuhn KP, Byrne DW, Arbogast PG *et al.* (2003) Outcome in 91 consecutive patients with pulmonary arterial hypertension receiving epoprostenol. *Am J Respir Crit Care Med*; **167**(4):580–586.

Lang I, Gomez-Sanchez M, Kneussl M *et al.* (2006) Efficacy of Long-term Subcutaneous Treprostinil Sodium Therapy in Pulmonary Hypertension. *Chest*; **129**(6):1636–1643.

Langleben D, Christman BW, Barst RJ *et al.* (2002) Effects of the thromboxane synthetase inhibitor and receptor antagonist terbogrel in patients with primary pulmonary hypertension. *Am Heart J*; **143**(5):E4.

Mathai SC, Girgis RE, Fisher MR *et al.* (2007) Addition of sildenafil to bosentan monotherapy in pulmonary arterial hypertension. *Eur Respir J*; **29**(3):469–475.

McKenna S, Doughty N, Meads D *et al.* (2006) The Cambridge Pulmonary Hypertension Outcome Review (CAMPHOR): A Measure of Health-Related Quality of Life and Quality of Life for Patients with Pulmonary Hypertension. *Qual Life Res*; **15**(1):103–115.

McLaughlin VV, Shillington A, Rich S. (2002) Survival in primary pulmonary hypertension: the impact of epoprostenol therapy. *Circulation*; **106**(12):1477–1482.

McLaughlin VV, Presberg KW, Doyle RL *et al.* (2004) Prognosis of Pulmonary Arterial Hypertension ACCP Evidence-Based Clinical Practice Guidelines. *Chest*; **126**, 78S–92S.

McLaughlin VV, Sitbon O, Badesch DB *et al.* (2005) Survival with first-line bosentan in patients with primary pulmonary hypertension. *Eur Respir J*; **25**(2):244–249.

McLaughlin VV, Oudiz RJ, Frost A *et al.* (2006) Randomized Study of Adding Inhaled Iloprost to Existing Bosentan in Pulmonary Arterial Hypertension. *Am J Respir Crit Care Med*; **174**(11):1257–1263.

Miyamoto S, Nagaya N, Satoh T *et al.* (2000) Clinical correlates and prognostic significance of six-minute walk test in patients with primary pulmonary hypertension. Comparison with cardiopulmonary exercise testing. *Am J Respir Crit Care Med*; **161**(2 Pt 1):487–492.

Nagaya N, Uematsu M, Okano Y *et al.* (1999) Effect of orally active prostacyclin analogue on survival of outpatients with primary pulmonary hypertension. *J Am Coll Cardiol*; **34**(4):1188–1192.

Olschewski H, Simonneau G, Galie N *et al.* (2002) Inhaled Iloprost in Severe Pulmonary Hypertension. *New Engl J Med*; **347**:322–329.

Olschewski H, Galie N, Ghofrani HA *et al.* (2006) A placebo-controlled efficacy and safety study of ambrisentan in patients with pulmonary arterial hypertension. *Am J Respir Crit Care Med*; **3**:A728.

Opitz CF, Wensel R, Winkler J *et al.* (2005) Clinical efficacy and survival with first-line inhaled iloprost therapy in patients with idiopathic pulmonary arterial hypertension. *Eur Heart J*; **26**(18):1895–1902.

Oudiz RJ, Torres F, Frost AE *et al.* (2007a) A placebo-controlled efficacy and safety study of ambrisentan in patients with pulmonary arterial hypertension. *Chest*; **132**(4S):

Oudiz RJ, Badesch DB, Rubin LJ *et al.* (2007b) ARIES-E: Long-term safety and efficacy of ambrisentan in pulmonary arterial hypertension. *Am J Respir Crit Care Med*; **175**:A300.

Paciocco G, Martinez F, Bossone E *et al.* (2001) Oxygen desaturation on the six-minute walk test and mortality in untreated primary pulmonary hypertension. *Eur Resp J*; **17**:647–652.

Partanen J, Nieminen, M, Luonmanmaki K, Rich S. (1993) Death in a patient with primary pulmonary hypertension after 20 mg of nifedipine. *New Engl J Med*; **329**:812.

Peacock A, Naeije R, Galie N, Reeves JT. (2004) End points in pulmonary arterial hypertension: the way forward. *Eur Respir J*; **23**(6):947–953.

Pepke-Zaba J, Brown M, Parpia T *et al.* (2005) The Impact of Sildenafil Citrate on Health-Related Quality of Life in Patients with Pulmonary Arterial Hypertension (PAH): Results of a Multicenter, Multinational, Randomized, Double-Blind, Placebo-Controlled Trial. *Proc Am Thor Soc*; **2**:A299.

Provencher S, Sitbon O, Humbert M *et al.* (2006) Long-term outcome with first-line bosentan therapy in idiopathic pulmonary arterial hypertension. *Eur Heart J*; **27**(5):589–595.

Rich S, Kaufmann E, Levy PS. (1992) The effect of high doses of calcium-channel blockers on survival in primary pulmonary hypertension. *New Engl J Med*; **327**(2):76–81.

Rubin LJ, Mendoza J, Hood M *et al.* (1990) Treatment of primary pulmonary hypertension with continuous intravenous prostacyclin (epoprostenol). Results of a randomized trial. *Ann Intern Med*; **112**(7):485–491.

Rubin LJ, Badesch DB, Barst RJ *et al.* (2002) Bosentan therapy for pulmonary arterial hypertension. *New Engl J Med*; **346**(12):896–903.

Rubin L, Burgess G, Parpia T, Simonneau G. (2005) Effects of Sildenafil on 6-Minute Walk Distance (6MWD) and WHO Functional Class (FC) after 1 Year of Treatment. *Proc Am Thor Soc*; **2**:A299.

Sastry BKS, Narasimhan C, Reddy NK, Raju BS. (2004) Clinical efficacy of sildenafil in primary pulmonary hypertension: A randomized, placebo-controlled, double-blind, crossover study. *Journal of the American College of Cardiology*; **43**(7):1149–1153.

Simonneau G, Barst RJ, Galie N *et al.* (2002) Continuous Subcutaneous Infusion of Treprostinil, a Prostacyclin Analogue, in Patients with Pulmonary Arterial Hypertension. A double-blind, randomized, placebo-controlled trial. *Am J Respir Crit Care Med*; **165**(6):800–804.

Simonneau G, Galie N, Rubin L *et al.* (2004) Clinical Classification of Pulmonary Arterial Hypertension. *J Am Coll Cardiol*; **43**:S5–S12.

Simonneau G, Rubin L, Galie N *et al.* (2007) Safety and Efficacy of Sildenafil-Epoprostenol Combination Therapy in Patients with Pulmonary Arterial Hypertension. *Am J Resp Crit Care Med*;**175**, A300.

Singh T, Rohit M, Grover A *et al.* (2006) A randomized, placebo-controlled, double-blind, crossover study to evaluate the efficacy of oral sildenafil therapy in severe pulmonary artery hypertension. *Am Heart J*; **151**(4):851.e1–851.e5.

Sitbon O, Humbert M, Nunes H *et al.* (2002) Long-term intravenous epoprostenol infusion in primary pulmonary hypertension: prognostic factors and survival. *J Am Coll Cardiol*; **40**(4):780–788.

Sitbon O, Badesch DB, Channick RN *et al.* (2003) Effects of the Dual Endothelin Receptor Antagonist Bosentan in Patients With Pulmonary Arterial Hypertension: A 1-Year Follow-up Study. *Chest*; **124**(1):247–254.

Sitbon O, Humbert M, Jais X *et al.* (2005a) Long-Term Response to Calcium Channel Blockers in Idiopathic Pulmonary Arterial Hypertension. *Circulation*; **111**(23):3105–3111.

Sitbon O, McLaughlin VV, Badesch DB *et al.* (2005b) Survival in patients with class III idiopathic pulmonary arterial hypertension treated with first line oral bosentan compared with an historical cohort of patients started on intravenous epoprostenol. *Thorax*; **60**(12): 1025–1030.

Stahl E, Lindberg A, Jansson SA *et al.* (2005) Health-related quality of life is related to COPD disease severity. *Health Qual Life Outcomes*; **3**(1):56.

11 Diagnosis and assessment of non-pulmonary arterial hypertension masquerading as idiopathic pulmonary arterial hypertension: Diastolic heart failure - evaluation and interactions

Mardi Gomberg-Maitland and Stuart Rich

Department of Medicine, University of Chicago, Chicago, USA

11.1 Definition of heart failure

The cardiac cycle encompasses systolic function, described as the ability of the ventricles to contract and eject, and diastolic function described as the ability to relax and fill (Leite-Moreira, 2006). Heart failure is a clinical syndrome resulting from abnormalities in systolic and/or diastolic function (Hunt *et al.*, 2005).

Pulmonary Arterial Hypertension, Edited by Robyn J. Barst
© 2008 John Wiley & Sons, Ltd

Diastolic heart failure, also known as heart failure with preserved ejection fraction, has emerged as a distinct entity, with clear differences in its pathophysiology, diagnostic evaluation and prognosis compared with heart failure with diminished systolic function (Leite-Moreira, 2006). The clinical syndrome of diastolic heart failure includes limitations in exercise capacity and fluid retention with peripheral edema, abdominal ascites and pulmonary congestion (Zile and Brutsaert, 2002a). Patient variability in presentation has led to the preferred term 'heart failure' rather than 'congestive heart failure' (Hunt *et al.*, 2005). However, there is no single diagnostic test for heart failure because it is largely a clinical diagnosis based on history and physical examination; diagnostic testing is a supplement.

11.2 Epidemiology

Heart failure is a growing public health problem, with a prevalence of approximately 5 million patients in the United States, and an incidence of more than 555,000 patients (AHA, 2005). The incidence of heart failure resulting from abnormalities of diastolic dysfunction with normal systolic function has increased to more than 50% of heart failure patients overall (Hogg, Swedberg and McMurray, 2004; Hunt *et al.*, 2005; Kitzman *et al.*, 2001; Owan and Redfield, 2005; Redfield *et al.*, 2003). Data suggest that patients with heart failure with preserved ejection fraction tend to be older females, and have a history of systemic hypertension, left ventricular hypertrophy, diabetes, myocardial ischemia or coronary artery disease and atrial fibrillation (Cohn and Johnson, 1990; Hunt *et al.*, 2005; Owan and Redfield, 2005; Redfield *et al.*, 2003). Although the prognosis for these patients was considered better than those with a reduced ejection fraction (Cohn and Johnson, 1990; Masoudi *et al.*, 2003; Redfield *et al.*, 2003; Smith *et al.*, 2003; Vasan *et al.*, 1999), recent data demonstrate otherwise (Bhatia *et al.*, 2006; Owan *et al.*, 2006). Owan and coworkers evaluated patients hospitalized for heart failure in Olmsted County, Minnesota from 1987 through 2001 and found an increased prevalence of normal ejection fraction heart failure patients (Bhatia *et al.*, 2006; Owan *et al.*, 2006). They found the prevalence of age > 65 years, systemic hypertension, atrial fibrillation and diabetes increased, with coronary artery disease remaining stable. These patients had a slightly higher survival compared with the patients with abnormal left ventricular systolic function (29% vs 32% at one year, 65% vs 68% at five years) which was maintained after adjustment (hazard ratio = 0.96; 0.92–1.00 95% CI) (Bhatia *et al.*, 2006; Owan *et al.*, 2006). Importantly, survival did not improve in the diastolic heart failure cohort during the course of the study but survival did in the comparator group.

Bhatia and coworkers also found an increased prevalence of diastolic heart failure with concomitant co-morbidities (Bhatia *et al.*, 2006; Owan *et al.*, 2006). The investigators found similar mortality (5% vs 7% at 30 days, $p = 0.08$; and 22% vs 26% at one year, $p = 0.07$) and morbidity (cardiac arrest, acute coronary syndromes, renal failure and intensive care unit admissions) between the two groups (Bhatia *et al.*, 2006; Owan *et al.*, 2006). Thus, it appears that diastolic dysfunction has become a separate and severe clinical entity since the late 1980s.

11.3   Physiology

Diastolic function is determined by myocardial relaxation and passive properties of the ventricular wall, such as myocardial stiffness, wall thickness and chamber size or volume (Leite-Moreira, 2006). Other factors not considered true causes of ventricular diastolic dysfunction include extrinsic structures surrounding the ventricle (e.g. pericardium), and disorders arising from the left atrium, the pulmonary veins or the mitral and aortic valves; the diagnosis requires their exclusion (Gaasch and Zile, 2004; Leite-Moreira, 2006)

Relaxation

Relaxation of the heart, the process by which the myocardium returns to an unstressed length and force comprises most of ventricular ejection, pressure fall and the initial part of rapid filling (Leite-Moreira, 2006). Relaxation is modulated by load (preload or afterload) and is dependent on the magnitude, duration and timing in the cardiac cycle (Brutsaert, Rademakers and Sys, 1984; Leite-Moreira *et al.*, 2000). In the normal heart, a mild to moderate increase in afterload will result in a compensatory response with a delay in the onset, and an accelerated rate, of pressure fall (Leite-Moreira and Correia-Pinto, 2001). However, a severe increase in afterload will accelerate the onset, and prolong the rate of pressure fall, often leading to an incomplete relaxation and thus an elevation in filling pressures. This will be further exacerbated if the preload is also elevated (Leite-Moreira and Correia-Pinto, 2001)

The underlying molecular mechanisms for relaxation include calcium homeostasis and myofilament cross-bridging cycling in the myocardium. Calcium extrusion from the cell is the dominant mechanism influenced by activity of the sarcoplasmic reticulum (SR) calcium adenosine triphosphate (ATP)ase pump (SERCA) and phospholamban, a SERCA-inhibitory protein (Leite-Moreira, 2006). Relaxation improves with β-adrenergic stimulation by increasing cyclic adenosine monophosphate (cAMP) or inhibition of cardiac phosphodiesterase, phosphorylating phospholamban, and thus halting its normal inhibition (Leite-Moreira, 2006). Hydrolysis of ATP is also needed for calcium dissociation from troponin-C, and for calcium uptake by the SR. If any of these proteins or processes is altered, diastolic function can diminish (Zile and Brutsaert, 2002b)

Relaxation requires uniform counteracting forces of re-extension and shortening. During isovolumeric relaxation, the ventricle remains isovolumic but changes its shape and displaces its volume (Leite-Moreira, 2006). Asynchronous early segment re-extension and regional non-uniform relaxation induce an early onset and slower rate of the ventricular pressure drop (Brutsaert and Sys, 1989; Leite-Moreira and Gillebert, 2000)

Passive properties

The ventricular wall is influenced by myocardial stiffness from the cardiomyocyte cytoskeleton and the extracellular matrix (ECM). Changes in the cytoskeleton microtubules (tubulin), intermediate filaments (desmin), microfilaments (actin) and endosarcomeric proteins (titin, α-actin, myomesin and M-protein) alter diastolic function (Zile and Brutsaert, 2002b). Most of the elastic force is attributed to titin, with tubulin and desmin contributing less than 10% at maximal sarcomere lengths (Kass, Bronzwaer and Paulus, 2004). Passive and active properties overlap with the post-translational modification of titan by calcium and phosphorylation (Kass, Bronzwaer and Paulus, 2004).

The ECM is composed of fibrillar proteins (collagen types I and III and elastin), proteoglycans and basement membrane proteins (collagen type IV, laminin and fibronectin) (Leite-Moreira, 2006). Fibrillar collagen contributes most to passive diastolic properties (Zile and Brutsaert, 2002b). Collagen synthesis and degradation is a complex interplay of processes. Transcription is regulated by physical (preload and afterload), neurohormonal (rennin-angiotensin, aldosterone and sympathetic nervous systems), and growth factors. Post-translation regulation occurs by collagen cross-linking and enzymatic degradation by matrix metalloproteinases (MMPs) (Zile and Brutsaert, 2002b). The quality of cross-linking and glycation determine stiffness (Kass, Bronzwaer and Paulus, 2004). Phosphorylation of myosin light chain 2 and troponin I myofilaments increases nitric oxide and cyclic guanosine monophosphate (cGMP), increasing resting diastolic cell length (Leite-Moreira and Correia-Pinto, 2001). In addition, endothelin-1 acutely decreases stiffness (Leite-Moreira et al., 2003)

Heart rate

Heart rate affects myocardial oxygen demand and coronary perfusion time (Leite-Moreira, 2006). In a hypertrophic myocardium, a rapid heart rate leads to relative ischemia within the myocardium in addition to a shortened diastolic time, thus preventing complete relaxation (Leite-Moreira, 2006; Zile and Brutsaert, 2002a). Increased filling pressures resulting in diastolic dysfunction often lead to volume overload states.

11.4 Evaluation of diastolic heart failure: Invasive and noninvasive techniques

Hemodynamic assessment of relaxation consists of the timing of pressure measurements of the cardiac cycle with left ventricular, aortic and left atrial tracings. The timing of the left ventricular pressure fall is measured by hemodynamic assessment, estimated from the time interval between end diastole and dP/dt_{min} or the time between aortic valve opening and closure (LVET). The rate of fall is measured as an instantaneous maximal value as dP/dt_{min}, as an isovolumic relaxation (IRT) time between aortic valve closure and mitral valve opening and/or the time constant of isovolumic relaxation, tau (Leite-Moreira and Gillebert, 2000). Tau is inversely related to the pressure fall and corresponds to the time it takes for the fall to be 36% of its initial value (Leite-Moreira, 2006) (Figure 11.1).

Assessment of left ventricular compliance/stiffness can by measured by evaluation of the end-diastolic pressure volume relationship (LV-EDPVR). This is done by examining multiple pressure–volume (PV) loops obtained at different preload conditions (Figure 11.2). The stiffness is determined by the slope of a tangent

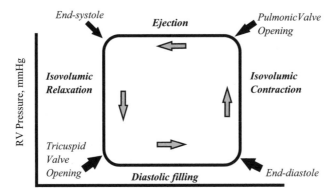

Figure 11.1   Ventricular Function: The PV loop. The hemodynamic assessment of the pressure volume relationship observed during the cardiac cycle.

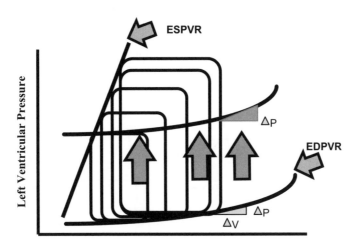

Left Ventricular Volume

Figure 11.2   Hemodynamic Evaluation of Diastolic Function: Sequential P/V loops. The operating stiffness at any point along a given end diastolic pressure volume relationship (EDPVR) is equal to the slope of a tangent drawn to the curve at that point ($\Delta P/\Delta V$). Operating stiffness changes with filling; stiffness is lower at smaller volumes and higher at larger volumes (volume dependent change in diastolic pressure and stiffness). When diastolic dysfunction occurs, the ejection fraction is preserved and end diastolic pressures are raised due to a left upward shift of the entire PV relation, reflecting a volume independent increase in chamber stiffness. (Depicted by orange arrows) Note that the slope of the end systolic pressure volume relationship (ESPVR) is preserved.

drawn to the curve at that point (*P/V*) (Leite-Moreira, 2006). Stiffness is lower at lower volumes, and with a higher compliance the curve shifts upward and leftward (Shapiro *et al.*, 2006). When this occurs, the relationship between pressure and volume becomes steeper, leading to a volume-independent increase in diastolic pressure and increase in stiffness (Leite-Moreira, 2006). Patients with impaired relaxation depend on left ventricular filling during atrial contraction. Unfortunately, this technique is imprecise because of the curvilinear nature of the relationship, and often requires additional analyses (Burkhoff, Mirsky and Suga, 2005).

Echocardiography is a validated technique used for assessment of diastolic function and filling pressures (Nishimura *et al.*, 1996; Ommen and Nishimura, 2003; Redfield *et al.*, 2003). The most common assessment is mitral inflow velocities, with the E wave corresponding to early flow during left ventricular relaxation and the A wave describing the contribution of atrial contraction (Angeja and Grossman, 2003). The E wave is greater than the A wave with normal function, but as the heart becomes less compliant, the atrial contraction contributes more to filling, with an A wave greater than the E wave and a prolonged deceleration of the E wave. With severe impairment, the atrium contributes little to filling and the E wave is again greater than the A wave, but there is a rapid deceleration first appearing as a pseudonormal pattern, (E > A) and then with a restrictive pattern (E twice A) (Angeja and Grossman, 2003). The pulmonary vein flow is measured in systole and diastole and with severe diastolic dysfunction, the pattern is diastolic dominant. More recently, additional indices derived from tissue Doppler velocity are now being used in conjunction with mitral and pulmonary vein velocity patterns to evaluate diastolic heart function (Zile and Brutsaert, 2002b) (Figure 11.3).

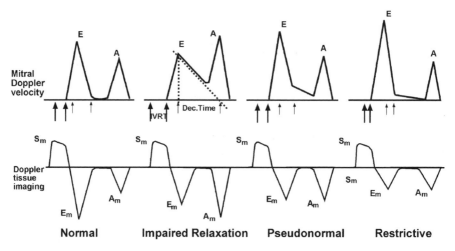

Figure 11.3 Echocardiographic evaluation of diastolic dysfunction. Mitral Doppler velocity tracings: E = early LV filling velocity; A = velocity of LV filling contributed by atrial contraction; IVRT = isovolumic relaxation time; Dec. Time = e-wave deceleration time. *Doppler Tissue imaging tracings:* Sm = myocardial velocity during systole. Em = myocardial velocity during early filling; Am = myocardial velocity during filling produced by atrial contraction.

11.5   Diagnosis and treatment of diastolic dysfunction

Diagnosis of heart failure with preserved left ventricular ejection fraction is based on the assessment of abnormal ventricular relaxation and a clinical diagnosis of heart failure (based on signs and symptoms) with no other etiology identified (Hunt *et al.*, 2005; Litwin and Grossman, 1993; Vasan, Benjamin and Levy, 1996).

These signs and symptoms (Hunt *et al.*, 2005) include:

- Incorrect diagnosis of heart failure (HF)
- Inaccurate measurement of left ventricular ejection fraction (LVEF)
- Primary valvular disease
- Restrictive (infiltrative) cardiomyopathies- Amyloidosis, sarcoidosis, hemochromatosis
- Pericardial constriction
- Episodic or reversible LV systolic dysfunction
- Systemic hypertension, myocardial ischemia
- HF associated with high metabolic demand (high-output states) - Anemia, thyrotoxicosis, arteriovenous fistulae
- Chronic pulmonary disease with right HF
- Pulmonary arterial hypertension associated with pulmonary vascular disorders
- Atrial myxoma
- Morbid obesity
- Diastolic dysfunction of uncertain origin
- Left ventricular ejection fraction

Current treatment is based on improvement of symptoms alone as there is little clinical trial data available. The control of systemic blood pressure with anti-hypertensive agents (beta blockers, angiotensin-converting enzyme inhibitors, angiotensin receptor blockers, calcium channel blockers), heart rate by either beta blocker or calcium channel blocker therapy and control of ischemia are recommended (Hunt *et al.*, 2005; Zile and Brutsaert, 2002b). Control of heart rate in patients with atrial fibrillation and restoration of sinus rhythm are also recommended (Hunt *et al.*, 2005). The goal of therapy is to reduce cardiac filling pressures at rest and with exertion, resulting in an improvement in functional capacity (Zile and Brutsaert, 2002a). Digoxin is not recommended and diuretics should be reserved for symptoms of congestion (Hunt *et al.*, 2005; Zile and Brutsaert, 2002a)

The CHARM-preserved trial is the only completed large-scale, placebo-controlled trial to date, assessing this patient population (Yusuf *et al.*, 2003). Patients with an ejection fraction > 40% were given either candesartan 32 mg or placebo. After a mean of 37 months follow-up, there was no difference in the primary combined end point of death by cardiovascular cause or admission for heart failure decompensation. The mortality rate was also not different but candesartan did decrease heart failure admissions (Yusuf *et al.*, 2003). Newer mechanistic approaches may lead to future therapies. Reports of ALT-711, alagebrium, a glucose cross-link breaker, resulted in a decrease in left ventricular mass and improved diastolic filling after 16 weeks of therapy, and data from a pilot study suggests that statins may decrease mortality (Fukuta *et al.*, 2005; Little *et al.*, 2005)

11.6   Pulmonary hypertension and diastolic dysfunction

Physiology

Progressive pulmonary hypertension leads to right ventricular pressure overload, with resultant right ventricular hypertrophy and dilatation. The interdependence of the right and left ventricles is such that the function of one affects the other (Visner *et al.*, 1983; Visner *et al.*, 1986). In chronic right ventricular pressure or volume overload, the motion of the interventricular septum can be asynchronous in both systole and diastole (Brutsaert, Rademakers and Sys, 1984). Impaired relaxation with a diminished E/A ratio and increased isovolumic relaxation time (IRT) and deceleration time are seen on echocardiographic studies on patients with idiopathic pulmonary arterial hypertension (IPAH) (Galie *et al.*, 2003; Louie, Rich and Brundage, 1986; Moustapha *et al.*, 2001; Stojnic *et al.*, 1992; Tutar *et al.*, 1999; Xie *et al.*, 1998). However, although most patients with IPAH have normal left ventricular end-diastolic pressures, it is clear that many do not. It has been proposed that this might be due to the significant right ventricular load, pericardial pressure and perhaps the left ventricular free wall (Dauterman *et al.*, 1995; Little, Badke and O'Rourke, 1984). However, pericardiotomy has not altered right or left ventricular filling pressures or cardiac output in patients with pulmonary hypertension as assessed by transesophageal echocardiography, suggesting an adaptation of the pericardium over time (Blanchard and Dittrich, 1992)

The hemodynamics of diastolic abnormalities in pulmonary arterial hypertension (PAH) patients is not well studied as clinical trials have most often excluded patients with an abnormally elevated wedge or left ventricular end-diastolic pressure. Many patients, despite severe right ventricular enlargement, have normal wedge pressure and left ventricular end-diastolic pressure. This observation is consistent with canine studies demonstrating reduced compliance of the left ventricle with no change in left ventricular pressure (Little, Badke and O'Rourke, 1984; Visner *et al.*, 1983; Visner *et al.*, 1986). In some patients, but not in all, the LVEDP is normal at rest but increases with exercise. Patients with chronic thromboembolic pulmonary hypertension have improved left ventricular diastolic compliance after thromboendarterectomy despite no fall in wedge pressure, again demonstrating the complexity in diagnosis and understanding of diastolic heart function (Dittrich, Chow and Nicod, 1989)

The increase in pulmonary vascular resistance in mitral stenosis, a classic model of pulmonary venous hypertension, although secondary to valvular disease, shares many similarities with pulmonary arterial hypertension. Pathologic comparison of patients with PAH associated with congenital heart disease, IPAH, and pulmonary hypertension associated with mitral stenosis demonstrate similar density of pulmonary arterial smooth muscle. However, in adult patients with mitral stenosis compared with children and the other categories, the density is replaced by a prominent contribution of collagen and edematous ground substance to the structure of the media (Wagenvoort and Wagenvoort, 1982). Pulmonary veno-occlusive disease, now categorized with PAH despite being a venous obstruction, also has similar pathology compared with patients with mitral stenosis. This suggests that elevated pulmonary artery pressure due to pulmonary venous hypertension thus triggers vascular changes similar to pulmonary arterial hypertension. The two etiologies may be more similar than once thought (Chazova *et al.*, 2000)

Diagnosis

Pulmonary venous hypertension is known to occur in diastolic dysfunction, (Kessler, Willens and Mallon, 1993; Willens and Kessler, 1993), and is often more severe than expected. These patients are thought to have a reactive pulmonary vasculature due to the elevated left ventricular filling pressure, leading to pulmonary hypertension and right ventricular dysfunction (Benza and Tallaj, 2006). As the pulmonary vascular disease progresses, the cardiac output declines, resulting in a lowering of right- and left-sided pressures, often making it difficult to assess diastolic dysfunction.

A history of conditions associated with diastolic abnormalities and evidence on diagnostic testing by electrocardiography, chest radiography, computed tomography, and/or echocardiography consistent with left heart disease, e.g. left atrial enlargement, left ventricular hypertrophy or infiltrative disease, should raise suspicion of diastolic heart failure. Testing with agents that increase inotropy, e.g. adenosine, dobutamine, dopamine, or exercise during cardiac catheterization, may uncover compliance abnormalities although no formal studies and/or recommendations are currently available. In addition, the transpulmonic gradient, i.e. the difference between the mean pulmonary artery pressure and the wedge pressure, and the pulmonary vascular resistance (the mean pulmonary artery pressure minus the wedge pressure/cardiac output L/min) may help differentiate PAH from pulmonary venous hypertension (Benza and Tallaj, 2006).

Treatment

Although patients with diastolic abnormalities and PAH can be treated with vasodilators, there is currently no evidence to support these therapies. There is a theoretical concern that successful therapies, i.e. those that result in an improvement in cardiac output, might increase the pulmonary capillary wedge pressure and induce left ventricular failure. Although some physicians are currently using endothelin-receptor antagonists, phosphodiesterase inhibitors and prostacyclins, randomized clinical trials have to date not been completed. Animal studies with endothelin-receptor blockers have yielded conflicting results. While some have shown they have potential to reduce hypertrophy-induced myocardial fibrosis (Yamamoto *et al.*, 2002; Yamamoto *et al.*, 2000) others have shown that myocardial ET-1 gene expression is necessary for normal cardiac function under physiologic stress (Zhao *et al.*, 2006). These data emphasize the need for caution when considering the use of these agents in clinical practice. Often in the setting of systemic hypotension, patients may benefit from increased systemic vascular resistance to improve coronary blood flow to the right ventricular myocardium. Agents used include phenylephrine and dopamine based on reducing right ventricular ischemia in the setting of severe pulmonary hypertension (Rich, Gubin and Hart, 1990; Vlhakes, Turley and Hoffman, 1981). Agents used to treat diastolic abnormalities may be helpful but physicians must remain aware that if the systemic blood pressure is low in the setting of elevated pulmonary pressures, a low cardiac output state may develop.

11.7 Conclusions

Diastolic dysfunction, also known as heart failure with preserved ejection fraction, is a distinct entity with significant morbidity and mortality. Although clinical evaluation has improved our ability to diagnose diastolic dysfunction, currently used diagnostic tools are less accurate in patients with concomitant pulmonary hypertension and right ventricular dysfunction. Right and left heart catheterization (including direct measurement of LVEDP) with and without provocative measures such as exercise, or intravenous loading during cardiac catheterization (if needed) should be performed if diastolic dysfunction is suspected.

In acute decompensation or severe chronic disease, patients develop right ventricular hypertrophy and dilatation, and owing to interventricular interdependence, right ventricular ischemia, right ventricular failure and, eventually, cardiogenic shock can develop. Agents such as dopamine and phenylephrine that decrease right ventricular ischemia (Rich, Gubin and Hart, 1990; Vlhakes, Turley and Hoffman, 1981) may be helpful in acute decompensation and late-stage disease. However, cardiogenic shock may develop if systemic blood pressure is significantly lowered in these patients and close monitoring of these patients is needed. Although new therapies appear promising in diastolic dysfunction, it remains unclear if they will provide benefit in patients with pulmonary hypertension. There is currently no data to support the use of any targeted PAH therapies in patients with diastolic heart failure.

References

Anjega, B. G., Grossman, W. (2003) Evaluation and management of diastolic heart failure. *Circulation*, **107**, 659–63.

AHA (2005) *Heart Disease and Stroke Statistics – 2005 Update*, American Heart Association, Dallas, TX.

Benza, R. and Tallaj, JA. (2006) Pulmonary hypertension out of proportion to left heart disease. *Adv Pulmon Hypertension*, **5**, 21–29.

Bhatia, R. S., Tu, J. V., Lee *et al.* (2006) Outcome of heart failure with preserved ejection fraction in a population-based study. *N Engl J Med*, **355**, 260–9.

Blanchard, D. G. and Dittrich, H. C. (1992) Pericardial adaptation in severe chronic pulmonary hypertension. An intraoperative transesophageal echocardiographic study. *Circulation*, **85**, 1414–22.

Brutsaert, D. L. and Sys, S. U. (1989) Relaxation and diastole of the heart. *Physiol Rev*, **69**, 1228–315.

Brutsaert, D. L., Rademakers , F. E. and Sys, S. U. (1984) Triple control of relaxation: implications in cardiac disease. *Circulation*, **69**, 190–6.

Burkhoff, D., Mirsky, I. and Suga, H. (2005) Assessment of systolic and diastolic ventricular properties via pressure-volume analysis: a guide for clinical, translational, and basic researchers. *Am J Physiol Heart Circ Physiol*, **289**, H501–12.

Chazova, I., Robbins, I., Loyd, J. *et al.* (2000) Venous and arterial changes in pulmonary venoocclusive disease, mitral stenosis and fibrosing mediastinitis. *Eur Respir J*, **15**, 116–22.

Cohn, J. N. and Johnson, G. (1990) Heart failure with normal ejection fraction. The V-HeFT Study. Veterans Administration Cooperative Study Group. *Circulation*, **81**(Suppl 2), 48–53.

Dauterman, K., Pak, P. H., Maughan, W. L. *et al.* (1995) Contribution of external forces to left ventricular diastolic pressure. Implications for the clinical use of the Starling law. *Ann Intern Med*, **122**, 737–42.

Dittrich, H. C., Chow, L. C. and Nicod, P. H. (1989) Early improvement in left ventricular diastolic function after relief of chronic right ventricular pressure overload. *Circulation*, **80**, 823–30.

Fukuta, H., Sane, D. C., Brucks, S. and Little, W. C. (2005) Statin therapy may be associated with lower mortality in patients with diastolic heart failure: a preliminary report. *Circulation*, **112**, 357–63.

Gaasch, W. H. and Zile, M. R. (2004) Left ventricular diastolic dysfunction and diastolic heart failure. *Annu Rev Med*, **55**, 373–94.

Galie, N., Hinderliter, A. L., Torbicki, A. *et al.* (2003) Effects of the oral endothelin-receptor antagonist bosentan on echocardiographic and doppler measures in patients with pulmonary arterial hypertension. *J Am Coll Cardiol*, **41**, 1380–6.

Hogg, K., Swedberrg, K., McMurray, J. (2004) Heart failure with preserved left ventricular systolic function; epidemiology, clinical characteristics, and prognosis. *J Am Coll Cardiol*, **43**, 317–27.

Hunt, S. A., Abraham, W. T., Chin *et al.* (2005) ACC/AHA 2005 Guideline Update for the Diagnosis and Management of Chronic Heart Failure in the Adult: a report of the American College of Cardiology/American Heart Association Task Force on Practice Guidelines (Writing Committee to Update the 2001 Guidelines for the Evaluation and Management of Heart Failure): developed in collaboration with the American College of Chest Physicians and the International Society for Heart and Lung Transplantation: endorsed by the Heart Rhythm Society. *Circulation*, **112**, e154–235.

Kass, D. A., Bronzwaer, J. G. and Paulus, W. J. (2004) What mechanisms underlie diastolic dysfunction in heart failure? *Circ Res*, **94**, 1533–42.

Kessler, K. M., Woillens, H. J. and Mallon, S. M. (1993) Diastolic left ventricular dysfunction leading to severe reversible pulmonary hypertension. *Am Heart J*, **126**, 234–5.

Kitzman, D. W., Gardin, J. M., Gottdiener *et al.* (2001) Importance of heart failure with preserved systolic function in patients > or = 65 years of age. CHS Research Group. Cardiovascular Health Study. *Am J Cardiol*, **87**, 413–9.

Leite-Moreira, A. F. (2006) Current perspectives in diastolic dysfunction and diastolic heart failure. *Heart*, **92**, 712–8.

Leite-Moreira, A. F. and Gillebert, T. C. (2000) The physiology of left ventricular pressure fall. *Rev Port Cardiol*, **19**, 1015–21.

Leite-Moreira, A. F. and Correia-Pinto, J. (2001) Load as an acute determinant of end-diastolic pressure-volume relation. *Am J Physiol Heart Circ Physiol*, **280**, H51–9.

Leite-Moreira, A. F., Correia-Pinto, J., de Hert, S. G. and Gillebert, T. C. (2000) Pressure relaxation of the left ventricle and filling pressures. *J Am Coll Cardiol*, **36**, 1438–9.

Leite-Moreira, A. F., Bras-Silva, C., Pedrosa, C. A. and Rocha-Sousa, A. A. (2003) ET-1 increases distensibility of acutely loaded myocardium: a novel ETA and Na+/H+ exchanger-mediated effect. *Am J Physiol Heart Circ Physiol*, **284**, H1332–9.

Little, W. C., Badke, F. R. and O'Rourke, R. A. (1984) Effect of right ventricular pressure on the end-diastolic left ventricular pressure-volume relationship before and after chronic right ventricular pressure overload in dogs without pericardia. *Circ Res*, **54**, 719–30.

Little, W. C., Zile, M. R., Kitzman *et al.* (2005) The effect of alagebrium chloride (ALT-711), a novel glucose cross-link breaker, in the treatment of elderly patients with diastolic heart failure. *J Card Fail*, **11**, 191–5.

Liytwin, S. E. and Grossman, W. (1993) Diastolic dysfunction as a cause of heart failure. *J Am Coll Cardiol*, **22**, 49A–55A.

Louie, E. K., Rich, S. and Brundage, B. H. (1986) Doppler echocardiographic assessment of impaired left ventricular filling in patients with right ventricular pressure overload due to primary pulmonary hypertension. *J Am Coll Cardiol*, **8**, 1298–306.

Masoudi, F. A., Havranek, E. P., Smith, G. *et al.* (2003) Gender, age, and heart failure with preserved left ventricular systolic function. *J Am Coll Cardiol*, **41**, 217–23.

Moustapha, A., Kaushik, V., Diaz, S. *et al* (2001) Echocardiographic evaluation of left-ventricular diastolic function in patients with chronic pulmonary hypertension. *Cardiology*, **95**, 96–100.

Nishimura, R. A., Appleton, C. P., Redfield, M. M. *et al.* (1996) Noninvasive doppler echocardiographic evaluation of left ventricular filling pressures in patients with cardiomyopathies: a simultaneous Doppler echocardiographic and cardiac catheterization study. *J Am Coll Cardiol*, **28**, 1226–33.

Ommen, S. R. and Nishimura, R. A. (2003) A clinical approach to the assessment of left ventricular diastolic function by Doppler echocardiography: update 2003. *Heart*, **89** (Suppl 3), 18–23.

Owan, T. E. and Redfield, M. M. (2005) Epidemiology of diastolic heart failure. *Prog Cardiovasc Dis*, **47**, 320–32.

Owan, T. E., Hodge, D. O., Herges, R. M. *et al.* (2006) Trends in prevalence and outcome of heart failure with preserved ejection fraction. *N Engl J Med*, **355**, 251–9.

Redfield, M. M., Jacobsen, S. J., Burnett, J. C., Jr. *et al.* (2003) Burden of systolic and diastolic ventricular dysfunction in the community: appreciating the scope of the heart failure epidemic. *JAMA*, **289**, 194–202.

Rich, S., Gubin, S. and Hart, K. (1990) The effects of phenylephrine on right ventricular performance in patients with pulmonary hypertension. *Chest*, **98**, 1102–06.

Shapiro, B., Nishimura, RA, McGoon, MD and Redfield, MM. (2006) Diagnostic dilemmas: diastolic heart failure causing pulmonary hypertension and pulmonary hypertension causing diastolic dysfunction. *Adv Pulmon Hypertension*, **5**, 13–20.

Smith, G. L., Masoudi, F. A., Vaccarino, V. *et al.* (2003) Outcomes in heart failure patients with preserved ejection fraction: mortality, readmission, and functional decline. *J Am Coll Cardiol*, **41**, 1510–8.

Stojnic, B. B., Brecker, S. J., Xiao, H. B. *et al.* (1992) Left ventricular filling characteristics in pulmonary hypertension: a new mode of ventricular interaction. *Br Heart J*, **68**, 16–20.

Tutar, E., Kaya, A., Gulec, S. *et al.* (1999) Echocardiographic evaluation of left ventricular diastolic function in chronic cor pulmonale. *Am J Cardiol*, **83**, 1414–7, A9.

Vasan, R. S., Benjamin, E. J. and Levy, D. (1996) Congestive heart failure with normal left ventricular systolic function. Clinical approaches to the diagnosis and treatment of diastolic heart failure. *Arch Intern Med*, **156**, 146–57.

Vasan, R. S., Larson, M. G., Benjamin, E. J. *et al.* (1999) Congestive heart failure in subjects with normal versus reduced left ventricular ejection fraction: prevalence and mortality in a population-based cohort. *J Am Coll Cardiol*, **33**, 1948–55.

Visner, M. C., Arentzen, C. E., O'Connor, M. J. *et al.* (1983) Alterations in left ventricular three-dimensional dynamic geometry and systolic function during acute right ventricular hypertension in the conscious dog. *Circulation*, **67**, 353–65.

Visner, M. C., Arentzen, C. E., Crumbley, A. J., III, *et al.* (1986) The effects of pressure-induced right ventricular hypertrophy on left ventricular diastolic properties and dynamic geometry in the conscious dog. *Circulation*, **74**, 410–9.

Vlhakes, G., Turley, K. and Hoffman, J. (1981) The pathophysiology of failure in acute right ventricular hypertension: hemodynamic and biochemical correlation. *Circulation*, **63**, 87–95.

Wagenvoort, C. A. and Wagenvoort, N. (1982) Smooth muscle content of pulmonary arterial media in pulmonary venous hypertension compared with other forms of pulmonary hypertension. *Chest*, **81**, 581–5.

Willens, H. J. and Kessler, K. M. (1993) Severe pulmonary hypertension associated with diastolic left ventricular dysfunction. *Chest*, **103**, 1877–83.

Xie, G. Y., Lin, C. S., Preston *et al.* (1998) Assessment of left ventricular diastolic function after single lung transplantation in patients with severe pulmonary hypertension. *Chest*, **114**, 477–81.

Yamamoto, K., Masuyama, T., Sakata, Y. *et al.* (2000) Prevention of diastolic heart failure by endothelin type A receptor antagonist through inhibition of ventricular structural remodeling in hypertensive heart. *Cardiovasc Res*, **47**, 274–83.

Yamamoto, K., Masuyama, T., Sakata, Y. *et al.* (2002) Roles of renin-angiotensin and endothelin systems in development of diastolic heart failure in hypertensive hearts. *J Hypertension*, **20**, 753–61.

Yusuf, S., Pfeffer, M. A., Swedberg, K. *et al.* (2003) Effects of candesartan in patients with chronic heart failure and preserved left-ventricular ejection fraction: the CHARM-Preserved Trial. *Lancet*, **362**, 777–81.

Zhao, X.S., Pan, W., Bekeredijian, R., and Shohet, R.V. (2006) Endogenous endothelin-1 is required for cardiomyocyte survival in vivo. *Circulation*, **114**, 830–7.

Zile, M. R. and Brutsaert, D. L. (2002a) New concepts in diastolic dysfunction and diastolic heart failure: Part I: diagnosis, prognosis, and measurements of diastolic function. *Circulation*, **105**, 1387–93.

Zile, M. R. and Brutsaert, D. L. (2002b) New concepts in diastolic dysfunction and diastolic heart failure: Part II: causal mechanisms and treatment. *Circulation*, **105**, 1503–8.

12 Treatment of pulmonary arterial hypertension: A look to the future

Lewis J. Rubin

San Diego School of Medicine, University of California, La Jolla, USA

Remarkable advances have been achieved in elucidating the pathogenesis of pulmonary arterial hypertension (PAH) since the mid-1990s, leading to the development of disease-targeted therapies for this condition (Figure 12.1). Despite these achievements, the response to therapy is often incomplete in many PAH patients, and survival remains poor. Accordingly, new treatment strategies must be developed for PAH that optimize the treatments currently available and capitalize on the identification of novel pathogenic pathways for PAH. This chapter will provide a glimpse into the future, based on recent developments in the field that hold promise for enhancing the treatment of this disease.

Identification of mutations in the bone morphogenetic protein receptor-2 (BMPR2) in the majority of cases of familial pulmonary arterial hypertension (FPAH) has been a major advance in the elucidation of the pathogenic sequence in PAH (Deng et al., 2000; Lane et al., 2000) (Figure 12.2). However, fewer than 20% of individuals

Pulmonary Arterial Hypertension, Edited by Robyn J. Barst
© 2008 John Wiley & Sons, Ltd

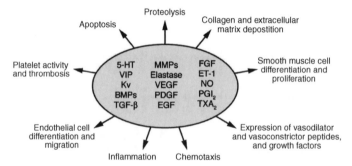

Figure 12.1   Postulated cellular and molecular pathobiology of pulmonary vascular remodeling in PAH. ET-1, endothelin 1; 5-HT, serotonin; Kv, potassium channel; PGI2, prostacyclin; TXA2, thromboxane A2; VIP, vasoactive intestinal peptide. Reproduced from Barst RJ (2005) PDGF Signaling in pulmonary arterial hypertension. *J Clin Invest;* **115**:2691–2694.

with a BMPR2 mutation develop FPAH, and most individuals with PAH do not have an identifiable mutation (Thomson *et al.*, 2000); accordingly, it is likely that other factors, including genes and environmental stimuli (a 'second hit'), are needed to initiate the pathological sequence that leads to vascular injury and the pulmonary hypertensive state. Both the role of these other factors in initiating the vascular injury and the mechanisms through which they interface with genetic abnormalities are unknown (Derynck and Zhang, 2003).

Various cellular pathway abnormalities have been described that may play important roles in the development and progression of PAH (Figure 3)

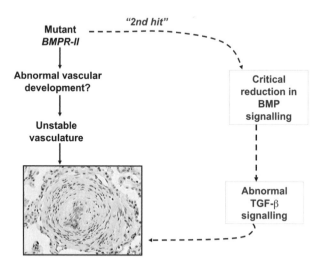

Figure 12.2   Potential role of BMPR2 mutations in PAH. (Personal communication Nicholas Morrell, MD.) There is a full-color version of this figure in the plate section of this book.

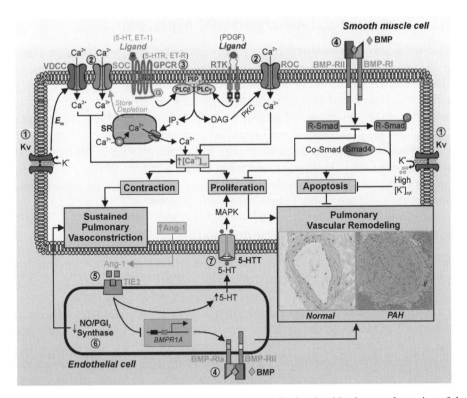

Figure 12.3 Cellular and molecular pathways potentially involved in the transformation of the normal to the hypertensive pulmonary vessel phenotype. These processes involve both endothelial and smooth muscle cell-dependent pathways, as well as interactions between the two cell types. According to this model, vasoconstriction, proliferation and altered apoptosis are involved, to varying degrees, in the pathologic transformation from normal to disease state. There is a full-color version of this figure in the color plate section of this book.

(Christman *et al.*, 1992; Tuder *et al.*, 1999; Yuan *et al.*, 1998; Mandegar, Remillard and Yuan, 2002; Eddhaibi *et al.*, 2001). These include altered synthesis of nitric oxide, prostacyclin and endothelin, impaired potassium channel and growth factor receptor function, altered serotonin transporter regulation, increased oxidant stress and enhanced matrix production. However, the relative importance of each of these processes is unknown, and the interactions between these various pathways need to be explored. Additionally, the intermediate steps involved in the transduction of signals related to BMPR2 are unknown; clarification of these pathways will lead to a more complete understanding of how impaired BMPR2 signaling, both inherited and acquired, leads to hypertensive pulmonary vascular disease (Du *et al.*, 2003; Krick *et al.*, 2001; Yuan and Rubin, 2005).

12.1 Therapy of pulmonary arterial hypertension

In the final years of the twentieth century, the treatment of PAH was based on a limited understanding of the disease pathogenesis and was largely empiric and usually ineffective. The treatment of PAH has advanced dramatically since then, with a number of well-designed clinical trials demonstrating the efficacy of several therapies that target specific abnormalities present in PAH (Barst *et al.*, 1996; Rubin *et al.*, 2002; Galie *et al.*, 2002; Olschewski *et al.*, 2002). Furthermore, the complexity of these treatments has evolved from continuous intravenous (IV) delivery to oral and inhaled modes of drug delivery. Future studies targeting newly identified alterations in endothelial and smooth muscle cell function may provide novel treatments. Several of the most promising targets are discussed below.

Serotonin receptor and transporter function

Serotonin (5-hydroxytryptamine, 5-HT) is a potent vasoconstrictor and mitogen that has long been suspected to play a pathogenic role in PAH (Fanburg and Lee, 1997). Recent work suggests that the $5HT2_B$ receptor may be upregulated in PAH, providing a novel therapeutic target since antagonists to this receptor have been developed. Others have shown that the serotonin transporter, a molecule that facilitates transmembrane transport of serotonin into the cell, is upregulated in PAH (Eddhaibi *et al.*, 2001); additionally, the fenfluramine anorexigens, which are known to increase the risk of developing PAH, produce an upregulation of the serotonin transporter *in vitro*, supporting a pathogenic mechanism for this system in PAH. Drugs that downregulate the serotonin transporter, such as the selective serotonin reuptake inhibitors (SSRIs), may be worth exploring as treatment options in the future.

Vasoactive intestinal polypeptide

Vasoactive intestinal polypeptide (VIP) is a substance that exerts cellular antiproliferative effects and is produced by a variety of cells. It is also a neuropeptide with potent vasodilating properties. Deficiency of VIP has been described in lung tissues from patients with idiopathic PAH (IPAH). In a preliminary open label case series, eight patients with IPAH who were treated with inhaled VIP at daily doses of 200 µg in four single inhalations showed marked clinical and hemodynamic improvement (Petkov *et al.*, 2003). Further studies confirming these encouraging preliminary findings and clarifying optimal dosing and long-term safety are being contemplated.

Rho kinase inhibitors

Rho kinase is part of a family of enzymes that is involved in the processes of cellular growth and, in particular, smooth muscle tone. Studies in animal models of pulmonary hypertension suggest that fasudil, an inhibitor of Rho kinase, may ameliorate the hemodynamic and pathologic severity of pulmonary vascular injury, and provide a rationale for clinical development of this agent in PAH (Oka *et al.*, 2007; Abe *et al.*, 2004).

Inhibitors of growth factor synthesis

Pulmonary arterial hypertension is characterized pathologically by uncontrolled angiogenesis, a process that is reminiscent of malignant transformation. In support of this concept, monoclonal expansion has been demonstrated in the plexiform lesion of IPAH. Published reports in which imatinib mesylate (ST1571), a tyrosine kinase inhibitor that is approved for the treatment of hematopoeitic malignancies, produced improvement in an animal model of pulmonary hypertension (Schermuly *et al.*, 2005) and a handful of PAH patients refractory of other available treatments (Ghofrani, Seeger and Grimminger, 2005) suggest that this novel approach may be of benefit in PAH and warrants further study (Figure 12.4).

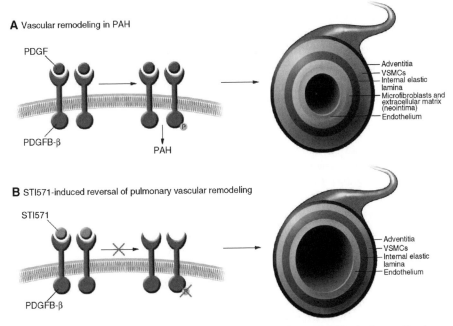

Figure 12.4   Schematic representation of pulmonary vascular remodeling in the small pulmonary arteries in PAH. (A) PDGF receptor (PDGFR) expression and phosphorylation (P) in pulmonary arteries are increased in PAH, which activates downstream signaling pathways that promote the abnormal proliferation and migration of vascular smooth muscle cells, as well as the formation of a layer of microfibroblasts and extracellular matrix (termed the neointima) between the internal elastic lamina and the endothelium. These changes underlie the structural and functional abnormalities in the vessel wall that lead to pulmonary vascular disease. (B) Schermuly and coworkers demonstrated that administration of the PDGF receptor antagonist STI571, i.e. imatinib mesylate, induces a reversal of the pulmonary vascular remodeling in two different animal models of pulmonary hypertension. STI571 prevents phosphorylation of the PDGF receptor and consequently suppresses activation of downstream signaling pathways associated with PAH. Reproduced from Barst RJ (2005) PDGF Signaling in pulmonary arterial hypertension. *J Clin Invest;* **115**:2691–2694. These is a full-color version of this figure in the color plate section of this book.

Adrenomedullin is a peptide that causes vasodilation and inhibits proliferation of pulmonary vascular smooth muscle cells (Nagaya and Kangawa, 2007; Said, 2006). Both intravenous and inhaled adrenomedullin lower pulmonary vascular resistance in patients with IPAH (von der Hardt *et al.*, 2004; Nagaya, 2000). Long-term data are not available but the substance has the potential of a promising future treatment for PAH (Said, 2006).

Cell-based Therapy

Several publications have demonstrated that infusions of endothelial progenitor cells in animal models of pulmonary hypertension attenuate the injury, particularly when these cells are transfected with nitric oxide synthase, the enzyme responsible for the generation of nitric oxide from L-arginine precursor (Zhao *et al.*, 2005). Thus, while cell-based therapies have yet to fulfill their promise in clinical studies, particularly in cardiovascular diseases, pilot safety and efficacy trials are now underway with progenitor cell infusions in patients with severe PAH refractory to medical therapy (Wang *et al.*, 2007).

Drugs currently marketed to treat other conditions may have effects that are beneficial in PAH as well. For example, the hydroxymethylglutaryl-coenzyme-A reductase inhibitors manifest pleiotropic effects that have been suggested to be responsible for a component of their benefit in arteriosclerotic disease (Indolfi *et al.*, 2000), and these agents attenuate the pulmonary arteriopathy induced by the administration of monocrotaline to experimental animals (Nishimura *et al.*, 2002; Nishimura *et al.*, 2003). Formal clinical studies with the statins may, therefore, be appropriate.

Similarly, currently available platelet inhibitors (e.g. aspirin) and newer antithrombotic agents may have a role in the treatment of PAH, in light of the beneficial effects (and inherent risks) of anticoagulation with warfarin in IPAH.

As with other diseases with a complex pathogenesis, targeting a single pathway in PAH is unlikely to be uniformly successful. With the development of several pathway-specific therapies, the opportunity exists for evaluating multidrug therapy in PAH. Uncontrolled, small trials have suggested that the addition of oral bosentan to patients failing oral or inhaled prostanoid therapy, with beraprost or iloprost, respectively, resulted in improved exercise capacity. Similarly, the addition of oral sildenafil to inhaled iloprost therapy resulted in potentiation of the clinical effects. Recently, randomized clinical trials have demonstrated that the addition of inhaled iloprost to background therapy with oral bosentan (McLaughlin *et al.*, 2006), or oral sildenafil to background IV epoprostenol therapy, resulted in further improvement in hemodynamics, exercise capacity and time-to-clinical-worsening (Simonneau *et al.*, 2007).

Unresolved questions exist regarding combination therapy for PAH:

• Which combinations are the most potent? Put another way, which pathways are the most relevant targets for treatment, and how many should be targeted?

- What is the optimal timing for combination therapy? Should combination therapy be initiated early in the course of the disease in order to maximize the response, or should it be considered only if monotherapy fails to achieve the desired clinical response?
- What are the appropriate criteria for assessing response to therapy?

12.2 Measuring outcomes and monitoring the course of therapy

The development of treatments for PAH has prompted the challenge of how to best assess and monitor the efficacy of long-term therapy. Because it is believed that randomized, placebo-controlled trials using survival as an end point would be unethical to perform in PAH, alternative strategies are required to measure and compare the relative effects of the available treatments. Similarly, noninvasive markers of disease severity, either biomarkers, imaging studies or physiological tests, are needed that can be widely applied to reliably monitor clinical course. Studies that assess the value of these outcome measures, alone or in combination, will enable physicians to time and select therapy in a more structured fashion. Furthermore, more attention needs to be focused on the state of right ventricular function in PAH, since this is arguably the single most important determinant of outcome (Voelkel *et al.*, 2006).

12.3 Conclusions

Although major advances in our understanding of the mechanism of disease development and in the treatment of PAH have been achieved over the past decade, substantial gaps in our knowledge remain. Bringing together physicians and scientists representing multiple disciplines and expertise, all sharing an interest in PAH, affords the opportunity to explore areas of mutual interest and collaboration that will, it is hoped, narrow these gaps of knowledge in the future.

References

Abe K, Shimokawa H, Morikawa K, *et al.* (2004) Long-term treatment with a Rho-kinase inhibitor improves monocrotaline-induced fatal pulmonary hypertension in rats. *Circ Res*; **94**:385-93.

Barst RJ, Rubin LJ, Long WA, *et al.* (1996) for the Primary Pulmonary Hypertension Study Group. A comparison of continuous intravenous epoprostenol (prostacyclin) with conventional therapy for primary pulmonary hypertension. *New Engl J Med*; **334**:296-301.

Barst RJ (2005) PDGF Signaling in pulmonary arterial hypertension. *J Clin Invest*; **115**:2691-2694.

Christman BW, McPherson CD, Newman JH, *et al.* (1992) An imbalance between the excretion of thromboxane and prostacyclin metabolites in pulmonary hypertension. *New Engl J Med*; **327**:70-5.

Deng Z, Morse JH, Slager SL, *et al.* (2000) Familial primary pulmonary hypertension (gene PPH1) is caused by mutations in the bone morphogenetic protein receptor-II gene. *Am J Hum Gen*; **67**:737–44.

Derynck R, Zhang YE (2003) TGF-beta-induced signalling pathways. *Nature*; **425**:581–3.

Du L, Sullivan CC, Chu D, *et al.* (2003) Signaling molecules in nonfamilial pulmonary hypertension. *New Engl J Med*; **348**:500–9.

Eddhaibi S, Humbert M, Fadel E, *et al.* (2001) Serotonin transporter overexpression is responsible for pulmonary artery smooth muscle hyperplasia in primary pulmonary hypertension. *J Clin Invest*; **108**:1141–50.

Fanburg BL, Lee SL (1997) A new role for an old molecule: serotonin as a mitogen. *Am J Physiol*; **272**:L795–806.

Galie N, Humbert M, Vachiery JL, *et al.* (2002) Effects of beraprost sodium, an oral prostacyclin analogue, in patients with pulmonary arterial hypertension: a randomized, double-blind, placebo-controlled trial. *J Am Coll Cardiol*; **39**:1496–502.

Ghofrani HA, Seeger W, Grimminger F (2005) Imatinib for the treatment of pulmonary arterial hypertension. *New Engl J Med*; **353**:1412–1413.

Indolfi C, Cioppa A, Stabile E, *et al.* (2000) Effects of hydroxymethylglutaryl coenzyme-A reductase inhibitor simvastatin on smooth muscle cell proliferation in vitro and neointimal formation in vivo after vascular injury. *J Am Coll Cardiol*; **35**:214–221.

Krick S, Platoshyn O, McDaniel SS, *et al.* (2001) Augmented K$^+$ currents and mitochondrial membrane depolarization in pulmonary artery myocyte apoptosis. *Am J Physiol Lung Cell Mol Physiol*; **281**:L887–94.

Lane KB, Machado RD, Pauciulo MW, *et al.* (2000) Heterozygous germline mutations in BMPR2, encoding a TGF-beta receptor, cause familial primary pulmonary hypertension. The International PPH Consortium. *Nat Genet*; **26**:81–4.

Mandegar M, Remillard CV, Yuan JX (2002) Ion channels in pulmonary arterial hypertension. *Prog Cardiovasc Dis*; **45**:81–114.

McLaughlin VV, Oudiz RJ, Frost A, *et al.* (2006) A Randomized, Double-Blind, Placebo-Controlled Study of Iloprost Inhalation as Add-On Therapy to Bosentan in Pulmonary Arterial Hypertension. *Am J Resp Crit Care Med*; **174**:1257-1263.

Nagaya N, Kangawa K (2007) Adrenomedullin in the treatment of pulmonary hypertension. *Peptides*; **25**:2013-2018

Nagaya N, Nishikimi T, Uematsua M, *et al.* (2000) Haemodynamic and hormonal effects of adrenomedullin in patients with pulmonary hypertension. *Heart*; **84**:653–658.

Nishimura T, Faul JL, Berry GJ, *et al.* (2002) Simvastatin attenuates smooth muscle neointimal proliferation and pulmonary hypertension in rats. *Am J Respir Crit Care Med*; **166**:1403–1408.

Nishimura T, Vaszar LT, Faul JL, *et al.* (2003) Simvastatin rescues rats from fatal pulmonary hypertension by inducing apoptosis in neointimal smooth muscle. *Circulation*; **108**: 1640–1645.

Oka M, Homma N, Taraseviciene-Stewart L, *et al.* (2007) Rho kinase-mediated vasoconstriction is important in severe occlusive pulmonary arterial hypertension in rats. *Circ Res*; **100**:923–9.

Olschewski H, Simonneau G, Galie N, *et al.* (2002) Inhaled iloprost for severe pulmonary hypertension. *New Engl J Med*; **347**:322–9.

Petkov V, Mosgeoller W, Ziesche, *et al.* (2003) Vasoactive intestinal polypeptide as a new drug for treatment of primary pulmonary hypertension. *J Clin Invest*; **111**:1339–46.

Rubin LJ, Badesch DB, Barst RJ, *et al.* (2002) Bosentan therapy for pulmonary arterial hypertension. *New Engl J Med*; **346**:896–903.

Said SI (2006) Mediators and modulators of pulmonary arterial hypertension. *Am J Physiol Lung Cell Mol Physiol*; **291**:547-558

Schermuly RT, Dony E, Ghofrani HA, *et al.* (2005) Reversal of experimental pulmonary hypertension by PDGF inhibition. *J Clin Invest*; **115**:2811–21.

Simonneau G, Rubin LJ, Galie N, *et al.* (2007) safety and efficacy of sildenafil-epoprostenol combination therapy in patients with pulmonary arterial hypertension. *Am J Resp Crit Care Med*; **175**:A300 (abstract).

Thomson JR, Machado RD, Pauciulo MW, *et al.* (2000) Sporadic primary pulmonary hypertension is associated with germline mutations of the gene encoding BMPR2, a receptor member of the TGF-beta family. *J Med Genet*; **37**:741–5.

Tuder RM, Cool CD, Geraci MW, *et al.* (1999) Prostacyclin synthase expression is decreased in lungs from patients with severe pulmonary hypertension. *Am J Respir Crit Care Med*; **159**: 1925–32.

Voelkel NF, Quaife RA, Leinwand LA, *et al.* (2006) Right ventricular function and failure: report of a National Heart, Lung, and Blood Institute working group on cellular and molecular mechanisms of right heart failure. *Circulation*; **114**:1883–1891.

von der Hardt K, Kandler MA, Chada M, *et al.* (2004) Brief adrenomedullin inhalation leads to sustained reduction of pulmonary artery pressure. *Eur Respir J*; **24**:615–623.

Wang XX, Zhang FR, Shang YP, *et al.* (2007) Transplantation of autologous endothelial progenitor cells may be beneficial in patients with idiopathic pulmonary arterial hypertension: a pilot randomized controlled trial. *J Am Coll Cardiol*; **49**:1566–1571

Yuan JX, Aldinger AM, Juhaszova M, *et al.* (1998) Dysfunctional voltage gated K$^+$ channels in pulmonary artery smooth muscle cells of patients with primary pulmonary hypertension. *Circulation*; **98**:400–6.

Yuan JXJ, Rubin LJ (2005) Pathogenesis of Pulmonary Artery Hypertension: Need for Multiple Hits. *Circulation*; **111**:534–538

Zhao YD, Courtman DW, Deng Y, *et al.* (2005) Rescue of monocrotaline-induced pulmonary arterial hypertension using bone marrow-derived endothelial-like progenitor cells: efficacy of combined cell and eNOS gene therapy in established disease. *Circ Res*; **96**:442–50.

Index

Note: Figures and Tables are indicated by *italic page numbers*. Abbreviations: CTEPH = chronic thromboembolic pulmonary hypertension; FPAH = familial pulmonary arterial hypertension; IPAH = idopathic pulmonary arterial hypertension; PAH = pulmonary arterial hypertension; PH = pulmonary hypertension

adenosine, in vasodilator testing   38, 49, 75
adrenomedullin   242
AIR study   *181*, 208, 210
altitude effects   *9*, 56–7
ambrisentan   3, 99–101
  clinical trials   99–101, *181*, 209
  in combination with sildenafil   141
  drug interactions   141
  exercise capacity affected by   99, *100*
  first approved for PAH treatment   2
  long-term studies   210, 211, 213
  survival data   *208*, 213
aminotransferases, elevation during ERA
    treatment   93, 96, 97, 98, 101, 102
anemia, sensitivity to   57
angina, in differential diagnosis   *11*
angiography *see* CT angiography; pulmonary
    angiography
anorexigen-induced PAH   1, 3, 240
  treatment with warfarin   53
  see also appetite suppressants

anticoagulant drugs, treatment of PAH
    with   35, 52–4, 214
antinuclear antibodies (ANA)   31
appetite suppressants
  effects on PAH risk   1, *12*
  see also anorexigen-induced PAH
ARIES-1 and ARIES-2 studies   99–101, 102, *181*
arterial blood gas measurements   33
aspergillus infection, in lung transplant
    patients   169
associated PAH (APAH)   *9*
  pulmonary function test   30
  risk profiles   *12*
  survival   2
  treatment with epoprostenol   70–4
  see also congenital heart disease; portal
    hypertension; connective tissue
    disease; HIV infection
atrial septostomy (AS)   4, 148–56, 172–3
  balloon dilation atrial septostomy (BDAS)
    149, 151, 152

Pulmonary Arterial Hypertension,   Edited by Robyn J. Barst
© 2008 John Wiley & Sons, Ltd